MRI and CT
of the Spine

Case Study Approach

MRI and CT of the Spine

Case Study Approach

Robert Kricun, M.D.
*Department of Radiology/Diagnostic
Medical Imaging
Lehigh Valley Hospital
Allentown, Pennsylvania*

*Clinical Associate Professor
of Diagnostic Radiology
Hahnemann University Hospital
Philadelphia, Pennsylvania*

Morrie E. Kricun, M.D.
*Professor of Radiology
Department of Radiology
Orthopedic Section
Hospital of the University of Pennsylvania
Philadelphia, Pennsylvania*

Raven Press ✒ New York

Raven Press, Ltd., 1185 Avenue of the Americas, New York, New York 10036

Made in the United States of America

Library of Congress Cataloging-in-Publication Data

Kricun, Robert.
    MR imaging and CT of the spine : case study approach / Robert Kricun, Morrie E. Kricun.
        p.   cm.
    Includes bibliographical references and index.
    ISBN 0-7817-0026-4
    1. Spine—Magnetic resonance imaging—Case studies.   2. Spine—Tomography—Case studies.   I. Kricun, Morrie E., 1938–
    II. Title.
    [DNLM: 1. Spinal Diseases—diagnosis—case studies.   2. Magnetic Resonance Imaging.   3. Tomography, X-Ray Computed.   WE 725 K92m 1993]
    RD768.K745   1993
    617.3′7507548—dc20
    DNLM/DLC
    for Library of Congress   93-16680
                                                                            CIP

The material contained in this volume was submitted as previously unpublished material, except in the instances in which some of the illustrative material was derived.

Great care has been taken to maintain the accuracy of the information contained in the volume. However, neither Raven Press nor the editors can be held responsible for errors or for any consequences arising from the use of the information contained herein.

Materials appearing in this book prepared by individuals as part of their official duties as U.S. Government employees are not covered by the above-mentioned copyright.

9   8   7   6   5   4   3   2   1

To our mother
Esther G. Kricun
and to the memory of our father
Dr. A. Alfred Kricun

To Stephanie, Ashley, and Bret
R. K.

To Ginny
M. E. K.

Contents

Foreword

Diagnostic imaging has undergone dramatic changes over the past decade. Technical developments have pushed magnetic resonance imaging (MRI) toward unforeseeable heights. The spine in particular has benefited from the technical revolution in noninvasive imaging during this time. This has occurred for several reasons, not the least of which is the large population that suffers from diseases of the spine. The advent of MRI has further improved upon the already exquisite anatomic display of the spine and its contents provided by computed tomography (CT). With more sophisticated software and hardware development, it is now uniformly accepted that MRI plays an important role in the diagnostic evaluation of this region.

The authors of this textbook provide the reader with a case presentation analysis of diseases of the spine. Both MRI and CT are utilized, and supplemental line drawings, as well as anatomic correlations, are presented. The chosen format is a proven and highly successful method of teaching imaging analysis of spinal diseases. The authors present examples of a wide spectrum of diseases affecting the spine and highlight relevant anatomy as well as pathoanatomic considerations for each case. The discussion of radiographic findings allows the reader to understand the rationale for formulating the diagnosis from the observations. Concise clinical relevance as well as the pertinent references have been selected for the reader.

In this volume, Doctors Robert Kricun and Morrie Kricun have once again produced a well-organized, highly informative, up-to-date textbook for anyone interested in diseases of the spine. The book is one that will appeal to the novice as well as the expert in spine imaging, whether they be physicians in clinical practice or residents in radiology, orthopedic surgery, neurosurgery, neurology, or rehabilitative medicine.

Scott W. Atlas, M.D.
Department of Radiology
Neuroradiology Section
Hospital of the University of Pennsylvania
Philadelphia, Pennsylvania

Preface

Magnetic resonance imaging and computed tomography are imaging modalities that provide invaluable diagnostic information in the evaluation of spinal disorders. This book will benefit those physicians interested in understanding and interpreting the images from MR and CT studies of the spine.

The case study approach used in this book offers the reader an opportunity to examine the case materials of "unknowns" and formulate a diagnostic opinion. On the page following each case presentation, the reader will find an in-depth discussion of the entity with special attention to the MRI and CT findings, use of MRI and CT in the evaluation of that particular disorder, and differential diagnosis. Additional images are also often presented to show the different appearances of the same disorder and the similar appearances of different entities. The cases are heavily illustrated with MR and CT images, and the images are liberally labeled to prevent any ambiguity in interpretation. Anatomic specimens and medical illustrations are also used to aid the reader in better understanding the anatomy and pathology of the spine. MR protocols change over time and vary with institutions and magnetic field strength; however, we provide sample protocols in the Appendix and discuss the use of various pulse sequences in the text. The use of gadopentetate dimeglumine in MR imaging is also described in the appropriate case discussions.

Cases have been grouped by general topics, such as disc disorders, spinal stenosis, infection, tumor, trauma, congenital disorders, the postoperative state, and so on. The reader should be cautioned, however, that "pitfalls" have been sprinkled throughout the book. Finally, up-to-date reference lists accompany the case material, allowing the reader to continue with further study.

MRI and CT of the Spine: Case Study Approach follows our book *Computed Tomography of the Spine: Diagnostic Exercises.* Whereas our first book emphasized the use of CT, this book is heavily weighted toward MR imaging. The majority of "unknowns" come from MR studies, although in some instances, for example when presenting a spinal fracture, we chose to present a CT study as the lead case.

Our goal is to provide the reader with diagnostic challenges and the knowledge needed to better utilize and interpret MR and CT images of the spine. We believe that the book's format, case material, and discussions accomplish this goal.

R. Kricun
M. Kricun

Acknowledgments

Many people have been instrumental in the preparation of this book. The authors wish to thank those who have given generously of their time, effort, and talent in this endeavor.

We thank Kathleen Moser for her tireless efforts preparing the manuscript. Carol Gagnon-Varma contributed the beautiful medical illustrations that add immeasurably to the quality of the book.

This type of book requires outstanding images and photographs. We are grateful to Steve Strommer and Juanitta James for their photographic assistance, and we appreciate the technical assistance of Eastman Kodak Company with the radiographic reproductions.

We thank the many MRI and CT technologists for the care and concern they gave our patients. In many instances, they spent extra time rephotographing images to produce optimal examples. The entire staff of the Lehigh Magnetic Imaging Center was cooperative and helpful. In particular, we thank Laurie Fleming for her help with the MR images and Lynn Fowler-Blatt for her role in obtaining optimal MR protocols.

We are especially indebted to Drs. Mark Osborne and Elliot Shoemaker who reviewed the manuscript and made valuable suggestions. Our many radiology colleagues gave needed support, and our referring physicians provided important clinical correlations. We are grateful to Dr. Scott Atlas for graciously contributing the Foreword.

At Raven Press, Craig Percy, Nicholas Radhuber, and Diana Andrews contributed significantly to the quality of the book.

We thank Steffi, Ashley, and Bret Kricun for providing assistance toward the completion of the book. Finally, we greatly appreciate the patience and encouragement of our families.

R. Kricun
M. Kricun

MRI and CT
of the Spine

Case Study Approach

CASE 1

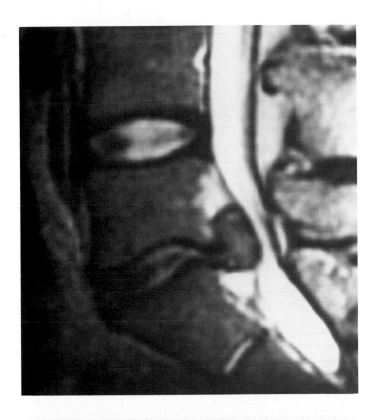

FIG. 1-1A. This 38-year-old man had magnetic resonance (MR) imaging of the lumbar spine because of low back pain which radiates into the left leg. Sagittal T2-weighted spin-echo (SE) MR image (2000/70).

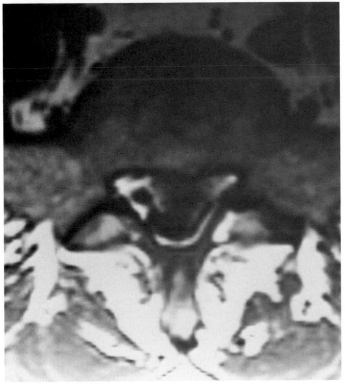

FIG. 1-1B. Axial T1-weighted SE MR image (700/14) obtained just caudad to the L5-S1 disc space.

1

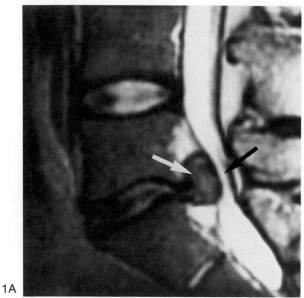 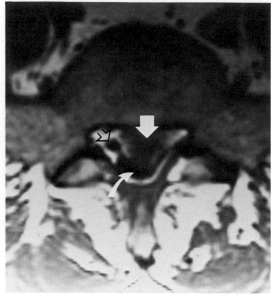

1A

1B

FIG. 1-1A. Disc herniation. There is a large disc herniation at L5-S1 (*white arrow*). The herniated disc is attached to and isointense with the intervertebral disc. Decreased signal intensity of the disc is caused by disc degeneration with decreased water content of the annulus fibrosus and the nucleus pulposus. There is marked compression of the high-signal cerebrospinal fluid (*black arrow*).

FIG. 1-1B. On the T1-weighted image the large disc herniation (*solid straight arrow*) is slightly hyperintense relative to the cerebrospinal fluid within the thecal sac. Compression of the thecal sac (*curved arrow*) and the left S1 nerve root is seen. Note normal right S1 nerve root (*open arrow*).

POSTEROLATERAL DISC HERNIATION

The sagittal and axial magnetic resonance (MR) images show focal posterior protrusion of the disc at L5-S1, causing compression of the anterior epidural fat, thecal sac, and left S1 nerve root (Fig. 1-1). This is a posterolateral disc herniation.

Various subtle differences in the terminology describing disc disease have been forwarded in the literature. We use the terms *bulging disc, herniated disc,* and *free disc fragment* as they have been described previously by other authors (1,3,9). The bulging disc is a uniform, generalized protrusion of the annulus fibrosus beyond the vertebral body margin. A herniated disc is present when a portion of the nucleus pulposus ruptures through a tear in the annulus fibrosus. Some authors classify disc herniation as *prolapsed disc* (with the nucleus still confined by some remaining fibers of the annulus) and *extruded disc* (complete tear of the annulus). We, like others (3), consider both of these subtypes as disc herniation. The terms *free disc fragment* or *sequestered disc* describe disc material that has ruptured through a tear of the annulus fibrosus and is separated from the parent disc. The free fragment may lie between the annulus and the posterior longitudinal ligament or between the posterior longitudinal ligament and the dura. Rarely, the free fragment lies within the thecal sac.

Both MR imaging and computed tomography (CT) are excellent methods of evaluating patients for lumbar disc herniation (2,6). Available techniques and protocols used with MR imaging of the spine are described for the interested reader in Appendix 1. MR protocols for imaging the spine may vary from one institution to another and are frequently revised as new technologic advances take place. Protocols also vary with the field strength of the magnet. Almost all images shown in this text were obtained with a 1.5 Tesla (T) magnet. In the evaluation for lumbar disc herniation, sagittal T1- and T2-weighted spin-echo (SE) images are obtained. Axial images are angled parallel to the disc spaces and T1-weighted spin-echo images are obtained. Additional axial T2-weighted fast spin-echo (FSE) images are optional.

When a central or posterolateral disc herniation is present, the disc can be seen extending posteriorly beyond the posterior vertebral body margin. Axial images show a focal herniation of the disc rather than the uni-

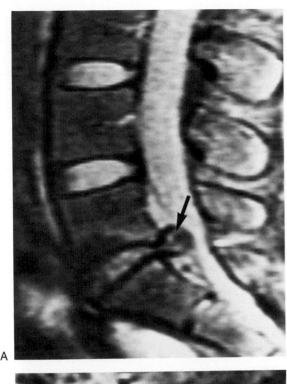

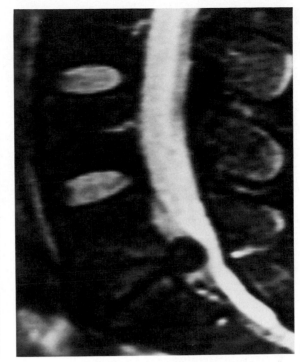

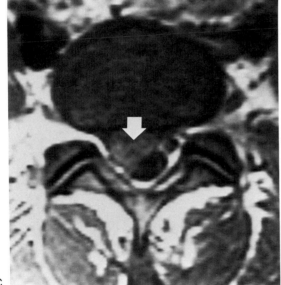

FIG. 1-2. Disc herniation at L5-S1. **A**: Sagittal proton density-weighted SE MR image (2000/30) shows a large disc herniation (*arrow*) at L5-S1, compressing the thecal sac. The herniated disc is isointense relative to the intervertebral disc and appears to remain attached to the intervertebral disc rather than being sequestered as a free fragment. **B**: Sagittal T2-weighted SE MR image (2000/70) shows marked hypointensity of the disc herniation caused by loss of water content within the disc. **C**: Axial T1-weighted SE MR image (600/15) shows the disc herniation (*arrow*), compressing the thecal sac and the right S1 nerve root. The disc herniation has intermediate signal intensity on this T1-weighted image and is slightly hyperintense relative to the thecal sac.

form generalized extension of the disc seen with a bulging annulus. Typically, the herniated portion of the disc is isointense or slightly hypointense relative to the nucleus pulposus on all SE images (Fig. 1-2), although occasionally it has higher signal intensity (2). Decreased signal intensity of the intervetebral disc seen on T2-weighted images is caused by disc degeneration and is best visualized in the sagittal plane (2,6). On the T2-weighted images, the degenerated disc is contrasted against the bright signal of the cerebrospinal fluid and thus the degree of thecal sac compression can be readily appreciated on these images. In some cases it is possible to visualize a tear in the posterior annulus fibrosus. T2-weighted FSE images can be obtained in less time than T2-weighted conventional SE images and provide images with high contrast between disc and cerebrospinal fluid (Fig. 1-3A). However, fat has bright signal intensity on T2-weighted FSE images and is less sharply contrasted to fluid. Fat suppression technique can be used with FSE imaging to increase the contrast between fat and cerebrospinal fluid. On T1-weighted SE images there is less contrast in signal intensity between disc and cerebrospinal fluid; however, there is good contrast between disc and epidural

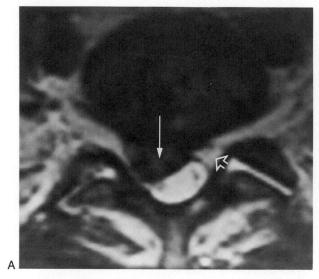 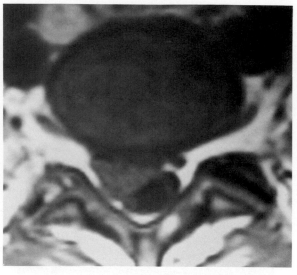

FIG. 1-3. Disc herniation at L5-S1 seen with T2-weighted fast spin-echo (FSE) and T1-weighted SE images. **A**: Axial T2-weighted FSE MR image (3000/100) shows a large disc herniation (*solid arrow*) on the right with low signal intensity. This is sharply contrasted to the bright signal of the cerebrospinal fluid within the compressed thecal sac. The epidural fat (*open arrow*) is moderately bright with this pulse sequence, but has less signal intensity than the cerebrospinal fluid. **B**: Axial T1-weighted SE MR image (600/14) shows the disc herniation with only slightly greater signal intensity than the low-signal cerebrospinal fluid. The epidural fat has bright signal intensity and is in sharp contrast to the disc herniation and the thecal sac. The left S1 nerve root is seen, whereas the disc herniation is compressing the right S1 nerve root.

fat (Fig. 1-3B). This is best appreciated on axial images and on sagittal images obtained lateral to the midline through the neural foramina.

Computed tomography is another excellent method of diagnosing lumbar disc herniation. There are two general methods of performing a lumbar CT scan. Both

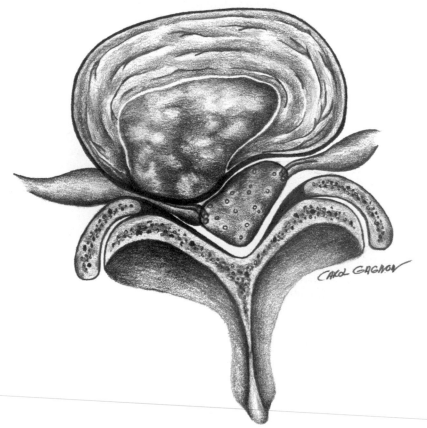

FIG. 1-4. Major characteristics of a posterolateral disc herniation. This drawing is a composite view of the intervertebral disc space and its adjacent levels. Posterolateral disc herniation compresses or displaces the nerve root, epidural fat, and the thecal sac.

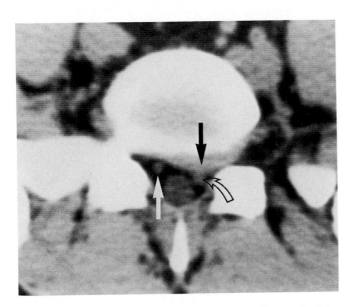

FIG. 1-5. Posterolateral disc herniation. Computed tomography scan shows focal protrusion of the disc on the left (*black arrow*), causing posterior displacement of the left S1 nerve root (*open arrow*) and obliteration of the anterior epidural fat. Compare with the normal position of the right S1 nerve root (*white arrow*) and presence of epidural fat on right.

methods begin with AP and lateral digital radiographs. The patient is in the supine position with the knees flexed. In one method the scans are obtained parallel to the disc space by appropriate angulation of the gantry. The examination includes scan slices that are 3 mm or 4 mm thick. These are obtained through and about the disc and include at least part of the surrounding pedicles. Approximately seven scans are obtained at each level. The L3-L4, L4-L5, and L5-S1 discs are typically studied in this fashion with individual gantry angulation. In the second general method of scanning, no attempt is made to scan parallel to the disc. Instead, contiguous scanning is performed from approximately the level of the L3 pedicle to the superior aspect of the sacrum using a 0-degree angulation of the gantry. Some investigators use contiguous scanning with additional angled scanning at the L5-S1 level. For the evaluation of disc herniation we prefer to obtain images that are parallel to the disc space; for the evaluation of suspected spinal stenosis we obtain contiguous images with 0-degree angulation of the gantry.

The most important CT features of disc herniation are focal protrusion of the disc altering the normal configuration of the disc margin, displacement or compression of the nerve root, displacement or compression of the thecal sac, and displacement or obliteration of the epidural fat (1,4,5,7,10) (Figs. 1-4, 1-5). The most common type of disc herniation is a "soft" herniation of the nucleus pulposus. A "hard" disc represents either a calcified disc herniation or an osteophyte and

may cause compression of the thecal sac and nerve root similar to a "soft" or noncalcified disc herniation. Differentiating a "hard" disc from a "soft" disc herniation is more readily accomplished with CT than with MR imaging.

Although MR imaging and CT are both excellent noninvasive methods of diagnosing lumbar disc herniation, in some cases computed tomographic myelography (CTM) may be performed, with a CT study obtained shortly after a myelogram using nonionic water-soluble contrast agents. The soft-tissue density of the disc is sharply contrasted to the increased density of the contrast-filled thecal sac and nerve root sleeves (Fig. 1-6). Compression and displacement of the thecal sac and nerve roots can be readily seen with this method.

Disc herniations may be described as posterolateral (60–85 percent), central (5–35 percent), or lateral (5–10 percent) (5,10). Posterolateral disc herniation may cause nerve root compression leading to back pain that progresses and radiates into the buttock, thigh, and leg in the distribution pattern of the involved nerve. A central disc herniation typically compresses the thecal sac while sparing an individual nerve root. This leads to low back pain due to sensory innervation to the meninges, posterior longitudinal ligament, and outer layers of the annulus fibrosus. Radiculopathy is usually absent unless the central disc herniation is so large that it compresses the cauda equina. A lateral disc herniation extends into or beyond the neural foramen, often with little or no impression on the dural sac. It may

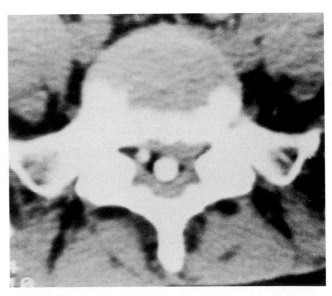

FIG. 1-6. Posterolateral disc herniation seen with computed tomographic myelography (CTM). The right S1 nerve root sleeve fills with contrast and is in normal position. On the left side the disc herniation fills the anterior epidural space and prevents filling of the nerve root sleeve.

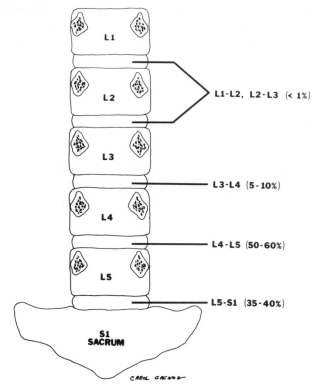

FIG. 1-7. Relative frequency of lumbar disc herniations. Data from refs. 5 and 8.

compress the nerve root as the nerve exits the neural foramen.

Almost all lumbar disc herniations occur at the lower three interspace levels (5,8) (Fig. 1-7). A routine CT examination for a patient with suspected lumbar disc herniation typically includes the last three intervertebral discs (and intervening structures) unless the clinical data suggest that other levels be examined. Using this protocol, the CT study will almost always include the level of disc herniation. However, the conus is not included on the routine CT examination, and occasionally a tumor of the conus has a clinical presentation that is similar to that of a disc herniation. Magnetic resonance imaging has an advantage over CT in that all lumbar levels are included on the study. The conus is well seen on MR images, and the diagnosis of a conus tumor can be made despite the clinical suspicion of disc herniation.

REFERENCES

1. Carrera GF, Williams AL, Haughton VM. Computed tomography in sciatica. *Radiology* 1980;137:433–7.
2. Edelman RR, Shoukimas GM, Stark DD, et al. High-resolution surface-coil imaging of lumbar disk disease. *AJNR* 1985;6:479–85, *AJR* 1985;144:1123–9.
3. Enzmann DR. Degenerative disc disease. In: Enzmann DR, DeLaPaz RL, Rubin JB, eds. *Magnetic resonance of the spine.* St. Louis: CV Mosby; 1990;437–509.
4. Firooznia H, Benjamin V, Kricheff II, et al. CT of lumbar spine disk herniation: correlation with surgical findings. *AJNR* 1984;5:91–6, *AJR* 1984;142:587–92.
5. Fries JW, Abodeely DA, Vijungco JG, et al. Computed tomography of herniated and extruded nucleus pulposus. *J Comput Assist Tomogr* 1982;6:874–87.
6. Modic MT, Masaryk T, Boumphrey F, et al. Lumbar herniated disk disease and canal stenosis: prospective evaluation by surface coil MR, CT, and myelography. *AJNR* 1986;7:709–17, *AJR* 1986;147:757–65.
7. Raskin SP, Keating JW. Recognition of lumbar disk disease: comparison of myelography and computed tomography. *AJR* 1982;139:349–55.
8. Salenius P, Laurent LE. Results of operative treatment of lumbar disc herniation: a survey of 886 patients. *Acta Orthop Scand* 1977;48:630–4.
9. Williams AL, Haughton VM, Daniels DL, et al. Differential CT diagnosis of extruded nucleus pulposus. *Radiology* 1983;148:141–8.
10. Williams AL, Haughton VM, Syvertsen A. Computed tomography in the diagnosis of herniated nucleus pulposus. *Radiology* 1980;135:95–9.

CASE 2

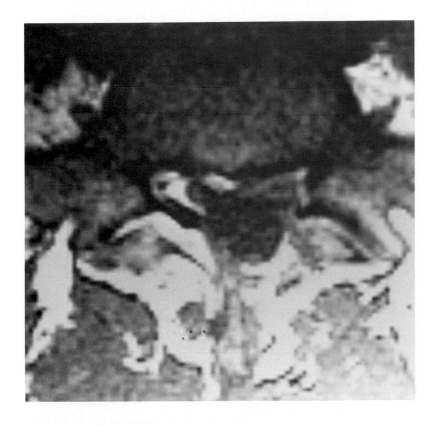

FIG. 2-1A. This 38-year-old man with left leg pain had previous surgery at L5-S1 for disc herniation 4 months ago. Axial T1-weighted SE MR image (600/15) obtained 10 mm caudad to the L5-S1 disc space.

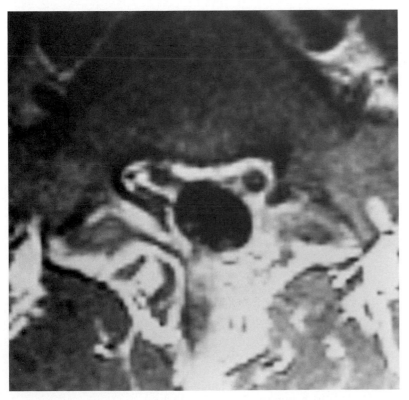

FIG. 2-1B. Axial T1-weighted SE MR image (600/15) obtained at the same level immediately after the intravenous injection of gadopentetate dimeglumine.

7

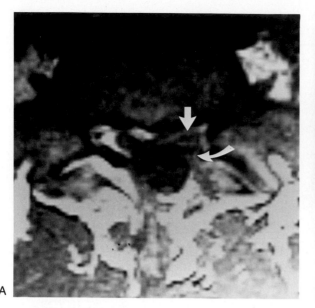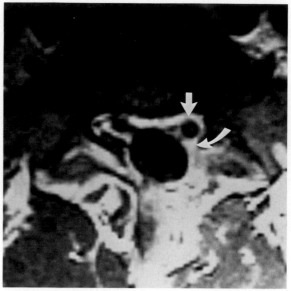

1A   1B

FIG. 2-1A. Fibrotic scar. The precontrast scan shows intermediate signal intensity in the left anterior epidural space (*straight arrow*) partially obliterating the epidural fat. The differential diagnosis includes fibrotic scar and recurrent disc herniation. Note the partial laminectomy on the left with scar (*curved arrow*) at the laminectomy site.

FIG. 2-1B. After gadopentetate dimeglumine injection there is marked enhancement of scar in the anterior epidural space (*straight arrow*) and at the laminectomy site (*curved arrow*). The left S1 nerve root is seen and is surrounded by scar.

POSTOPERATIVE FIBROTIC SCAR

In this case the unenhanced T1-weighted MR image shows abnormal signal intensity in the anterior epidural space that could be caused by postoperative scar or disc herniation (Fig. 2-1A). The patient was given an intravenous injection of gadopentetate dimeglumine (formerly called Gd-DTPA), which caused marked enhancement of fibrotic scar (Fig. 2-1B). There was no disc herniation seen on the postcontrast images.

In a study of the failed back surgery syndrome reported in 1981, recurrent or persistent disc herniation was the primary factor in 12–16 percent of cases, and epidural fibrosis was the cause in 6–8 percent (6). The differentiation of disc herniation from scar is clinically important since reoperation for disc herniation is often successful, whereas reoperation for fibrosis is discouraged as it leads to further scar.

Imaging of the failed back surgery syndrome is, therefore, frequently directed toward determining whether disc herniation or scar is present. Myelography is not a reliable method of distinguishing between disc herniation and fibrotic scar in the postoperative patient. There also may be difficulty in making this differentiation by CT. Both disc herniation and scar may appear as soft-tissue density obliterating epidural fat and obscuring the margins of the thecal sac and

ipsilateral nerve root. The diagnosis of a scar may be suggested on CT if the density is linear or strandlike, contours itself around the thecal sac, or retracts the sac toward the soft-tissue density (19). However, approximately 15 percent of scars have a nodular shape simulating a disc herniation (16). Typically, a disc herniation does not follow the contour of the thecal sac and does not cause retraction of the sac, but instead compresses the thecal sac or displaces a nerve root (19).

Scars often extend above or below the disc space and may not appear contiguous to the posterior disc margin, whereas herniated discs are typically at the disc space level and are contiguous with the disc margin. However, an extruded disc with a free fragment is likely to extend cephalad or caudad and is separated from the posterior disc margin by fat in 50 percent of the cases (8,22). It is suggested that fibrosis typically has a lower CT density measurement than disc herniation; however, there is overlap in their range of attenuation values.

Prior to the advent of MR imaging, some investigators recommended the use of intravenous injection of iodinated contrast medium in an effort to distinguish disc from scar (2,16,19). With this method disc material characteristically does not enhance, whereas scar may enhance significantly. Studies with light and electron microscopy show that the size of the extracellular space and the gap junction status are more important than vascular density in determining the degree of contrast enhancement (5). Scar that is 1 year old or less enhances more intensely than older scar and tends to have leaky junctional complexes (5).

With the advent of surface-coil MR imaging of the spine, investigators began studying the ability of MR to examine the postoperative spine. Unenhanced MR imaging of the lumbar spine has been reported to have an accuracy of 79–89 percent in the differentiation of fibrotic scar from recurrent or persistent disc herniation in patients with failed back surgery syndrome (4,5, 11,17). This accuracy is similar to that obtained from intravenous contrast-enhanced CT (2,5,17). Some authors have found unenhanced MR imaging to be more accurate than contrast-enhanced CT and favored MR as the modality of choice in diagnosing the cause of recurrent postoperative sciatica (9). The unenhanced MR parameters for differentiating scar from herniated disc include morphology, mass effect, and often signal intensity. Recurrent disc herniation tends to be smooth and polypoid, whereas scar has irregular, unsharp margins (10). In one study (4), scars in the anterior epidural space or lateral recess were hypointense or isointense relative to the annulus on T1-weighted images and hyperintense on T2-weighted images. The frequency with which scar appears hyperintense on T2-weighted images appears to vary with the location of the scar. In another study (5), the percentage of scar that was hyperintense on T2-weighted images was reported to be: anterior, 82 percent; lateral recess, 70 percent; lateral, 47 percent; and posterior, 20 percent. Disc herniations are contiguous with the disc margin and are usually either isointense or hypointense with the annulus on all imaging sequences (4). Free disc fragments tend to be well circumscribed and exert mass effect. Relative to the annulus they are isointense or hyperintense on T1-weighted images and hyperintense on T2-weighted images (4). Thus, if free disc fragments are compared to scar, the disc fragments tend to be slightly hyperintense on T1-weighted images and of similar intensity on T2-weighted images.

In an effort to improve the diagnostic accuracy of MR imaging in patients with the failed back surgery syndrome, investigators have studied the use of gadopentetate dimeglumine as a contrast agent and have found that it increases diagnostic accuracy (3,13,18). Excellent correlation with surgical pathology has been found in the initial studies. In one study (13), contrast-enhanced MR imaging was 96 percent accurate in predicting the presence of scar, disc herniation, or combined scar and disc. Gadopentetate dimeglumine is a stable paramagnetic metal ion chelate. Paramagnetic substances have a permanent magnetic moment because of the presence of one or more unpaired electrons (15). This property can be used to enhance the appearance of tissue with adequate vascular supply, a route for contrast to move out of the vasculature, and an interstitial space for sequestering the contrast material (12). When gadopentetate dimeglumine is sequestered in a particular tissue, it changes the magnetic field of the surrounding water protons, shortening their T1 and T2 relaxation times (15). By using T1-weighted pulse sequences (e.g., TR = 400–600 msec, TE = 15–30 msec), the effect of T1 shortening by gadopentetate dimeglumine can be maximized. This leads to increased signal intensity in the affected area. Gadopentetate dimeglumine is injected intravenously in doses of 0.1 mmol/kg body weight. At these low concentrations, the shortening of the T1 relaxation time predominates over the T2 shortening effect. Using the recommended dosage, gadopentetate dimeglumine, which is excreted by the kidneys, has been safely used in clinical trials (7,21). Caution should be exercised in patients with severely impaired renal function. Very rarely, a serious anaphylactoid reaction may occur (20).

Axial and sagittal T1-weighted images are obtained within minutes of the intravenous injection of gadopentetate dimeglumine and compared with the T1-weighted precontrast images (see Appendix 1). Clinical trials have found that scar has maximum enhancement 5 minutes after intravenous injection of gadopentetate dimeglumine (Fig. 2-2) (12). Enhancement slowly diminishes with time, being only slightly decreased 30 minutes after injection and further reduced but still present 58 minutes after injection (12). The contrast enhancement of fibrotic scar is inhomogeneous on the early postcontrast studies and becomes more homogeneous on delayed images. However, in one study (3), qualitative and quantitative evaluation of fibrotic scar enhancement revealed a variable degree of enhancement, from inconspicuous to marked.

Typically, a herniated disc does not show contrast enhancement on images obtained shortly after contrast injection (Fig. 2-3) (12). Often, on these early images, the disc herniation is unenhanced and is surrounded by an enhanced scar (Fig. 2-4). However, a disc herniation, when surrounded by scar, may enhance on delayed images obtained more than 30 minutes after the intravenous injection of contrast (12). In one study (11), enhancement of disc herniation occurred in nine of twelve patients examined with delayed images. In all but one of these cases the herniated disc was associated with scar. The mechanism for enhancement is not known, but may be caused by the diffusion of contrast into the disc from the surrounding scar (12). Thus, it is critical to obtain images as soon as possible after contrast injection so that in most cases scar enhances and disc remains unenhanced. Disc herniations consis-

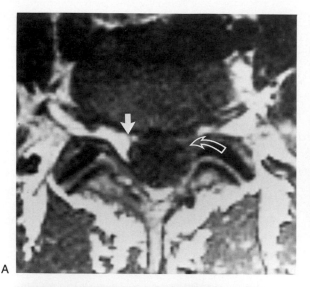

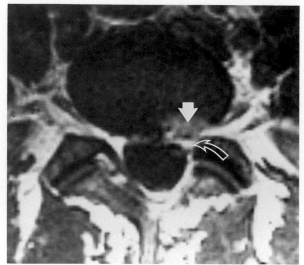

A

B

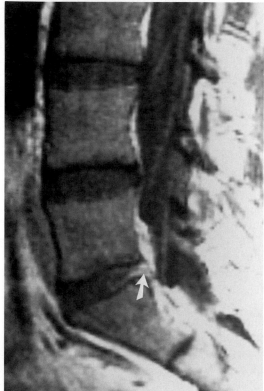

C

FIG. 2-2. Postoperative fibrotic scar, same patient as shown in Fig. 2-1. **A**: Axial T1-weighted MR image (600/15) obtained at the L5-S1 disc level, 10 mm cephalad to Fig. 2-1A. Scar (*curved arrow*) in the left anterior epidural space obscures the anterior epidural fat. Compare to normal bright-signal fat on the right (*straight arrow*). **B**: Axial T1-weighted MR image (600/15) after gadopentetate dimeglumine injection shows enhancement of scar (*curved arrow*) and the posterior aspect of the disc at the discectomy site (*straight arrow*). **C**: Sagittal T1-weighted MR image (600/15) after gadopentetate dimeglumine injection shows enhancement of the posterior aspect of the disc (*arrow*) that is thought to be caused by scar and granulation tissue at the site of discectomy.

tently produce mass effect; however, scar alone may also produce mass effect and thus the presence or absence of a mass effect is a secondary consideration when compared to the presence or absence of contrast enhancement with MR imaging (13).

Several pitfalls of contrast-enhanced MR imaging should be mentioned. As noted, a false negative diagnosis of disc herniation may be given when granulation tissue extends into the margin of a herniated disc and leads to enhancement of the disc (13). Scar tissue has even been seen in association with disc herniation in previously unoperated patients and can enhance simi-

lar to scar in postoperative patients (14). Importantly, a study of successfully decompressed asymptomatic patients examined in the early postoperative period has shown residual mass effect on the nerve roots with peripheral rim enhancement that may simulate a disc fragment during the first 3–6 months postoperatively (1). This observation suggests that additional caution is warranted in the study of patients in the early postoperative period.

It is also important to be aware of the enhancement characteristics of normal structures. Some reports state that nerve roots do not enhance (due to the pres-

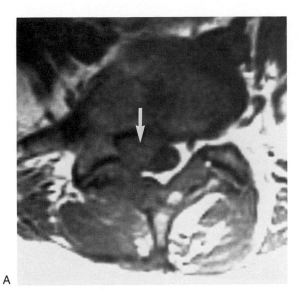
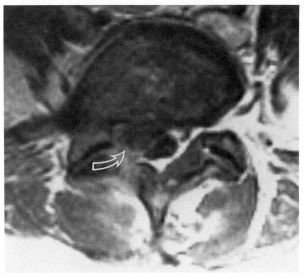

A

B

FIG. 2-3. Large recurrent disc herniation at L4-L5 in a 47-year old woman with right leg pain and a history of previous laminectomy for disc herniation. **A**: Axial precontrast T1-weighted MR image (700/15) shows a large rounded area of intermediate signal (*arrow*) compressing the thecal sac and the right S1 nerve root and obscuring anterior epidural fat. **B**: Axial T1-weighted MR image (817/15) obtained after gadopentetate dimeglumine injection reveals moderate rim enhancement (*arrow*) with the major portion of the disc herniation remaining unenhanced.

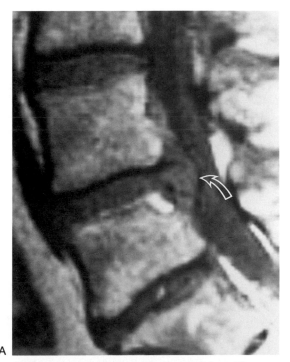
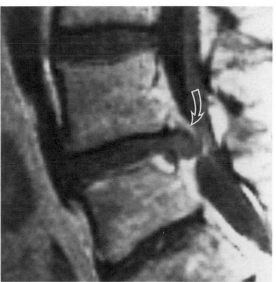

A

B

FIG. 2-4. Recurrent disc herniation with surrounding scar in a patient with left leg pain and a history of previous surgery. **A**: Sagittal T1-weighted MR image (600/15) obtained prior to contrast injection raises the question of recurrent disc herniation and/or scar at L4-L5 (*arrow*). **B**: Sagittal T1-weighted MR image (600/15) obtained approximately 10 minutes after intravenous injection of gadopentetate dimeglumine reveals an unenhanced disc herniation compressing the thecal sac. Bright enhancement of surrounding scar (*arrow*) now has signal intensity similar to epidural fat and could not be differentiated from fat without the ability to compare to pre-enhancement images.

ence of a blood-nerve barrier) whereas a dorsal root ganglion located within the neural foramen does enhance (due to the lack of a blood-nerve barrier) (3). Others have shown enhancement of intradural and extradural nerve roots in most asymptomatic postoperative patients examined 3 weeks after surgery (1). Enhancement of extradural nerve roots is still seen in about one-third of these patients studied 6 months postoperatively. In addition, the epidural venous plexus enhances and should not be confused with a pathologic process. Enhancement at the site of discectomy may be seen and is thought to be caused by scar and granulation tissue that forms at the discectomy site (see Figs. 2-2B, 2-2C).

REFERENCES

1. Boden SD, Davis DO, Dina TS, et al. Contrast-enhanced MR imaging performed after successful lumbar disk surgery: prospective study. *Radiology* 1992;182:59–64.
2. Braun IF, Hoffman JC Jr, David PC, et al. Contrast enhancement in CT differentiation between recurrent disk herniation and postoperative scar: prospective study. *AJNR* 1985;6:607–12, *AJR* 1985;145:785–90.
3. Breger RK, Williams AL, Daniels DL, et al. Contrast enhancement in spinal MR imaging. *AJNR* 1989;10:633–7, *AJR* 1989; 153:387–91.
4. Bundschuh CV, Modic MT, Ross JS, et al. Epidural fibrosis and recurrent disk herniation in the lumbar spine: MR imaging assessment. *AJNR* 1988;9:169–78, *AJR* 1988;150:923–32.
5. Bundschuh CV, Stein L, Slusser JH, et al. Distinguishing between scar and recurrent herniated disk in postoperative patients: value of contrast-enhanced CT and MR imaging. *AJNR* 1990;11:949–58.
6. Burton CV, Kirkaldy-Willis WH, Yong-Hing K, et al. Causes of failure of surgery on the lumbar spine. *Clin Orthop* 1981;157: 191–9.
7. Carr DH, Brown J, Bydder GM, et al. Gadolinium-DTPA as a contrast agent in MRI: initial clinical experience in 20 patients. *AJR* 1984;143:215–24.
8. Dillon WP, Kaseff LG, Knackstedt VE, et al. Computed tomography and differential diagnosis of the extruded lumbar disc. *J Comput Assist Tomogr* 1983;7:969–75.
9. Frocrain L, Duvauferrier R, Husson J-L, et al. Recurrent postoperative sciatica: evaluation with MR imaging and enhanced CT. *Radiology* 1989;170:531–3.
10. Hochhauser L, Kieffer SA, Cacazorin ED, et al. Recurrent postdiskectomy low back pain: MR-surgical correlation. *AJNR* 1988; 9:769–74, *AJR* 1988;151:755–60.
11. Hueftle M, Modic MT, Ross JS, et al. Lumbar spine: postoperative MR imaging with Gd-DTPA. *Radiology* 1988;167:817–24.
12. Ross JS, Delamarter R, Hueftle MG, et al. Gadolinium-DTPA-enhanced MR imaging of the postoperative lumbar spine: time course and mechanism of enhancement. *AJNR* 1989;10:37–46, *AJR* 1989;152:825–34.
13. Ross JS, Masaryk TJ, Schrader M, et al. MR imaging of the postoperative lumbar spine: assessment with gadolinium dimeglumine. *AJNR* 1990;11:771–6, *AJR* 1990;155:867–72.
14. Ross JS, Modic MT, Masaryk TJ, et al. Assessment of extradural degenerative disease with Gd-DTPA-enhanced MR imaging: correlation with surgical and pathologic findings. *AJNR* 1989;10:1243–9, *AJR* 1990;154:151–7.
15. Runge VM, Schaible TF, Goldstein HA, et al. Gd-DTPA: Clinical efficacy. *RadioGraphics* 1988;8:147–59.
16. Schubiger O, Valavanis A. Postoperative lumbar CT: technique, results, and indications. *AJNR* 1983;4:595–7.
17. Sotiropoulos S, Chafetz NI, Lang P, et al. Differentiation between postoperative scar and recurrent disk herniation: prospective comparison of MR, CT, and contrast-enhanced CT. *AJNR* 1989;10:639–43.
18. Sze G, Bravo S, Krol G. Spinal lesions: quantitative and qualitative temporal evolution of gadopentetate dimeglumine enhancement in MR imaging. *Radiology* 1989;170:849–56.
19. Teplick JG, Haskin ME. CT of the postoperative lumbar spine. *Radiol Clin North Am* 1983;21:395–420.
20. Tishler S, Hoffman JC Jr. Anaphylactoid reactions to IV gadopentetate dimeglumine. *AJNR* 1990;11:1167.
21. Valk J. Gd-DTPA in MR of spinal lesions. *AJNR* 1988;9:345–50, *AJR* 1988;150:1163–8.
22. Williams AL, Haughton VM, Daniels DL, et al. Differential CT diagnosis of extruded nucleus pulposus. *Radiology* 1983;148: 141–8.

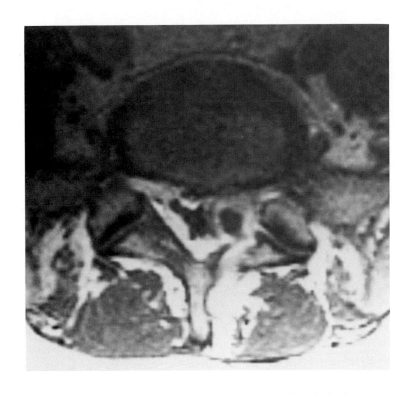

FIG. 3-1A. Axial MR imaging at L5-S1 in a 42-year-old man with pain radiating into the left leg. He had a previous laminectomy at this level 1 year ago. T1-weighted SE MR image (700/15).

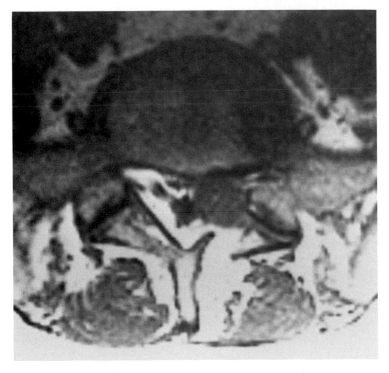

FIG. 3-1B. Axial T1-weighted SE MR image (700/15) at the same level as Fig. 3-1A, obtained after the intravenous injection of gadopentetate dimeglumine.

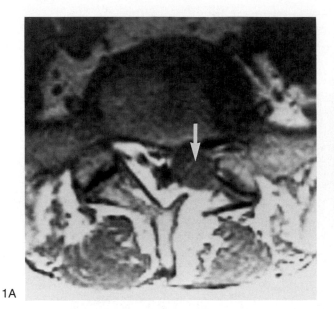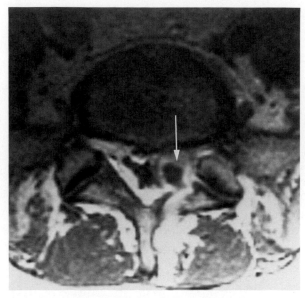

1A   1B

FIG. 3-1A. Free disc fragment in a postoperative patient. A large rounded area of intermediate to low signal intensity (*arrow*) fills the left side of the spinal canal and obscures the normal bright signal of the anterior epidural fat. Note laminectomy defect on the left.

FIG. 3-1B. After the intravenous injection of gadopentetate dimeglumine there is rim enhancement of peripheral scar (*arrow*). A large unenhanced free disc fragment is clearly seen and is causing compression of the thecal sac and left S1 nerve root.

FREE DISC FRAGMENT

There is abnormal signal intensity in the epidural space on the left at L5-S1 seen on the axial T1-weighted MR image (Fig. 3-1A). After the intravenous injection of gadopentetate dimeglumine, rim enhancement of scar surrounds an unenhanced free disc fragment (Fig. 3-1B). Sagittal T1-weighted images before and after contrast enhancement further display this abnormality (Fig. 3-2).

A free disc fragment (sequestered fragment) represents a disc herniation that has extended through a tear in the annulus and has separated from the parent disc. It may extend through or around the posterior longitudinal ligament and may be displaced cephalad or caudad to the intervertebral disc of origin. Often the disc fragment lies free in the anterior epidural space, or rarely posterior to the thecal sac (8) or in the intradural compartment (3). The anterior epidural space is a fairly well-defined space, delimited posteriorly by the posterior longitudinal ligament and laterally by membranes attached to this ligament (11). A midline septum separates the anterior epidural space into left and right compartments and can be identified by MR imaging. Most free fragments are found to the side rather than in the midline because of the presence of this septum (11) (Fig. 3-3). A disc fragment is said to be contained if it remains confined by the posterior longitudinal ligament

and lateral membranes and is noncontained if it has broken this complex.

A free disc fragment can be diagnosed by both MR imaging and CT. The MR diagnosis of a free disc fragment relies on both morphology and signal intensity (7,9). With MR imaging, the free disc fragment appears as a soft-tissue mass which is separate from the parent intervertebral disc (9). The separation of the fragment from the parent disc is best seen on T2-weighted sagittal images. When a disc is extruded but remains attached to the parent disc, the adjoining pedicle can be seen as a high-signal attachment on T2-weighted sagittal images. Interestingly, free disc fragments often show increased signal intensity on T2-weighted images (7,9). The parent disc, on the other hand, frequently has low signal intensity on T2-weighted images because of degeneration.

In one study of twenty patients with surgically proved free disc fragments, 80 percent had MR findings of an extradural mass that had intermediate signal on T1-weighted images, increased signal on T2-weighted images, and distinct separation from the parent disc (9) (Fig. 3-4). The other 20 percent had MR findings of an extradural mass that had low signal intensity on T2-weighted images similar to that of the degenerated disc of origin. It should be noted that disc herniations that

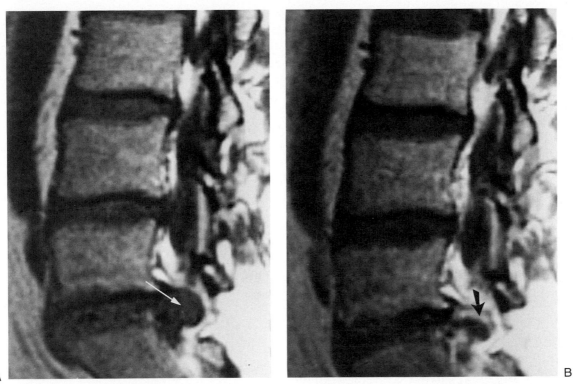

FIG. 3-2. Free disc fragment. Same patient as Fig. 3-1. **A**: Sagittal T1-weighted SE MR image (700/15) obtained 1 cm to the left of the midline before contrast enhancement. Large free disc fragment (*arrow*) is isointense relative to parent disc. **B**: Sagittal T1-weighted SE MR image (700/15) obtained 1 cm to the left of the midline after contrast enhancement. After injection of gadopentelate dimeglumine there is rim enhancement of scar (*arrow*) surrounding a free disc fragment.

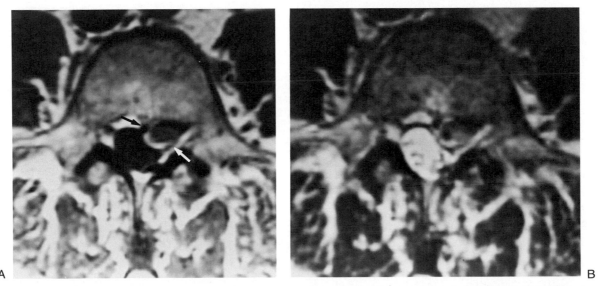

FIG. 3-3. Free disc fragment with MR demonstration of the anatomy of the anterior epidural space. **A**: Axial T1-weighted SE MR image (600/14) at level of the mid-L4 vertebral body. There is a free disc fragment on the left that was proven at surgery to have been displaced caudad from the L3-L4 disc space. The disc fragment is nearly isointense relative to the thecal sac with this pulse sequence. Note the posterior longitudinal ligament/midline septum complex (*black arrow*) and thin lateral membrane (*white arrow*) that demarcate the anterior epidural space. **B**: Axial T2-weighted FSE MR image (2800/100) again shows the midline septum and the lateral membrane that demarcate the anterior epidural space. The free disc fragment has intermediate signal and is hypointense relative to the bright signal of cerebrospinal fluid within the thecal sac.

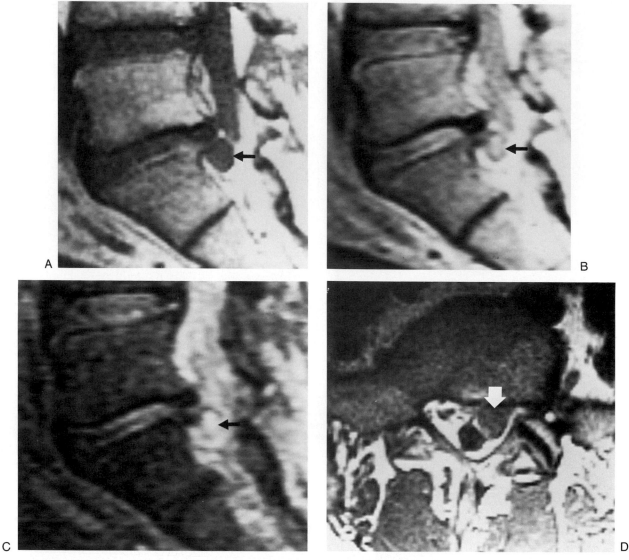

FIG. 3-4. Free disc fragment at L5-S1. **A**: Sagittal T1-weighted SE MR image (600/15) obtained to the left of the midline reveals a free disc fragment (*arrow*) displaced caudad to the L5-S1 intervertebral disc space. **B**: Proton density-weighted SE MR image (2000/35) reveals high signal intensity of the free disc fragment (*arrow*). **C**: T2-weighted SE MR image (2000/70). The disc fragment (*arrow*) has bright signal intensity and is difficult to identify on this pulse sequence because of the adjacent high-signal cerebrospinal fluid. The disc fragment is of higher signal than the parent L5-S1 intervertebral disc, and appears to be separate from it. **D**: Axial T1-weighted SE MR image caudad to the L5-S1 disc space shows the disc fragment (*arrow*) compressing the thecal sac and the left S1 nerve root.

remain attached to the parent disc may occasionally have high signal intensity on T2-weighted images; however, their continuity with the disc of origin can be seen on these T2-weighted sagittal studies (9). Using this criteria, the ability to distinguish a free disc fragment from other types of disc herniation was studied and found to have sensitivity of 89 percent, specificity of 82 percent, and accuracy of 85 percent (9).

In another study (7), 12 percent of disc herniations identified by MR imaging showed a free disc fragment that was hyperintense on T2-weighted sagittal images. Others (10) have obtained both sagittal and axial T2-

weighted images that have shown high signal intensity within surgically confirmed free disc fragments.

The cause for the high signal intensity of free disc fragments on T2-weighted images is not known, although several theories have been suggested (7). For example, it is possible that the extruded disc fragment may absorb water, which results in an increased signal intensity on T2-weighted images. Another suggestion is that the free fragment represents complete extrusion of the nucleus pulposus, which is the portion of the disc with the greatest water content and therefore shows increased signal intensity on the T2-weighted images.

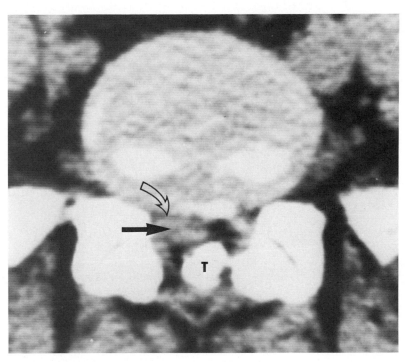

FIG. 3-5. Free disc fragment in postoperative patient. CTM at L5-S1 shows a large free disc fragment (*straight arrow*) that fills the anterior epidural space on the right. There is partial obliteration of the anterior epidural fat and compression of the contrast-filled thecal sac (*T*). The posteriorly displaced fragment is separated from the posterior margin of the disc by a thin layer of fat (*curved arrow*). There is a bilateral laminectomy defect.

The signal intensity characteristics described are not specific for an extruded disc fragment, but should be used in conjunction with the lack of continuity between the disc fragment and the parent disc in the MR evaluation.

Computed tomography is also useful in the diagnosis of a free fragment. The original CT studies of free fragments defined an extruded disc as representing nuclear material that protrudes through a tear in the annulus fibrosus and extends through or around the posterior longitudinal ligament (2,12). The portion of the disc that has extruded beyond the ligament may remain solidly attached to the parent disc or may be displaced and lie as a free fragment within the vertebral canal or neural foramen. An extruded disc can be diagnosed with CT when a free fragment is seen displaced into the canal and separated from the disc margin by epidural fat (Fig. 3-5), a finding that occurs in only 50 percent of the cases (4,12). In CT examination of the other half of the cases, the extruded disc is contiguous with the posterior margin and may be indistinguishable from a focal subligamentous herniation, particularly when the contour is smooth and curvilinear. An extruded disc may be considered if the soft-tissue mass has a polypoid or irregular shape. A free disc fragment may migrate superiorly, inferiorly, or in both directions, and may be as far as 15–30 mm from the intervertebral disc space (Fig. 3-6). In one study, superior and inferior migration occurred with equal frequency (11). An extruded fragment has been reported to lie 6 mm or more from the center of the disc space in 85 percent of cases of disc extrusion (4). The fragment may appear

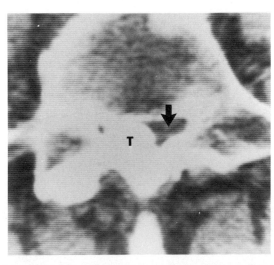

FIG. 3-6. Free disc fragment in patient with previous surgery. CTM obtained 12 mm caudad to the L4-L5 disc. The extruded disc fragment (*arrow*) is within the lateral recess on the left and displaces the contrast-filled thecal sac (*T*) to the right.

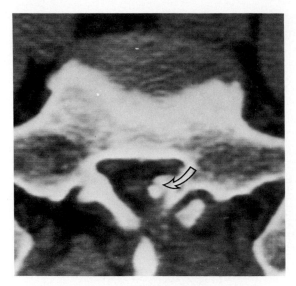

FIG. 3-7. Postoperative bone fragment within the spinal canal. A partial left laminectomy and discectomy had been performed. Increased intensity of pain in the immediate postoperative period led to this CT study at L5-S1. There is a large free bone fragment within the spinal canal (*arrow*) abutting the thecal sac. An additional bone fragment is seen posterior to the remaining left lamina.

larger in the cephalad or caudad direction than at the disc level, a finding not present in patients with subligamentous herniation (4). It is important to study CT scans above and below the disc space, since approximately 10 percent of disc extrusions are associated with a normal posterior disc margin and would go undetected if evaluation were limited to the disc itself (4,12). Extruded discs tend to be larger than subligamentous herniations. In one study, the maximum AP diameter of the herniated disc was compared to the anticipated normal sagittal diameter of the dural sac. In patients in whom the ratio was less than one half, 10 percent had an extruded disc at surgery. In patients with a ratio of one half or more, 90 percent had an extruded disc (5).

The MR imaging and CT diagnosis of a free disc fragment is important. It alerts the surgeon to the presence and location of the fragmented disc and suggests a less favorable outcome should chymopapain chemonucleolysis be attempted (1,6).

In some postoperative patients, a free fragment of bone rather than disc may be found. One such patient had a partial left laminectomy and discectomy for disc herniation at L5-S1, and had increased intensity of pain in the immediate postoperative period which led to evaluation with CT (Fig. 3-7). A large bone fragment was identified within the spinal canal, and reoperation was performed. CT is particularly well suited for evaluation of bony or calcific structures.

REFERENCES

1. Benoist M, Deburge A, Busson J, et al. Treatment of lumbar disc herniation by chymopapain chemonucleolysis. *Spine* 1982; 7:613–7.
2. Carrera GF, Williams AL, Haughton VM. Computed tomography in sciatica. *Radiology* 1980;137:433–7.
3. Ciappetta P, Delfini R, Cantore GP. Intradural lumbar disc hernia: description of three cases. *Neurosurgery* 1981;8:104–7.
4. Dillon WP, Kaseff LG, Knackstedt VE, et al. Computed tomography and differential diagnosis of the extruded lumbar disc. *J Comput Assist Tomogr* 1983;7:969–75.
5. Fries JW, Abodeely DA, Vijungco JG, et al. Computed tomography of herniated and extruded nucleus pulposus. *J Comput Assist Tomogr* 1982;6:874–87.
6. Gentry LR, Strother CM, Turski PA, et al. Chymopapain chemonucleolysis: correlation of diagnostic radiographic factors and clinical outcome. *AJR* 1985;145:351–60.
7. Glickstein MF, Burke DL Jr, Kressel HY. Magnetic resonance demonstration of hyperintense herniated discs and extruded disc fragments. *Skeletal Radiol* 1989;18:527–30.
8. Lutz JD, Smith RR, Jones HM. CT myelography of a fragment of a lumbar disk sequestered posterior to the thecal sac. *AJNR* 1990;11:610–1.
9. Masaryk TJ, Ross JS, Modic MT, et al. High-resolution MR imaging of sequestered lumbar intervertebral disks. *AJNR* 1988; 9:351–8, *AJR* 1988;150:1155–62.
10. Modic MT, Masaryk T, Boumphrey F, et al. Lumbar herniated disk disease and canal stenosis: prospective evaluation by surface coil MR, CT, and myelography. *AJNR* 1986;7:709–17, *AJR* 1986;147:757–65.
11. Schellinger D, Manz HJ, Vidic B, et al. Disk fragment migration, *Radiology* 1990;175:831–6.
12. Williams AL, Haughton VM, Daniels DL, et al. Differential CT diagnosis of extruded nucleus pulposus. *Radiology* 1983;148: 141–8.

CASE 4

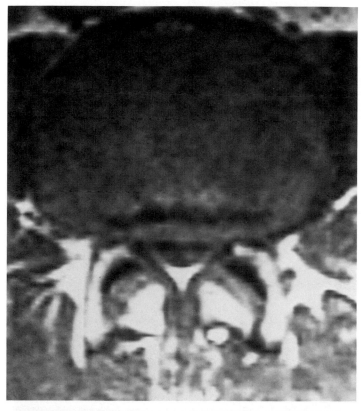

FIG. 4-1A. This 63-year-old man had right leg pain and a disc herniation at L4-L5 on the right. What is the diagnosis at L2-L3? Axial T1-weighted SE MR image (767/20) at L2-L3.

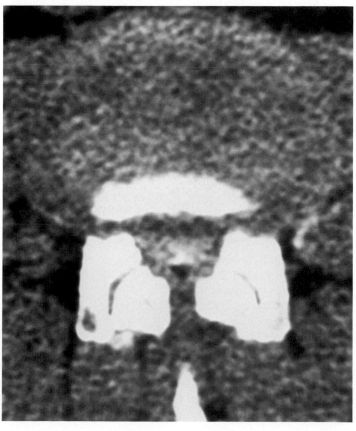

FIG. 4-1B. Axial CTM scan at L2-L3.

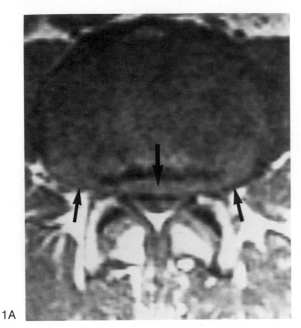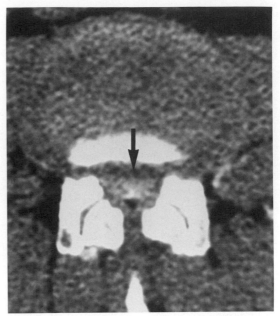

1A   1B

FIG. 4-1A. Bulging annulus. There is generalized bulging of the annulus fibrosus (*arrows*) without focal disc herniation. There is compression of the thecal sac.

FIG. 4-1B. The contrast-filled thecal sac is markedly compressed by the bulging annulus (*arrow*).

BULGING ANNULUS

There is bulging of the annulus fibrosus which protrudes in a generalized fashion beyond the vertebral body (Fig. 4-1). MR imaging and CT can be used to accurately diagnose bulging of the annulus fibrosus and differentiate it from herniation of the nucleus pulposus (5,14,16,17). A bulging annulus is seen as a generalized, usually symmetric extension of the disc margin beyond the vertebral body, with disc protruding posteriorly, laterally, and anteriorly (Fig. 4-2). There is no focal protrusion of the disc margin as occurs with herniation of the nucleus pulposus (16,17). The posterior margin of a bulging disc is most often convex but infrequently may remain concave because of reinforcement of the central portion of the annulus by the posterior longitudinal ligament (16,17). Gas within the disc and calcification of the outer annulus may be present.

Patients with generalized bulging of the disc are unlikely to have nerve root compression. However, in some instances a bulging disc may be associated with thickening of the ligamenta flava, prominent laminae and hypertrophied articular processes (6). This combination of abnormalities may lead to spinal stenosis with nerve root compression that is predominantly related to bony and ligamentous encroachment (13).

Pathologically, several biochemical and biomechanical factors may lead to generalized bulging of the disc with aging (16,17). Gradual desiccation of the nucleus

pulposus leads to decreased nuclear turgor, permitting a decrease in disc space height. In addition, the annulus fibrosus develops fissuring, hyalin degeneration, and increased pigmentation. The annulus loses elasticity and bulges in a generalized fashion beyond the adjacent vertebral body margins (16,17). The inner fibers of the annulus fibrosus may tear; however, it has been thought that the outer fibers remain intact, preventing any nuclear material from herniating (17). More recently, it has been suggested that disc bulging may be associated with tears that extend from the nucleus to the surface of the annulus (18,20).

Three types of tears of the annulus have been described: concentric, radial, and transverse (20). Concentric tears are characterized by fluid-filled spaces between adjacent lamellae. These tears are found commonly in cadaver specimens, but are not effectively demonstrated on MR images and are thought to have no clinical significance.

Radial tears are characterized by rupture of all layers in the annulus, with fissures extending from the nucleus pulposus to the surface of the annulus. These tears are most often found at L4-L5 and L5-S1 in individuals over 40 years of age (20). T2-weighted sagittal MR images may reveal increased signal intensity within a radial tear of the annulus (14,20). The tear may have a globular configuration extending from the

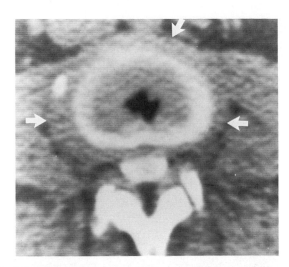

FIG. 4-2. Bulging annulus. Computed tomographic myelography at L3-L4. The annulus bulges in a generalized fashion anteriorly, posteriorly, and laterally (*arrows*). The anterior aspect of the thecal sac is flattened by the bulging annulus. There is calcification within the periphery of the annulus on the right. Note low density gas in the disc (vacuum disc phenomenon) indicating degeneration of the disc.

nucleus to the surface of the annulus. Enhancement of a radial tear can be seen on T1-weighted images after the intravenous injection of gadopentetate dimeglumine (14). This is thought to be related to vascularized granulation tissue within the annulus. In one study there were more radial tears seen on T1-weighted contrast-enhanced images than on T2-weighted studies, suggesting that enhanced images may be more sensitive (14). A study of lumbar spine cadaver specimens found that 84 percent of discs with radial tears had disc bulging greater than 2.5 mm (18). Those authors believe that disc bulging is associated with radial tears of the annulus and that the tears may play a primary role in disc degeneration. In addition, some authors believe that these tears may be a clinically significant cause of pain (14).

The third type of tear of the annulus is a transverse tear. These tears are due to rupture of Sharpey's fibers in the periphery of the annulus near the ring apophysis. Transverse tears are the most common type of tear of the annulus, most often occur in the anterior portion of the disc, and are thought to be clinically insignificant (20). Magnetic resonance imaging can show these transverse tears on T2-weighted images as small linear areas of increased signal intensity in the region of the torn Sharpey's fibers.

In summary, MR imaging can show generalized bulging of the annulus fibrosus and can also show radial tears of the annulus on T2-weighted images and on contrast-enhanced T1-weighted images. Although clinical importance of showing a radial tear needs further evaluation, it is possible that these tears may be associated with discogenic pain (chronic back pain related to leakage of the nucleus pulposus into the outer annulus or epidural canal without herniation) (14).

The intervertebral disc is made up of an outer annulus fibrosus and a more central nucleus pulposus. The annulus is composed of circular fibrous lamellae that surround the nucleus and attach it to the vertebral bodies. The nucleus is a remnant of embryonic notochord tissue and is made up of fibrous strands within a gelatinous matrix (10). Several stages of maturation and degeneration of the nucleus pulposus have been identified (19). The nucleus may be considered immature (up to 2 years of age), transitional (teenage years), adult, early degenerated, and severely degenerated. The immature nucleus has a translucent appearance, is sharply demarcated from the surrounding annulus, and is associated with an intact annulus fibrosus. The transitional nucleus has a fibrous structure within the central portion of the annulus and nucleus. The transitional nucleus usually has an intact annulus, although concentric tears may sometimes be present (19). The adult nucleus has increased fiber content. A horizontal intranuclear cleft is a normal anatomic structure which is a constant feature in adults over 30 years of age (1). The adult nucleus may be associated with an intact annulus, but more frequently concentric or transverse tears are present. These tears appear to be incidental findings (19). An early degenerated nucleus is associated with disc space narrowing and a reduced amount of fibrocartilage within the nucleus. A radial tear of the annulus is found in 92 percent of patients with an early degenerated nucleus (19). There is associated loss of disc space height and decreased signal intensity within the disc on T2-weighted images. With severely degenerated discs there is replacement of the normal nuclear fibrocartilage with amorphous fiber and cystic spaces. The severely degenerated nucleus is associated with complete disruption of the annulus (19).

Magnetic resonance imaging is the most sensitive method of detecting early degenerative changes of the disc. In the normal young adult lumbar spine, the nucleus pulposus is 85–90 percent water, whereas the annulus fibrosus is 78 percent water (8). With aging and/or disc desiccation, the water content becomes approximately 70 percent for both the nucleus and the annulus. The decreased water content of the disc, along with other biochemical changes that may occur, leads to readily identifiable decreased signal intensity of the disc on T2-weighted MR images (Fig. 4-3).

Another feature of degenerative disc disease (primary intervertebral osteochondrosis) is the common presence of gas within the disc (vacuum disc phenomenon). With advancing age, clefts form in the nucleus pulposus and later progress to involve the fibers of the annulus fibrosus (12). Gas is released from surrounding tissues and accumulates within the fissures of the disc (3). This gas is approximately 90 percent nitrogen and 10 percent a combination of other gases (3). The vacuum disc phenomenon can be identified with conventional radiography, especially when the patient is studied in spinal extension. With MR imaging, the gas appears as an area of signal void within the disc on both sagittal T1- and T2-weighted images (Fig. 4-4). This is more readily identified on T1-weighted images because of the contrast between the signal void of gas and the intermediate signal of the disc with this pulse sequence (4). On the T2-weighted images the degenerated disc has low signal intensity and does not afford a favorable contrast to the gas. The signal void of gas has been described as a thin line, a thick irregular line, or having a mottled pattern and can be found in the middle of the disc or along the adjacent vertebral body endplates (4).

There are several pitfalls to the diagnosis of a vacuum phenomenon studied with MR imaging (4). When gas is adjacent to either cortical endplate, it may be difficult to visualize because both gas and cortical bone have very low signal intensity. A vacuum phenomenon

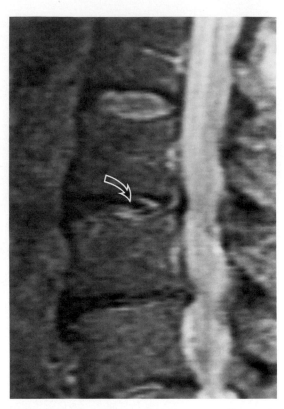

FIG. 4-4. Vacuum disc phenomenon. Sagittal T2-weighted SE MR image (2000/70) of the lumbar spine. Signal void within the disc (*arrow*) is caused by gas in a degenerated disc.

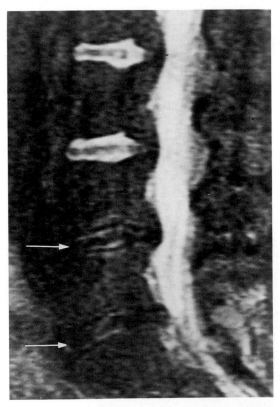

FIG. 4-3. Degenerative disc disease. Sagittal T2-weighted SE MR image (2500/80) shows degenerative disc disease at L4-L5 and L5-S1 with very low signal intensity of the discs (*arrows*) caused by decreased water content of the annulus fibrosus and nucleus pulposus. Normally hydrated discs such as at L2-L3 and L3-L4 have bright signal intensity on T2-weighted images. Note the normal cleft within the center of these discs.

that is located adjacent to the superior endplate of the inferior vertebral body may be obscured by chemical shift artifact which is known to give a thicker appearance to this cortex than is seen along the inferior endplate of the superior vertebra. Finally, calcifications within the disc can produce signal void (Fig. 4-5). However, signal void caused by disc calcification is more typically nodular (4). Calcification that is scattered throughout the disc may go undetected by MR imaging.

Although MR imaging may be more accurate than conventional radiography in detecting a vacuum phenomenon, CT appears to be more accurate than either method (4). Gas is readily found within the disc on CT (see Fig. 4-2) and is seen in 50 percent of patients over 40 years of age and 75 percent of patients over 60 years (7). A vacuum phenomenon may also be seen in patients with secondary intervertebral osteochondrosis associated with calcium pyrophosphate dihydrate crystal deposition disease, alkaptonuria, tumor, or trauma (7,12,15).

Abnormal signal intensity of the vertebral body endplates as seen with MR imaging is not uncommon with degenerative disc disease. Altered signal intensity of the endplates has been found in 50 percent of degenerated discs (2). Three patterns of degenerative changes of the endplates have been described (2,9). Type I de-

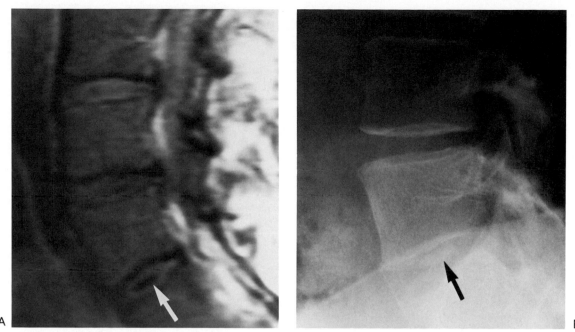

FIG. 4-5. Calcification within the disc. **A**: Proton density-weighted MR image (2000/35) of the lumbar spine shows globular-shaped signal void (*arrow*) within the L5-S1 disc. **B**: Conventional radiograph of the lower lumbar spine shows calcification within the disc (*arrow*) corresponding to the area of low signal on the MR study.

generative changes have decreased signal intensity on T1-weighted images and increased signal intensity on T2-weighted images (2,9,11) (Fig. 4-6). In one study, this pattern was found in 4 percent of patients with low back pain (11). This pattern is associated with disruption and fissuring of the endplates and vascularized

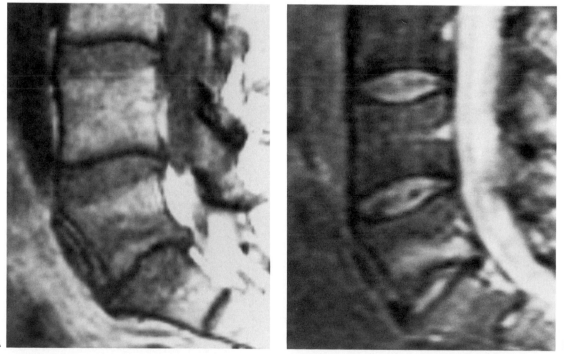

FIG. 4-6. Type I degenerative changes of the vertebral body endplates. **A**: Sagittal T1-weighted SE MR image (700/15) of the lumbar spine shows decreased signal intensity of the inferior endplate of L5 and superior endplate of S1. There is narrowing of the L5-S1 disc space. **B**: Sagittal T2-weighted SE MR image (2000/70) shows increased signal intensity of the vertebral endplates adjacent to the L5-S1 disc space.

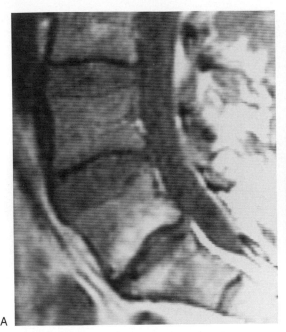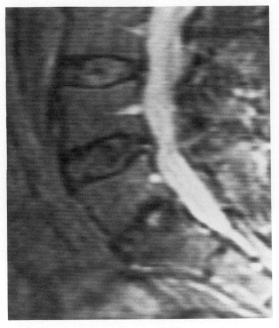

FIG. 4-7. Type II degenerative changes of the vertebral body endplates. **A**: Sagittal T1-weighted SE MR image (700/15) shows increased signal intensity of the vertebral endplates at L5-S1. **B**: Sagittal T2-weighted SE MR image (2000/70) shows isointensity of the vertebral endplates at L5-S1 relative to the other vertebrae.

fibrous tissue (11). It is hypothesized that there is a relative increase in water of the bone marrow which could reflect local inflammation or ischemia (2). Type II degenerative changes of the endplates have increased signal intensity on the T1-weighted images and similar or slightly increased intensity relative to normal vertebral endplates on T2-weighted images (2,9,11) (Fig. 4-7). This is seen in 16 percent of patients with low back pain and is thought to be caused by conversion of red marrow to yellow marrow (11). The presence of increased lipid content within the vertebral body marrow has been documented by chemical shift imaging (11). These changes may reflect local stress and ischemia associated with degenerative disc disease (2). In one study, conversion of a Type I pattern to a Type II pattern was seen in five of six patients evaluated over a period of between 14 months and 3 years (11). The Type II pattern, on the other hand, appears to remain stable. There is a Type III pattern which has decreased signal intensity on both T1- and T2-weighted images. This appears to correlate with extensive bony sclerosis on conventional radiographs (9). This is the least common type of endplate pattern associated with degenerative disc disease. In a study of degenerated discs with adjacent abnormal marrow patterns, 14 percent were Type I, 83 percent Type II, and 3 percent Type III (2).

REFERENCES

1. Aguila LA, Piraino DW, Modic MT, et al. The intranuclear cleft of the intervertebral disk: magnetic resonance imaging. *Radiology* 1985;155:155–8.
2. de Roos A, Kressel H, Spritzer C, et al. MR imaging of marrow changes adjacent to end plates in degenerative lumbar disk disease. *AJR* 1987;149:531–4.
3. Ford LT, Gilula LA, Murphy WA, et al. Analysis of gas in vacuum lumbar disc. *AJR* 1977;128:1056–7.
4. Grenier N, Grossman RI, Schiebler ML, et al. Degenerative lumbar disk disease: pitfalls and usefulness of MR imaging in detection of vacuum phenomenon. *Radiology* 1987;164:861–5.
5. Haughton VM, Eldevik OP, Magnaes B, et al. A prospective comparison of computed tomography and myelography in the diagnosis of herniated lumbar disks. *Radiology* 1982;142:103–10.
6. Kieffer SA, Sherry RG, Wellenstein DE, et al. Bulging lumbar intervertebral disk: myelographic differentiation from herniated disk with nerve root compression. *AJR* 1982;138:709–16.
7. Lardé D, Mathieu D, Frija J, et al. Spinal vacuum phenomenon: CT diagnosis and significance. *J Comput Assist Tomogr* 1982; 6:671–6.
8. Lipson SJ, Muir H. 1980 Volvo award in basic science: proteoglycans in experimental intervertebral disc degeneration. *Spine* 1981;6:194–210.
9. Modic MT, Masaryk TJ, Ross JS, et al. Imaging of degenerative disk disease. *Radiology* 1988;168:177–86.
10. Modic MT, Pavlicek W, Weinstein MA, et al. Magnetic resonance imaging of intervertebral disk disease: clinical and pulse sequence considerations. *Radiology* 1984;152:103–11.
11. Modic MT, Steinberg PM, Ross JS, et al. Degenerative disk disease: assessment of changes in vertebral body marrow with MR imaging. *Radiology* 1988;166:193–9.
12. Resnick D, Niwayama G, Guerra J Jr, et al. Spinal vacuum phe-

nomena: anatomical study and review. *Radiology* 1981;139: 341–8.

13. Roberson GH, Llewellyn HJ, Taveras JM. The narrow lumbar spinal canal syndrome. *Radiology* 1973;107:87–97.

14. Ross JS, Modic MT, Masaryk TJ. Tears of the anulus fibrosus: assessment with Gd-DTPA-enhanced MR imaging. *AJNR* 1989; 10:1251–4, *AJR* 1990;154:159–69.

15. Schabel SI, Moore TE, Rittenberg GM, et al. Vertebral vacuum phenomenon: a radiographic manifestation of metastatic malignancy. *Skeletal Radiol* 1979;4:154–6.

16. Williams AL. CT diagnosis of degenerative disc disease: the bulging annulus. *Radiol Clin North Am* 1983;21:289–300.

17. Williams AL, Haughton VM, Meyer GA, et al. Computed tomographic appearance of the bulging annulus. *Radiology* 1982;142: 403–8.

18. Yu S, Haughton VM, Sether LA, et al. Anulus fibrosus in bulging intervertebral disks. *Radiology* 1988;169:761–3.

19. Yu S, Haughton VM, Sether LA, et al. Criteria for classifying normal and degenerated lumbar intervertebral disks. *Radiology* 1989;170:523–6.

20. Yu S, Sether LA, Ho PSP, et al. Tears of the anulus fibrosus: correlation between MR and pathologic findings in cadavers. *AJNR* 1988;9:367–70.

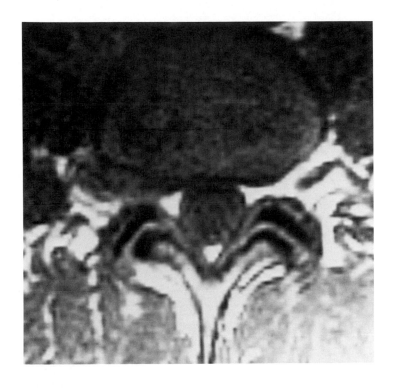

FIG. 5-1A. This 36-year-old man with back and right hip pain had an MR examination of lumbar spine. Axial T1-weighted SE image (600/15) cephalad to the L4-L5 disc space.

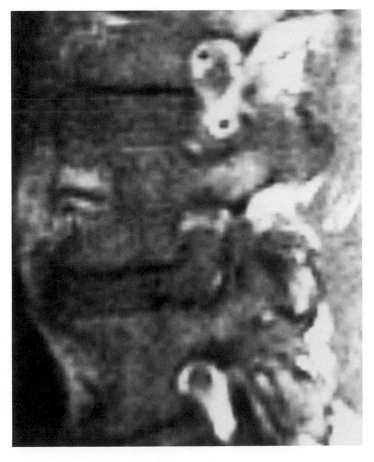

FIG. 5-1B. Parasagittal T1-weighted SE image (600/15) through the plane of the right neural foramina.

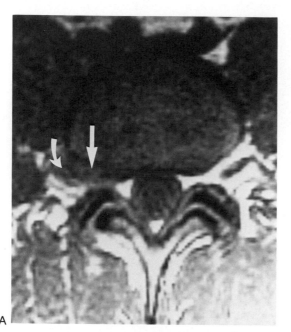
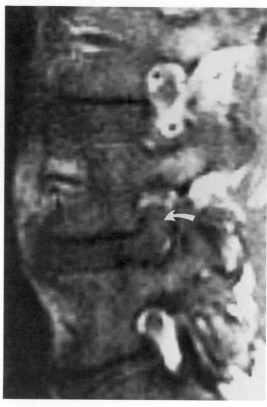

1A

1B

FIG. 5-1A. Lateral disc herniation. A disc herniation (*straight arrow*) is seen extending laterally on the right. The herniated disc is compressing the right L4 nerve root (*curved arrow*) and is obscuring the perineural fat. Compare with the normal left side that has a clearly seen nerve root surrounded by the bright signal of fat. Note the lack of thecal sac compression because of the lateral location of the disc herniation.

FIG. 5-1B. The lateral disc herniation (*arrow*) is isointense relative to the disc of origin. It extends cephalad into the intervertebral foramen and compresses the exiting L4 nerve root. Compare to the foramina above and below that have normal bright signal of fat and intermediate signal of the nerve root.

LATERAL DISC HERNIATION

Magnetic resonance imaging and CT make an important contribution to the diagnosis of disc disease with their ability to depict far lateral disc herniations that might otherwise go undetected by myelography or limited surgical exploration (3,4,6,9,10,15). In this case there is focal protrusion of the disc margin at L4-L5 far laterally on the right, causing obliteration of perineural fat within the neural foramen (Fig. 5-1). The L4 nerve root exits through the upper half of the neural foramen located beneath the L4 pedicle. A lateral disc herniation at L4-L5 may compress the exiting L4 nerve root if the disc is displaced cephalad.

The most frequent MR and CT findings associated with lateral disc herniation include focal protrusion of disc within or lateral to the neural foramen, displacement of fat within the foramen, and absence of dural sac deformity (10,15). Less frequently, disc herniation

may protrude to a greater extent and appears as a large soft tissue mass within or lateral to the foramen (Fig. 5-2). The CT density of herniated disc material is about the same or slightly less than the intervertebral disc and almost always greater than that of the thecal sac (3,12). Occasionally, calcification or gas may be seen within the herniated lateral disc. Magnetic resonance imaging has the advantage of showing the lateral disc herniation in the sagittal plane as well as the axial plane. Parasagittal images obtained through the plane of the neural foramen normally show the exiting nerve root in the upper half of the foramen surrounded by abundant perineural fat that appears bright on T1-weighted images. When a lateral disc herniation extends into the foramen it can be seen replacing the high signal fat and compressing the nerve root.

Approximately 5 percent of all lumbar disc hernia-

28

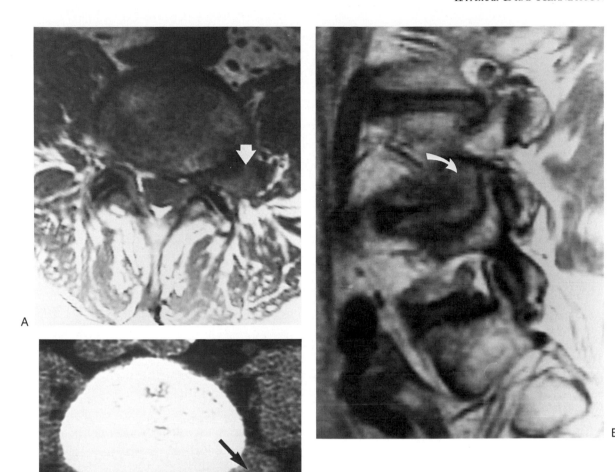

FIG. 5-2. Lateral disc herniation. A: Axial T1-weighted SE MR image (750/20) above the L4-L5 disc space shows a large lateral disc herniation on the left (*arrow*) in this patient with left leg pain. B: Parasagittal T1-weighted SE MR image (600/20) obtained 20 mm to the left of the midline through the plane of the intervertebral foramina. The lateral disc herniation (*arrow*) compresses the exiting L4 nerve root and obscures the perineural fat. C: Axial CT scan cephalad to the L4-L5 disc shows the large lateral disc herniation (*arrow*) extending into the intervertebral foramen.

tions diagnosed by CT are far lateral (2,9,15). Lateral disc herniations can be divided into intraforaminal (located in the foramen anterior to the superior facet of the inferior vertebra), extraforaminal (located beyond the facet), or mixed (5). With MR imaging, the location can be assessed on axial, sagittal, or oblique coronal images. The latter can be obtained by angling 15–30 degrees caudally and anteriorly, following the course of the nerve roots from the foramina (5). In one series of lateral disc herniations, 30 percent were intraforaminal, 24 percent extraforaminal, and 46 percent mixed (5). In another series, 50 extraforaminal disc herniations were evaluated by CT and/or MR (10). An intraforaminal component was found in 82 percent of the extraforaminal disc herniations, whereas an associated intraspinal component was present in only 26 percent. The location of a lateral disc fragment may influence the surgical approach. Cephalad migration of disc fragments is found in 50–71 percent of cases (5,10). While approximately 90 percent of central and posterolateral disc herniations occur at L4-L5 and L5-S1, lateral disc herniations frequently occur at the higher lumbar levels (Fig. 5-3).

Lateral disc herniation is a known cause of false negative myelograms (4,13,14). Unlike MR imaging and CT with their direct anatomic visualization, myelography relies on indirect evidence of disease by showing extrinsic compression of the thecal sac and nerve roots. With myelography performed with water-soluble contrast, the nerve root sheaths can be visualized

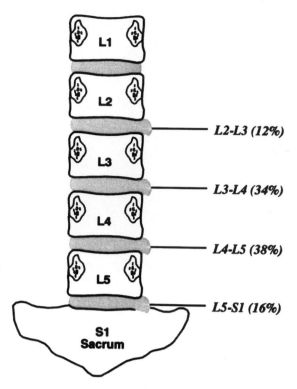

FIG. 5-3. Relative frequency of lateral lumbar disc herniation. Data from ref. 10.

L2-L3 (12%)

L3-L4 (34%)

L4-L5 (38%)

L5-S1 (16%)

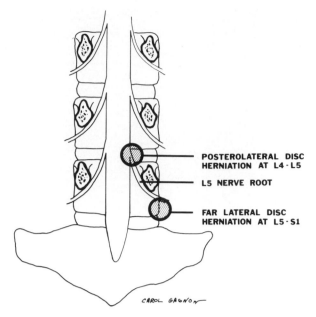

FIG. 5-5. Effect of posterolateral disc herniation at L4-L5 and far lateral disc herniation at L5-S1 on the same L5 nerve root.

POSTEROLATERAL DISC HERNIATION AT L4-L5

L5 NERVE ROOT

FAR LATERAL DISC HERNIATION AT L5-S1

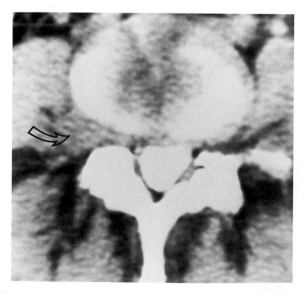

FIG. 5-4. Far lateral disc herniation. Computed tomographic myelography performed after myelography with water-soluble contrast. There is a large far lateral disc herniation (*arrow*) at L4-L5. Despite the size of the disc herniation, a myelogram with water-soluble contrast was unremarkable because the herniation was lateral to the myelographically visualized portion of the nerve root sheath.

to their termination near the dorsal root ganglion within the neural foramen. Disc herniation that is located lateral to the ganglion may therefore go undetected with myelography. An example of a far lateral disc herniation at L4-L5 is shown in a patient who presented with right radiculopathy and had a normal myelographic examination performed with water-soluble contrast (Fig. 5-4).

Information gained by MR imaging and CT may be of great benefit in the surgical management of patients with lateral disc herniation. The specific compromised nerve root can often be suggested by the pain distribution, physical examination, and electromyography (1). However, it must be kept in mind that a far lateral disc herniation compromises the same nerve root as does a typical posterolateral disc herniation at the next higher level (Table 5-1, Fig. 5-5). When the far lateral position of a disc herniation is not appreciated preoperatively, initial surgical exploration may be unrewarding (8) (Fig. 5-6).

The differential diagnosis of lateral disc herniation with CT includes schwannoma and soft tissue involvement by lymphoma, metastatic disease, or infection (3,12,15). Cystic nerve root sleeve dilatation and conjoined nerve root sheath anomaly may also be considered. A schwannoma located in the intervertebral foramen may have a sharp border similar to lateral disc herniation but may cause widening of the neural foramen. Metastasis and lymphoma usually have attenuation values similar to or slightly less than a herniated lateral disc. However, these neoplasms are likely to

TABLE 5-1. *Effect of posterolateral and far lateral herniation of the nucleus pulposus on the lumbar nerve root*

Nerve root	Posterolateral HNP	Far lateral HNP	Diminished or absent reflex	Pain and parethesias
L3	L2-L3	L3-L4	Knee	Anterior thigh and knee
L4	L3-L4	L4-L5	Knee	Anterior thigh and knee, medial leg
L5	L4-L5	L5-S1	± Ankle	Hip, posterolateral thigh, lateral calf, dorsal foot, 1st or 2nd and 3rd toes
S1	L5-S1		Ankle	Midgluteal, posterior thigh, posterior calf to heel, outer plantar foot, 4th and 5th toes

Data from ref. 1.

have irregular, indistinct margins with an infiltrative appearance and may cause widening of paraspinal soft tissues (3,12). Metastasis is usually associated with bone destruction of the adjacent pedicle or vertebral body. Similarly, soft tissue infection has indistinct margins and may be associated with adjacent bone destruction. Cystic dilatation of the nerve root sleeve is isodense with the thecal sac because it contains cerebrospinal fluid. Unlike a lateral disc herniation, the density of a conjoined nerve root sheath is similar to or only slightly greater than the thecal sac. Serial scans may show the derivation of the conjoined nerve roots from the dural sac and the asymmetry of the nerve roots (7). Other pitfalls that may lead to the incorrect diagnosis of lateral disc herniation include pseudoherniation of the disc caused by scoliosis and volume averaging of an adjacent dense structure such as an osteophyte or articular process (16).

With MR imaging, a lateral disc herniation must be differentiated from several entities. Schwannomas may widen the neural foramen and show enhancement after the intravenous injection of gadopentetate dimeglumine. It should be noted, however, that occasionally a disc herniation may show some enhancement, especially if postinjection scanning is delayed. This enhancement is thought to be related to vascular granulation tissue (11). Metastatic disease or lymphoma may be accompanied by adjacent bone destruction which typically leads to decreased signal intensity of the bone marrow on T1-weighted images. Increased signal intensity may be seen on T2-weighted images. Cystic dilatation of the nerve root sleeve has similar signal intensity to the cerebrospinal fluid within the thecal sac. Enlargement of foraminal veins can be mistaken for a lateral disc herniation and has been reported as a cause of false positive MR diagnosis of lateral disc

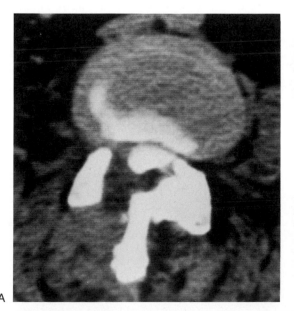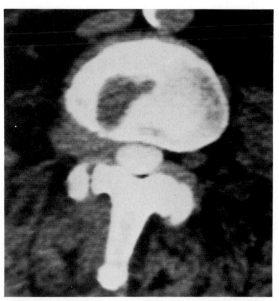

FIG. 5-6. Far lateral disc herniation in a patient who remained symptomatic after surgery. **A:** Postoperative CTM obtained at the L3-L4 intervertebral disc level. Note right laminectomy. **B:** Cephalad to the disc level there is a large lateral disc herniation that is compressing the L3 dorsal root ganglion on the right. The far lateral extent of the disc herniation had not been appreciated prior to initial surgery. Information gained from CT was used to guide reoperation.

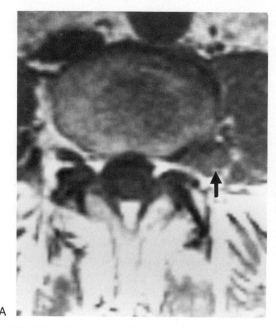
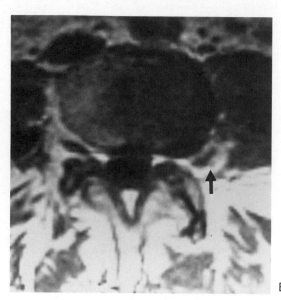

A

B

FIG. 5-7. Prominent dorsal root ganglion. **A**: Axial T1-weighted MR image obtained prior to contrast injection. A prominent dorsal root ganglion (*arrow*) is present on the left and has an appearance that is similar to a lateral disc herniation. **B**: An axial T1-weighted MR image obtained after the intravenous injection of gadopentetate dimeglumine shows considerable enhancement of the dorsal root ganglion in the left intervertebral foramen (*arrow*).

herniation (5). A prominent dorsal root ganglion must also be differentiated from a lateral disc herniation (Fig. 5-7).

REFERENCES

1. Adams RD, Victor M. *Principles of neurology.* 3rd ed. New York: McGraw-Hill; 1985.
2. Fries JW, Abodeely DA, Vijungco JG, et al. Computed tomography of herniated and extruded nucleus pulposus. *J Comput Assist Tomogr* 1982;6:874–87.
3. Gado M, Patel J, Hodges FJ III. Lateral disk herniation into the lumbar intervertebral foramen: differential diagnosis. *AJNR* 1983;4:598–600.
4. Godersky JC, Erickson DL, Seljeskog EL. Extreme lateral disc herniation: diagnosis by computed tomographic scanning. *Neurosurgery* 1984;14:549–52.
5. Grenier N, Gréselle J-F, Douws C, et al. MR imaging of foraminal and extraforaminal lumbar disk herniations. *J Comput Assist Tomogr* 1990;14:243–9.
6. Haughton VM, Eldevik OP, Magnaes B, et al. A prospective comparison of computed tomography and myelography in the diagnosis of herniated lumbar disks. *Radiology* 1982;142:103–10.
7. Helms CA, Dorwart RH, Gray MG. The CT appearance of con-
joined nerve roots and differentiation from a herniated nucleus pulposus. *Radiology* 1982;144:803–7.
8. Macnab I. Negative disc exploration: an analysis of the causes of nerve-root involvement in sixty-eight patients. *J Bone Joint Surg Am* 1971;53A:891–903.
9. Novetsky GJ, Berlin L, Epstein AJ, et al. The extraforaminal herniated disk: detection by computed tomography. *AJNR* 1982;3:653–5.
10. Osborn AG, Hood RS, Sherry RG, et al. CT/MR spectrum of far lateral and anterior lumbosacral disk herniations. *AJNR* 1988;9:775–8.
11. Quencer RM, Atlas SW, Batnitzky S, et al. Advances in neuroradiology: highlights of the 27th annual meeting of the American Society of Neuroradiology. Orlando, March 19–24, 1989. *AJNR* 1989;10:851–66.
12. Schubiger O, Valavanis A, Hollmann J. Computed tomography of the intervertebral foramen. *Neuroradiology* 1984;26:439–44.
13. Shapiro R. *Myelography.* 4th ed. Chicago: Year Book Medical Publishers; 1984.
14. Strother CM. Lumbar examination. In: Sackett JF, Strother CM, eds. *New techniques in myelography.* Philadelphia: Harper and Row; 1979:69–89.
15. Williams AL, Haughton VM, Daniels DL, et al. CT recognition of lateral lumbar disk herniation. *AJNR* 1982;3:211–3, *AJR* 1982;139:345–7.
16. Winter DDB, Munk PL, Helms CA, et al. CT and MR of lateral disc herniation: typical appearance and pitfalls of interpretation. *Can Assoc Radiol J* 1989;40:256–9.

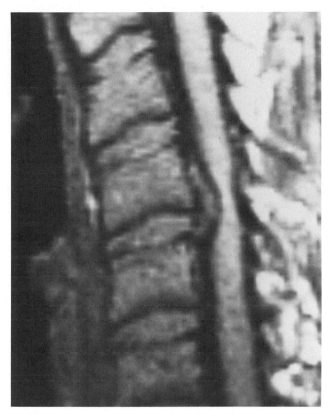

FIG. 6-1A. This 27-year-old man was examined because of neck pain and heaviness in the right arm. Sagittal T1-weighted SE MR image (700/15) of the midcervical spine.

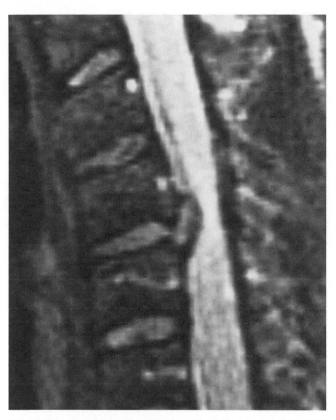

FIG. 6-1B. Sagittal T2-weighted SE MR image (2182/70) of the midcervical spine.

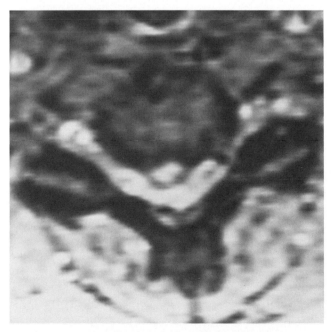

FIG. 6-1C. Axial gradient-echo (GRE) MR image [gradient recalled acquisition in the steady state (GRASS), 24/13 with 8-degree flip angle] obtained at C4-C5.

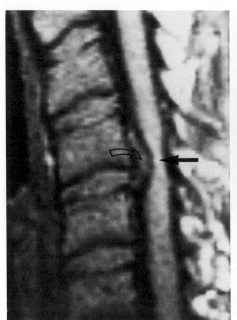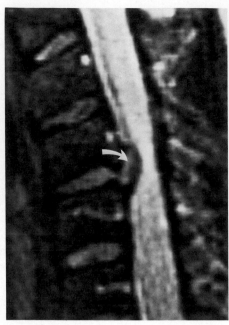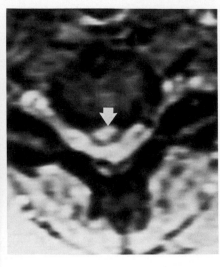

1A

1B

1C

FIG. 6-1A. Cervical disc herniation. There is a large disc herniation (*curved arrow*) causing extradural compression of the anterior subarachnoid space and the spinal cord (*straight arrow*) at C4-C5.

FIG. 6-1B. The T2-weighted image further shows spinal cord compression caused by the large disc herniation (*arrow*). The disc herniation extends cephalad from the disc space.

FIG. 6-1C. The GRE image shows bright signal of the disc herniation (*arrow*). Spondylosis would typically have low signal intensity with this pulse sequence.

CERVICAL DISC HERNIATION

In this case there is a large cervical disc herniation causing compression of the anterior subarachnoid space and the spinal cord (Fig. 6-1). Most cervical disc herniations are posterolateral or lateral to the disc space. Often they cause neck pain and radiculopathy (neurologic deficit caused by nerve root compression). Central disc herniations are associated with more variable clinical presentations. Patients may complain of vague neck pain or there may be intermittent signs of radiculopathy or myelopathy (neurologic deficit caused by spinal cord compression). The clinical signs and symptoms of cervical nerve root irritation and compression are summarized in Table 6-1 (13).

In the evaluation of patients with cervical radiculopathy, early MR investigators (9) found that CTM and MR imaging were equally capable of determining the level of abnormality; however, CTM was more specific in differentiating disc herniation from osteophyte. Others (1,10) believe that CTM is unnecessary in most cases. They argue that MR imaging should be used in conjunction with conventional radiography of the cervical spine to efficiently diagnosis disc herniation and spondylosis, obviating the need for an invasive

procedure such as myelography and CTM in most cases. Computed tomographic myelography can then be reserved for those cases in which MR imaging and conventional radiography fail to determine the cause of radiculopathy.

Disc herniation is frequently associated with radiculopathy; spondylosis is frequently associated with myelopathy. However, in one series 23 percent of patients with cervical disc herniation presented with myelopathy, and 22 percent of patients with bony canal stenosis presented with radiculopathy (1). This suggests that the imaging modality chosen should be capable of evaluating patients with either radiculopathy or myelopathy. When patients with cervical radiculopathy or myelopathy were studied, surgically proved lesions were correctly predicted by MR imaging in 88 percent, CTM in 81 percent, myelography in 58 percent, and conventional CT without contrast in 50 percent (1).

One potential pitfall with MR imaging is in differentiating an osteophyte from disc herniation, as osteophytes have variable signal intensity related to differences in marrow content. Another pitfall is the occasional cervical disc herniation that extends into

34

TABLE 6-1. *Signs and symptoms of cervical radiculopathy by disc level and nerve root involved*

Disc level	Nerve root	Signs and symptoms
C2-3	C3	Pain and numbness in back of neck; no upper-extremity weakness or reflex changes
C3-4	C4	Pain and numbness in back of neck radiating along levator scapula muscle; no upper-extremity weakness or reflex changes
C4-5	C5	Pain radiating from side of neck to top of shoulder; numbness over mid-deltoid muscle; weakness of arm and shoulder extension; atrophy of deltoid muscle; no reflex changes
C5-6	C6	Pain radiating down lateral side of arm and forearm, often into thumb and index finger; numbness in tip of thumb or over first dorsal interosseous muscle; weakness of biceps muscle; depression of biceps reflex
C6-7	C7	Pain radiating down medial aspect of forearm, usually to middle finger; weakness of triceps muscle; depression of triceps reflex
C7-T1	C8	Pain down medial aspect of forearm to ring and small finger with numbness in those fingers; weakness of triceps and small muscles of hand; no reflex changes

From ref. 13, with permission.

the intervertebral foramen and may be a source of a false negative MR scan (1). The use of gradient-echo (GRE) imaging, which will be discussed later, may improve the ability of MR imaging to show this abnormality.

Magnetic resonance imaging of the cervical spine is performed with a surface coil. There are several methods available for obtaining good quality studies of the cervical spine, and different centers have their preferred protocols (Appendix 1). Sagittal T1-weighted SE images are obtained with a short TR and short TE pulse sequence (e.g., 600/20). Sagittal proton density- and T2-weighted SE images can be obtained with a long TR and short (proton density-) and long (T2-weighted) TE pulse sequence (e.g., 2000/35, 70); however, the MR image may be hindered by cerebrospinal fluid flow artifact. Methods of reducing these artifacts include cardiac gating combined with some form of velocity compensation such as flow compensation (gradient moment nulling technique) and spatial presaturation (3–7,11,12,16). The interested reader may refer to the cited references for details of these techniques.

Until this point, only SE techniques have been considered. In the evaluation of cervical radiculopathy, many investigators obtain GRE images in the sagittal

and axial planes, replacing the long TR SE sequence. The use of partial flip angles and GRE techniques can produce images with high object contrast in significantly less time than with conventional SE techniques (2,8,15–17). With some GRE techniques, data are collected sequentially in single slices. Such techniques as GRASS (gradient recalled acquisition in the steady state), FLASH (fast low-angle shot) and FISP (fast imaging with steady state procession) are GRE techniques of various manufacturers that use a flip angle of less than 90 degrees. For example, a flip angle of 5–20 degrees coupled with a short repetition time of 10–75 msec can be used to produce images with bright cerebrospinal fluid signal. A drawback to low flip-angle GRE technique is its extreme sensitivity to inhomogeneities in the magnetic field (17). Another technique, referred to by one manufacturer as MPGR (multiplanar gradient recalled) is a GRE technique that excites multiple slices within one repetition time, allowing multisliced interleaved images to be obtained. With the selection of certain parameters (e.g., 200–800/10–20; flip angle of 10–30 degrees), the cerebrospinal fluid will appear bright. This technique provides increased signal and increased contrast resolution compared to single-slice technique because of the longer TR. The use of low flip angles permits contiguous images with minimal crosstalk between slices. Cardiac gating and flow compensation can be used. Gradient-echo images may also be helpful in differentiating cervical disc herniation (Fig. 6-2) from cervical spondylosis (Fig. 6-3). Osteophytes tend to be of lower signal intensity than disc with this method.

Cervical spondylosis can be readily identified with CT or CTM (Fig. 6-4). Although conventional CT obtained without myelographic contrast is an adequate examination for the evaluation of cervical spondylosis and lumbar disc herniation, it is not an adequate study for evaluation of cervical disc herniation. This is because in the cervical spine there is less epidural fat to contrast with the disc margin, the disc spaces are narrower, thinner slice sections are needed leading to decreased resolution, and artifact may be present when scanning through the plane of the shoulders. Computed tomographic myelography, however, is an excellent method of evaluating patients for cervical disc herniation. Intrathecal contrast enhances the visualization of the subarachnoid space, nerve roots, and spinal cord, and permits excellent appreciation of spinal cord and nerve root compression (Figs. 6-5, 6-6). A disadvantage of CTM is its invasive nature which is related to the need for a lumbar puncture. Therefore, the evaluation of cervical radiculopathy should begin, in most cases, with MR imaging. If the clinical problem is satisfactorily resolved, then no further study is needed. If a clinically significant problem is not resolved, then CTM should be performed.

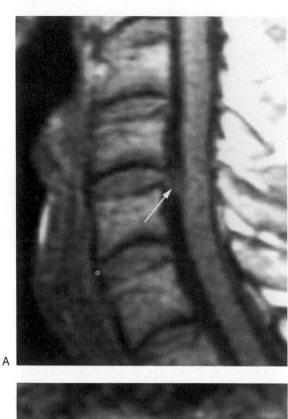

A

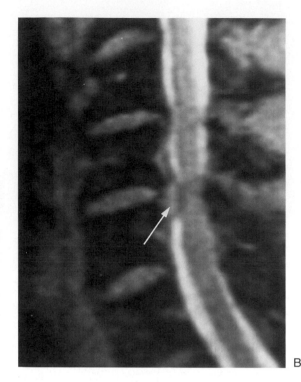

B

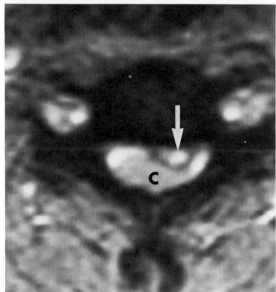

C

FIG. 6-2. Cervical disc herniation. **A**: Sagittal T1-weighted SE MR image (550/12) of the cervical spine obtained slightly to the left of midline. There is a disc herniation at C5-C6 (*arrow*). Compression of the anterior subarachnoid space and spinal cord is seen. **B**: Sagittal GRE MR image [multiplanar gradient recalled (MPGR), 500/15 with 15-degree flip angle] obtained slightly to the left of midline. The disc herniation is well seen with this GRE sequence. **C**: Axial GRE MR image (MPGR, 600/20 with 20-degree flip angle) shows bright signal intensity disc herniation (*arrow*) to the left of midline, compressing the anterior subarachnoid space and the left anterolateral aspect of the spinal cord (*C*).

When evaluating patients with MR imaging and CTM, caution should be exercised when attributing clinical symptoms to identified structural abnormalities. In one study, *asymptomatic* patients were evaluated with T1-weighted sagittal and axial MR images, and many were found to have structural abnormalities (14). The presence of these abnormalities increased with the age of the patient. For example, disc protrusion was found in 20 percent of asymptomatic individuals aged 45–54 years and in 57 percent of those older than 64 years (14). Individuals under age 65 had MR demonstration of osteophytes in 16 percent and spinal cord impingement in 16 percent. Spinal cord impingement was defined as a concave defect in the spinal cord at the site of disc protrusion or osteophyte without obliteration of the subarachnoid space posterior to the cord. Asymptomatic patients aged 65 or older had disc protrusion in 57 percent, osteophytes in 37 percent, and spinal cord impingement in 26 percent of cases. Spinal cord compression (concave defect in the spinal

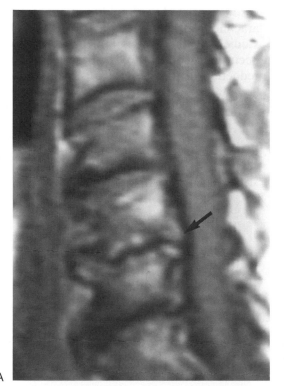

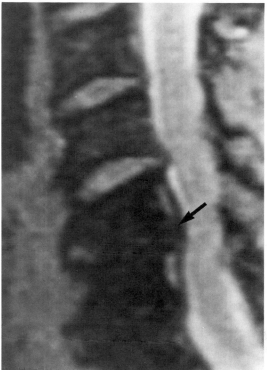

A

B

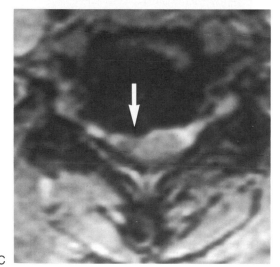

C

FIG. 6-3. Cervical spondylosis. **A**: Sagittal T1-weighted SE MR image (500/12) of the cervical spine. There are posterior vertebral osteophytes at C5-C6 (*arrow*). The osteophytes have moderately bright signal caused by fatty marrow. **B**: Sagittal GRE MR image (MPGR, 500/15 with 15-degree flip angle) of the cervical spine. With this pulse sequence the osteophytes (*arrow*) have very low signal intensity. **C**: Axial GRE MR image (MPGR, 600/20 with 20-degree flip angle) obtained at C5-C6. The very low signal intensity of an osteophyte (*arrow*) seen with this GRE sequence can be helpful in differentiating cervical spondylosis from disc herniation.

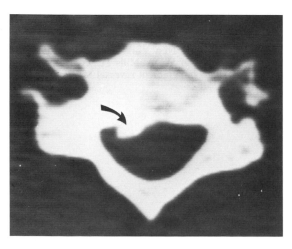

FIG. 6-4. Cervical osteophyte. This patient has an osteophyte (*arrow*) on the right at C5-C6. CT can readily distinguish an osteophyte from a soft disc herniation.

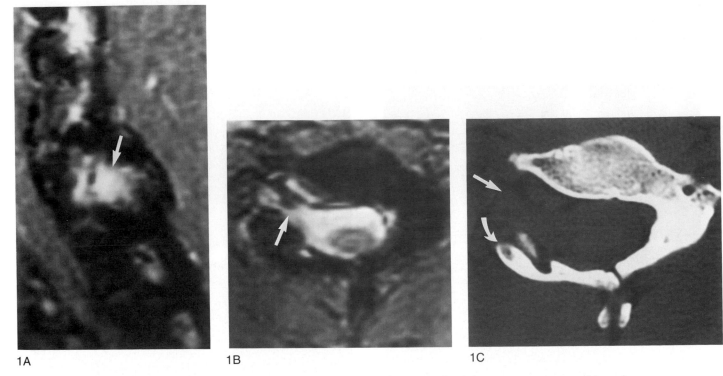

1A   1B   1C

FIG. 7-1A. Congenital absence of the pedicle. The intervertebral foramen appears widened (*arrow*) and a C7 pedicle cannot be seen. The articular processes are dorsally positioned. Compare with vertebral levels below.

FIG. 7-1B. There is absence of the right pedicle of C7 (*arrow*). Vascular, neural, and fatty structures are seen within the widened foramen with no evidence of tumor.

FIG. 7-1C. There is absence of the right pedicle of C7 (*straight arrow*). Abnormal articular processes are dorsally positioned (*curved arrow*) and the foramen is wide.

CONGENITAL ABSENCE OF THE PEDICLE

The parasagittal MR image shows an apparent malposition or malalignment of the articular processes at C6-C7 on the right (Fig. 7-1A). There is widening of the intervertebral foramen. Axial MR and CT images show absence of the right pedicle of C7, multiple developmental abnormalities of the articular processes on the right, widening of the intervertebral foramen and vascular, neural, and fatty tissues within the widened foramen (Figs. 7-1B, 7-1C). These are the typical features of congenital absence of the pedicle (Fig. 7-2).

Congenital absence of a pedicle is rare. It is found in the lumbar, cervical, and thoracic spine in decreasing order of frequency (4). Most cases of congenital absence of the pedicle are discovered fortuitously and the patient's signs and symptoms are rarely due to the absent pedicle (5). Pedicle defects may be associated with genitourinary and other congenital abnormalities (6) and rarely occur in neurofibromatosis (5).

Congenital absence of the pedicle should not be mistaken for a pedicle destroyed by tumor. With congenital absence of the pedicle, there are usually associated bony alterations. CT may show hypoplasia or absence of the ipsilateral superior articular process, dorsal displacement and malformation of the ipsilateral pillar, absence of the dorsal portion of the transverse process, and apparent widening of the intervertebral foramen (1–3,6). In addition, there may be hypertrophy and sclerosis of the contralateral pedicle and vertebral arch caused by added bony stress (3). In comparison, destruction of the pedicle by tumor or infection is not associated with bony alterations of hypertrophy, sclerosis, or hypoplasia that are found with congenital absence of the pedicle. Instead, pedicle destruction is likely to be associated with a soft tissue mass or additional destruction of adjacent bone.

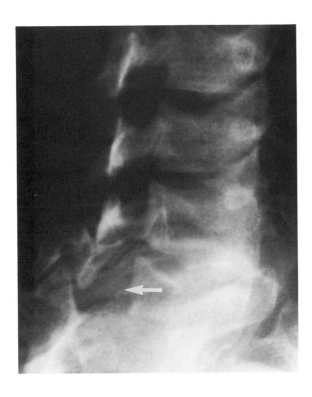

FIG. 7-2. Congenital absence of the pedicle. Conventional oblique radiograph of the cervical spine in the same patient shown in Fig. 7-1. The pedicle of C7 is absent (*arrow*), there is widening of the foramen, and abnormal articular processes are dorsally positioned.

REFERENCES

1. Cox HE, Bennett WF. Computed tomography of absent cervical pedicle: case report. *J Comput Assist Tomogr* 1984;8:537–9.
2. Edwards MG, Wesolowski D, Matasar K. Imaging of the absent cervical pedicle. *Skeletal Radiol* 1991;20:325–8.
3. Maldague BE, Malghem JJ. Unilateral arch hypertrophy with spinous process tilt: a sign of arch deficiency. *Radiology* 1976;121:567–74.
4. Manaster BJ, Norman A. CT diagnosis of thoracic pedicle aplasia: case report. *J Comput Assist Tomogr* 1983;7:1090–1.
5. Wortzman G, Steinhardt MI. Congenitally absent lumbar pedicle: a reappraisal. *Radiology* 1984;152:713–8.
6. Yousefzadeh DK, El-Khoury GY, Lupetin AR. Congenital aplastic-hypoplastic lumbar pedicle in infants and young children. *Skeletal Radiol* 1982;7:259–65.

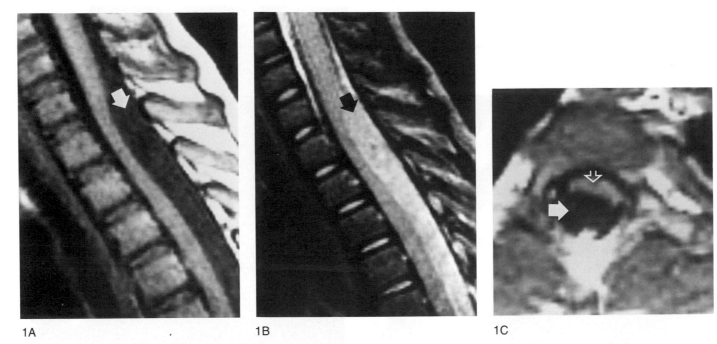

1A   1B   1C

FIG. 9-1A. Arachnoid cyst. There is a large arachnoid cyst (*arrow*) located posterior to the spinal cord. This is isointense relative to the cerebrospinal fluid on the T1-weighted image. Spinal cord compression is evident.

FIG. 9-1B. The arachnoid cyst (*arrow*) is hyperintense to the spinal cord, but of lower signal intensity than the adjacent cerebrospinal fluid. This cyst extends from the superior aspect of C7 to the midthoracic spine.

FIG. 9-1C. The axial image shows the arachnoid cyst (*closed arrow*), causing severe compression of the spinal cord (*open arrow*).

ARACHNOID CYST

This 7-year-old girl experienced discomfort in the neck for 4 months. Magnetic resonance imaging shows a cystic extradural fluid collection posteriorly, causing compression of the spinal cord. The cyst, which extends throughout multiple cervical and thoracic levels, is isointense with cerebrospinal fluid on T1-weighted images (Fig. 9-1A) and is slightly hypointense relative to cerebrospinal fluid on T2-weighted images (Fig. 9-1B). Axial images further show spinal cord compression (Fig. 9-1C). Images after gadopentetate dimeglumine showed no enhancement. This is a typical appearance of an arachnoid cyst.

Over the years there has been some confusion in the literature concerning the appropriate terminology to describe spinal meningeal cysts. Nabors et al. (6) have proposed a classification that is based on operative and histologic examination. This classification divides meningeal cysts into three categories: extradural cysts without nerve root fibers, extradural cysts with nerve root fibers, and intradural cysts (Table 9-1).

Spinal meningeal cysts are thought to be congenital diverticulae of the spinal meningeal sac, nerve root sheath, or arachnoid (6). Extramedullary intraspinal cysts containing cerebrospinal fluid can occur as a primary lesion or may occur as a sequelae of chronic inflammation, surgery, or trauma (1,5,8). Some authors

TABLE 9-1. *Classification of spinal meningeal cysts*

Type	Description
I	extradural meningeal cysts without spinal nerve root fibers
IA	extradural meningeal cyst (extradural arachnoid cyst)
IB	sacral meningocele (occult sacral meningocele)
II	extradural meningeal cysts with spinal nerve root fibers (Tarlov's perineurial cyst, spinal nerve root diverticulum)
III	spinal intradural meningeal cysts (intradural arachnoid cyst)

From ref. 6, with permission.

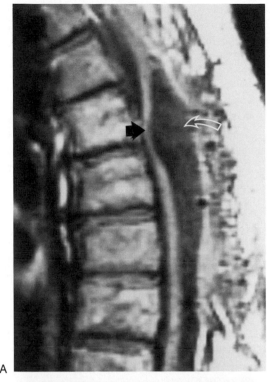

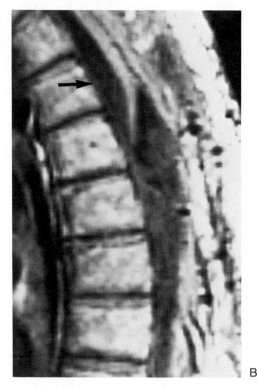

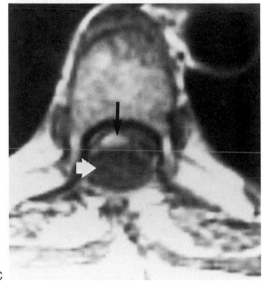

FIG. 9-2. Recurrent arachnoid cyst. **A**: Sagittal T1-weighted MR image (800/20) obtained near the midline in the mid-thoracic spine. There is a recurrent arachnoid cyst (*curved arrow*) which is displacing and compressing an atrophic spinal cord (*straight arrow*). Note postoperative changes posterior to the arachnoid cyst. **B**: Sagittal T1-weighted MR image (800/20) located 4 mm to the left of Fig. 9-2A. In addition to the posterior arachnoid cyst, there is an anterior component (*arrow*) which is further compressing the spinal cord. **C**: Axial T1-weighted MR image (800/20) obtained at the T6 level. The arachnoid cyst (*white arrow*) fills the spinal canal and markedly compresses the spinal cord (*black arrow*). Note posterior postoperative changes.

have used the term *arachnoid cyst* for the primary lesions and *subarachnoid cyst* for the acquired lesions (8). Arachnoid cysts may be intradural or extradural (5). An extradural arachnoid cyst is a rare developmental anomaly thought to occur either from arachnoid protrusion through a small congenital dural defect or as a congenital diverticulum of the dura (1). Extradural arachnoid cysts most frequently occur in the posterior or posterolateral spinal canal and may extend for several vertebral segments, as in our case. They may cause compression of the spinal cord or nerve root leading to pain, parasthesias, or neurologic symptoms that may have remissions and exacerbations simulating

multiple sclerosis (1). The cyst may be single or multiple and frequently extends into a neural foramen (1).

Conventional radiography and CT may show the effects of chronic pressure on the adjacent osseous structures: posterior vertebral body scalloping, erosion of the pedicles and laminae, and neural foraminal enlargement (1,3,5). Computed tomographic myelography may show contrast within the cyst which indicates communication between the cyst and the subarachnoid space (5). Magnetic resonance imaging shows an extradural fluid collection with signal intensity similar to cerebrospinal fluid causing obliteration of epidural fat and compression of the spinal cord. The extradural location produces a sharp interface with the cord and displacement of the subarachnoid space. The cyst may be surrounded by a low signal septation or membrane (1). As would be anticipated, there is no enhancement of the cysts after intravenous injection of gadopentetate dimeglumine (7). Magnetic resonance imaging may also be useful in identifying associated abnormalities such as spinal cord atrophy or myelomalacia which may impact on the degree of neurologic recovery (1).

Acquired subarachnoid cysts occur secondary to previous chronic inflammation, surgery, or trauma (Fig. 9-2). Magnetic resonance imaging is more accurate than myelography or CTM in diagnosing these cysts (8). The subarachnoid location is suggested by mass effect on the spinal cord, indentation and irregularity of the cord surface, and widening of the corresponding subarachnoid space (8). These cysts may be loculated without direct communication with the subarachnoid space or they may communicate freely. The cysts are hypointense on T1 and have a variable intensity on T2-weighted images. Some authors suggest examining these patients without the use of cardiac gating or motion suppression technique (8). Under these circumstances, the T2-weighted images may show hyperintensity of the cysts that are loculated and thus nonpulsatile, and relative hypointensity of the cysts that freely communicate with the subarachnoid space and are subject to cerebrospinal fluid pulsation. Septations may be seen within the cyst in approximately half of the cases (8). In some cases, it may be difficult to differentiate a subarachnoid cyst from an atrophic spinal cord that is adherent to the dura and has an enlarged subarachnoid space (8).

Several factors influence the MR signal intensity of a cystic collection when compared to cerebrospinal fluid. These factors include protein content, the presence of paramagnetic material, and motion effects (2,4,8). In a study of cystic intracranial lesions (4), a correlation was found between MR signal intensity and the contents of the cyst. Arachnoid and postoperative cysts are isointense to cerebrospinal fluid. Protein-

aceous cysts, such as inflammatory cysts or nonhemorrhagic neoplastic cysts, have an intermediate pattern. The high protein content shortens both T1 and T2 relaxation times, leading to a slight increase in signal intensity on T1-weighted images compared to cerebrospinal fluid (4). However, with the most commonly used T2-weighted pulse sequences, proteinaceous cysts appear brighter than cerebrospinal fluid, even though the T2 relaxation time is shortened. This is because the effect of the shortened T1 relaxation time increases the signal intensity and has more of an effect on the signal with the pulse sequences commonly used in clinical practice (4). Paramagnetic substances, including blood degradation products from old hemorrhage, may alter signal intensity. As described above, pulsatile cerebrospinal fluid motion may have lower signal intensity than stationary fluid. This is because of signal-voids and ghost images found with pulsatile motion (2).

REFERENCES

1. Gray L, Djang WT, Friedman AH. MR imaging of thoracic extradural arachnoid cysts. *J Comput Assist Tomogr* 1988;12:646–8.
2. Hackney DB, Grossman RI, Zimmerman RA, et al. Low sensitivity of clinical MR imaging to small changes in the concentration of nonparamagnetic protein. *AJNR* 1987;8:1003–8.
3. Kim KS, Weinberg PE. Magnetic resonance imaging of a spinal extradural arachnoid cyst. *Surg Neurol* 1986;26:249–52.
4. Kjos BO, Brant-Zawadzki M, Kucharczyk W, et al. Cystic intracranial lesions: magnetic resonance imaging. *Radiology* 1985;155: 363–9.
5. Mirich DR, Hall JT, Carrasco CH. MR imaging of traumatic spinal arachnoid cyst: case report. *J Comput Assist Tomogr* 1988; 12:862–5.
6. Nabors MW, Pait TG, Byrd EB, et al. Updated assessment and current classification of spinal meningeal cysts. *J Neurosurg* 1988;68:366–77.
7. Pierot L, Dormont D, Oueslati S, et al. Gadolinium-DTPA enhanced MR imaging of intradural neurenteric cysts. *J Comput Assist Tomogr* 1988;12:762–4.
8. Sklar E, Quencer RM, Green BA, et al. Acquired spinal subarachnoid cysts: evaluation with MR, CT myelography, and intraoperative sonography. *AJNR* 1989;10:1097–104, *AJR* 1989;153: 1057–64.

CASE 10

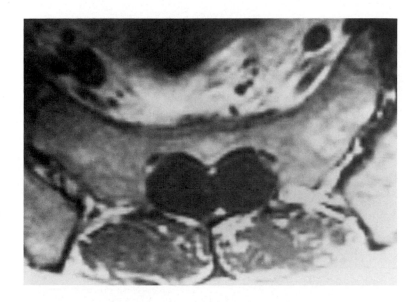

FIG. 10-1A. A 37-year-old woman was examined because of low back pain. Axial T1-weighted SE MR image (800/20) obtained at the level of the second sacral segment.

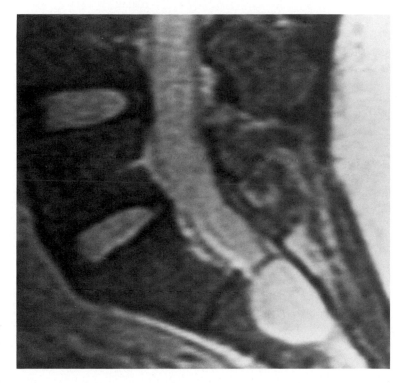

FIG. 10-1B. Sagittal T2-weighted SE MR image (2000/70) of the lumbosacral spine.

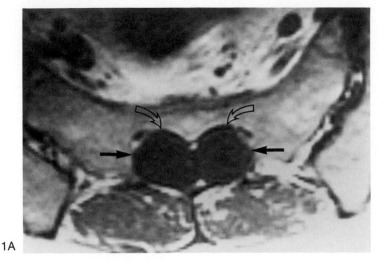 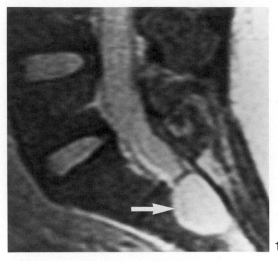

1A   1B

FIG. 10-1A. Tarlov (perineurial) cysts. Tarlov cysts (*straight arrows*) are seen as large round fluid collections at the S2 level. Posterior scalloping of the sacrum is noted (*curved arrows*).

FIG. 10-1B. In the sagittal projection, one of the Tarlov cysts is seen (*arrow*) and has high signal intensity on the T2-weighted image. The fluid in the cyst appears brighter than the cerebrospinal fluid within the thecal sac. This may be caused by increased protein content of the fluid within the cyst and a lack of cerebrospinal fluid motion effects. Posterior sacral scalloping is again noted.

TARLOV CYST

The T1- and T2-weighted MR images show large cystic fluid collections at the S2 level, causing scalloping of the posterior margin of the sacrum (Fig. 10-1). These are Tarlov (perineurial) cysts.

As the normal nerve root emerges from the thecal sac and traverses toward the neural foramen, it is covered by arachnoid and the intervening subarachnoid space. The continuation of the arachnoid at and beyond the level of the dorsal root ganglion is termed the *perineurium* (7). Typically, water-soluble myelographic contrast fills the subarachnoid space to the level of the dorsal root ganglion. A potential space is present beneath the perineurium, which usually does not fill with contrast. Tarlov cysts occur at the level of the dorsal root ganglion and contain neural elements in their wall (7). Tarlov, who studied perineurial cysts with Pantopaque myelography, found a lack of filling of the cyst during the initial myelogram, although delayed myelographic filling was seen in some cases (7). With the advent of water-soluble contrast, filling of sacral perineurial cysts has been shown on the initial myelographic and CTM studies (6). This is thought to occur because of communication between the subarachnoid space and the potential space beneath the perineurium (7). Tarlov cysts are classified as type II meningeal cysts (spinal extradural meningeal cysts with spinal nerve fibers) (3) and may occasionally cause symptoms which are relieved by surgery.

The perineurial cyst is well seen with CT as a cyst of low attenuation, occurring most frequently in the sacral levels (8). These sacral cysts can attain large size, causing sacral canal enlargement and osseous erosion (6) (Fig. 10-2). Magnetic resonance imaging shows a fluid collection with low signal intensity on T1-weighted images and high signal intensity on T2-weighted images. The fluid within the cyst may have brighter signal on the T2-weighted images than does the cerebrospinal fluid within the thecal sac. This could be caused by higher protein content of the cyst or absence of cerebrospinal fluid motion effects.

Cystic Nerve Root Sleeve Dilatation

Not infrequently, MR imaging or CT may reveal cystic nerve root sleeve dilatation (CNRSD), which occurs when there is enlargement of the subarachnoid space that surrounds the exiting nerve root. The etiology is not known but may be related to increased hydrostatic pressure of the cerebrospinal fluid. Dilatation of the nerve root sleeve is located proximal to the dorsal root ganglion, permitting intrathecal contrast to communicate freely with the cystic structure during myelography (5,7). Dilatation may be tubular or saccular (2), the latter sometimes being termed a *meningeal diverticulum* (5). Cystic nerve root sleeve dilatation may be

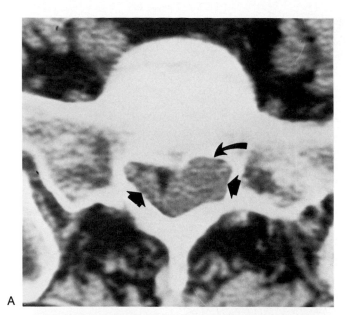

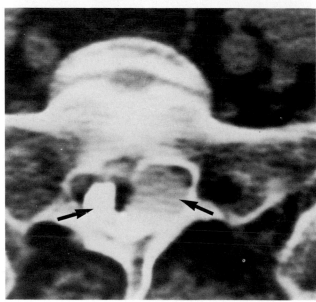

FIG. 10-2. Sacral perineurial cysts. **A**: Axial CT scan of the superior sacrum. There are bilateral perineurial cysts (*straight arrows*). The larger cyst on the left is causing pressure erosion of the posterior aspect of the sacrum (*curved arrow*). **B**: Water-soluble contrast filling the large bilateral sacral cysts (*arrows*) revealed by CTM.

seen in as many as 18 percent of lumbar myelograms performed for low back pain or sciatica but is usually not a cause of symptoms (2).

With MR imaging, CNRSD is seen as a round cystic mass in the region of the neural foramen, isointense to cerebrospinal fluid with low signal intensity on T1- and high signal on T2-weighted images (Fig. 10-3). Computed tomography attenuation measurements reveal CNRSD to be isodense with the thecal sac (Fig. 10-

4A). Cystic nerve root sleeve dilatation causes asymmetry of the perineural fat and may cause enlargement of the neural foramen. Scalloping of the adjacent vertebral body, pedicle, or pedicular-laminar junction may occur (1,4,5). Multilevel involvement and dural ectasia are other features of this entity (2,5). The most frequent sites of CNRSD are S1 and S2 (2). When intrathecal contrast is introduced, filling of the dilated nerve root sleeve is readily apparent (Figs. 10-4B, 4C).

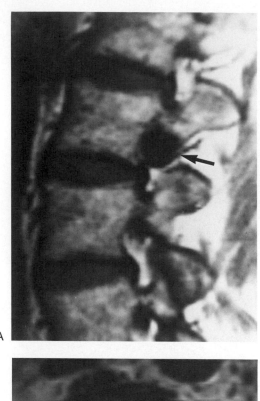

A

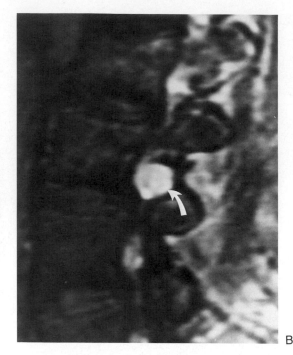

B

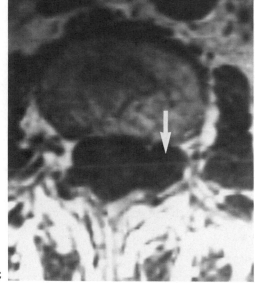

C

FIG. 10-3. Cystic nerve root sleeve dilatation seen with MR imaging. **A**: Sagittal T1-weighted SE image (700/20) through the plane of the left intervertebral foramina reveals cystic dilatation of the nerve root sleeve at L2-L3 (*arrow*), seen as a round lesion within the neural foramen having signal intensity similar to cerebrospinal fluid. **B**: Sagittal T2-weighted SE image (2000/70) obtained just medial to Fig. 10-3A. Enlarged nerve root sleeve (*arrow*) has bright signal intensity on T2-weighted image similar to cerebrospinal fluid. **C**: Axial T1-weighted image at L2-L3. The signal of the dilated nerve root sleeve (*arrow*) is isointense relative to the thecal sac. The perineural fat within the foramen is obscured on the left side. Compare to the normal right foramen.

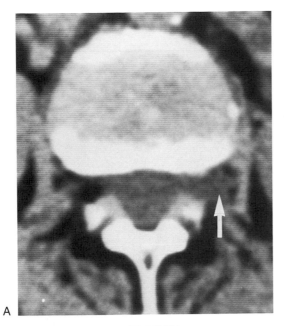

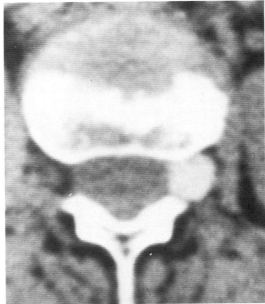

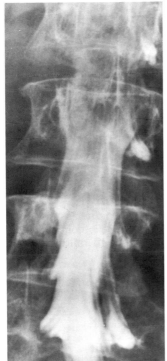

FIG. 10-4. Cystic nerve root sleeve dilatation. **A**: Axial CT scan at the L1-L2 intervertebral disc shows cystic dilatation of the nerve root sleeve (*arrow*) within the left neural foramen, which appears rounded and isointense relative to the thecal sac. This measured 14 HU. Note that the perineural fat is obliterated. **B**: Myelogram performed with water-soluble contrast shows CNRSD at multiple lumbar levels. **C**: Computed tomographic myelography performed after the myelogram shows contrast within the dilated nerve root sleeve that has a smooth, rounded configuration.

REFERENCES

1. Eisenberg D, Gomori JM, Findler G, et al. Symptomatic diverticulum of the sacral nerve root sheath: case note. *Neuroradiology* 1985;27:183.
2. Larsen JL, Smith D, Fossan G. Arachnoidal diverticula and cyst-like dilatations of the nerve-root sheaths in lumbar myelography. *Acta Radiol Diagn* 1980;21:141–5.
3. Nabors MW, Pait TG, Byrd EB, et al. Updated assessment and current classification of spinal meningeal cysts. *J Neurosurg* 1988;68:366–77.
4. Naidich TP, McLone DG, Harwood-Nash DC. Arachnoid cysts, paravertebral meningoceles, and perineurial cysts. In: Newton TH, Potts DG, eds. *Computed tomography of the spine and spinal cord*. San Anselmo, Calif: Clavadel Press; 1983:383–96.
5. Neave VCD, Wycoff RR. Computed tomography of cystic nerve root sleeve dilatation: case report. *J Comput Assist Tomogr* 1983; 7:881–5.
6. Siqueira EB, Schaffer L, Kranzler LI, et al. CT characteristics of sacral perineurial cysts: report of two cases. *J Neurosurg* 1984; 61:596–8.
7. Tarlov IM. Spinal perineurial and meningeal cysts. *J Neurol Neurosurg Psychiatry* 1970;33:833–43.
8. Willinsky RA, Fazl M. Computed tomography of a sacral perineural cyst: case report. *J Comput Assist Tomogr* 1985;9:599–601.

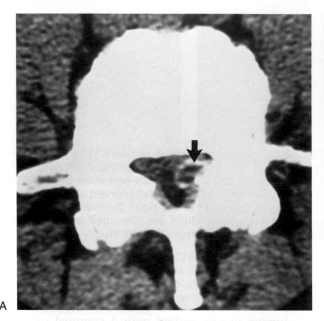

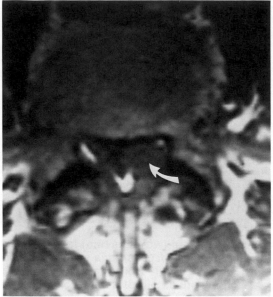

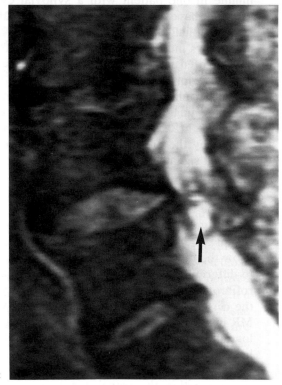

FIG. 12-3. Synovial cyst at L4-L5 in a 55-year-old man. **A**: Computed tomography examination without intravenous or intrathecal contrast shows a dense rim (*arrow*) surrounding a synovial cyst that is located medial to the facet joint on the left. Osteoarthritic changes of the facet joints are noted, although they were better visualized on the images obtained with bone window settings. **B**: Axial T1-weighted SE MR image (850/15) obtained caudad to the L4-L5 disc shows a large round synovial cyst (*arrow*) in the left side of the spinal canal compressing the thecal sac. The cyst is of slightly higher signal intensity than the cerebrospinal fluid within the thecal sac. **C**: Sagittal T2-weighted SE MR image (2000/70) of the lower lumbar spine. The synovial cyst (*arrow*) has bright signal surrounded by a rim of low signal intensity.

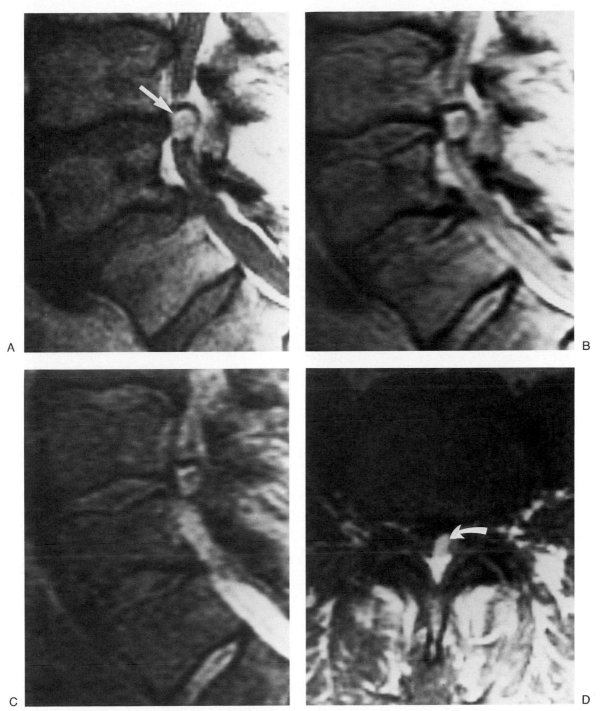

FIG. 12-4. Hemorrhagic cyst in a 48-year-old man with pain in both legs. **A**: Sagittal T1-weighted SE MR images of the lower lumbar spine shows a high signal intensity hemorrhagic cyst (*arrow*) with a low intensity rim at the L3-L4 level. The central portion of the cyst has high signal intensity on all SE pulse sequences, indicating the presence of extracellular (free) methemoglobin. The low signal intensity rim could be caused by calcification or hemosiderin. At L4-L5 there is grade I spondylolisthesis and spinal stenosis. **B**: Proton density-weighted SE MR images showing hemorrhagic cyst (*arrow*) as in Fig. 12-4A. **C**: T2-weighted SE MR images showing hemorrhagic cyst (*arrow*) as in Fig. 12-4A. **D**: Axial T1-weighted SE MR image (800/15) at L3-L4. A high signal intensity hemorrhagic cyst (*arrow*) is seen to the left of the midline and is compressing the thecal sac.

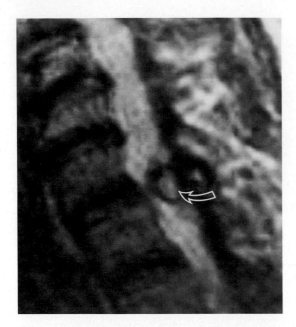

FIG. 12-5. Synovial cyst at C7-T1. Sagittal T2-weighted SE MR image (2553/70) obtained to the left of the midline shows a synovial cyst (*arrow*) with a low signal intensity rim. Spinal cord compression could be seen on the sagittal and axial images in this patient with left arm pain.

to degenerative spinal stenosis. A patient with synovial cyst may have pain related to pressure effect from the cyst or to facet joint arthropathy (8). The neurologic examination is frequently abnormal. A review of reported cases (11) found motor deficits in 44 percent, sensory deficits in 28 percent, and reflex changes in 31 percent, while no neurologic deficit was present in 39 percent of patients. Patients with synovial cyst of the cervical spine may have myelopathy and spastic paraparesis (14).

Synovial cysts may regress spontaneously, although in some cases surgical intervention may be necessary (5,6,10). An alternative to surgery is CT-guided needle placement of corticosteroids into the facet joint with a synovial cyst (4). This treatment, however, depends on the presence of communication between the facet joint and the cyst. Direct CT-guided needle aspiration biopsy of an intraspinal synovial cyst has also been reported (1).

REFERENCES

1. Abrahams JJ, Wood GW, Eames FA, et al. CT-guided needle aspiration biopsy of an intraspinal synovial cyst (ganglion): case report and review of the literature. *AJNR* 1988;9:398–400.
2. Awwad EE, Martin DS, Smith KR Jr, et al. MR imaging of lumbar juxtaarticular cysts. *J Comput Assist Tomogr* 1990;14:415–7.
3. Bhushan C, Hodges FJ III, Wityk JJ. Synovial cyst (ganglion) of the lumbar spine simulating extradural mass. *Neuroradiology* 1979;18:263–8.
4. Bjorkengren AG, Kurz LT, Resnick D, et al. Symptomatic intraspinal synovial cysts: opacification and treatment by percutaneous injection. *AJR* 1987;149:105–7.
5. Casselman ES. Radiologic recognition of symptomatic spinal synovial cysts. *AJNR* 1985;6:971–3.
6. Conrad MR, Pitkethly DT. Bilateral synovial cysts creating spinal stenosis: CT diagnosis. *J Comput Assist Tomogr* 1987;11:196–7.
7. Gorey MT, Hyman RA, Black KS, et al. Lumbar synovial cysts eroding bone. *AJNR* 1992;13:161–3.
8. Hemminghytt S, Daniels DL, Williams AL, et al. Intraspinal synovial cysts: natural history and diagnosis by CT. *Radiology* 1982;145:375–6.
9. Jackson DE Jr, Atlas SW, Mani JR, et al. Intraspinal synovial cysts: MR imaging. *Radiology* 1989;170:527–30.
10. Kurz LT, Garfin SR, Unger AS, et al. Intraspinal synovial cyst causing sciatica. *J Bone Joint Surg* 1985;67A:865–71.
11. Liu SS, Williams KD, Drayer BP, et al. Synovial cysts of the lumbosacral spine: diagnosis by MR imaging. *AJNR* 1989;10:1239–42, *AJR* 1990;154:163–6.
12. Maupin WB, Naul LG, Kanter SL, et al. Synovial cyst presenting as a neural foraminal lesion: MR and CT appearance. *AJR* 1989;153:1231–2.
13. Nijensohn E, Russell EJ, Milan M, et al. Case report: calcified synovial cyst of the cervical spine: CT and MR evaluation. *J Comput Assist Tomogr* 1990;14:473–6.
14. Quaghebeur G, Jeffree M. Synovial cyst of the high cervical spine causing myelopathy. *AJNR* 1992;13:981–2.
15. Rosenblum J, Mojtahedi S, Foust RJ. Synovial cysts in the lumbar spine: MR characteristics. *AJNR* 1989;10:S94.
16. Schulz EE, West WL, Hinshaw DB, et al. Gas in a lumbar extradural juxtaarticular cyst: sign of synovial origin. *AJR* 1984;143:875–6.
17. Silbergleit R, Gebarski SS, Brunberg JA, et al. Lumbar synovial cysts: correlation of myelographic, CT, MR, and pathologic findings. *AJNR* 1990;11:777–9.
18. Spencer RR, Jahnke RW, Hardy TL. Dissection of gas into an intraspinal synovial cyst from contiguous vacuum facet. *J Comput Assist Tomogr* 1983;7:886–8.

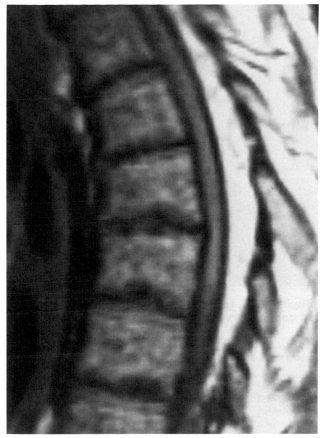

FIG. 13-1A. This 58-year-old woman was examined because of progressive myelopathy. Sagittal T1-weighted SE MR image (800/20) of the thoracic spine.

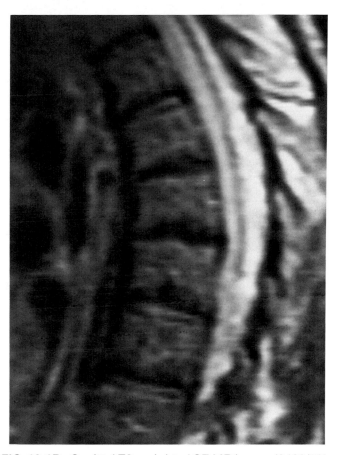

FIG. 13-1B. Sagittal T2-weighted SE MR image (2400/70).

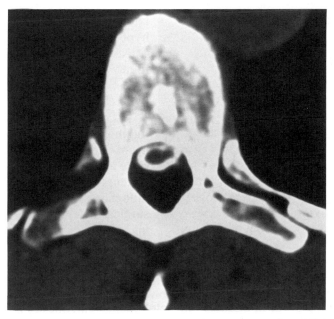

FIG. 13-1C. Computed tomographic myelography of the thoracic spine.

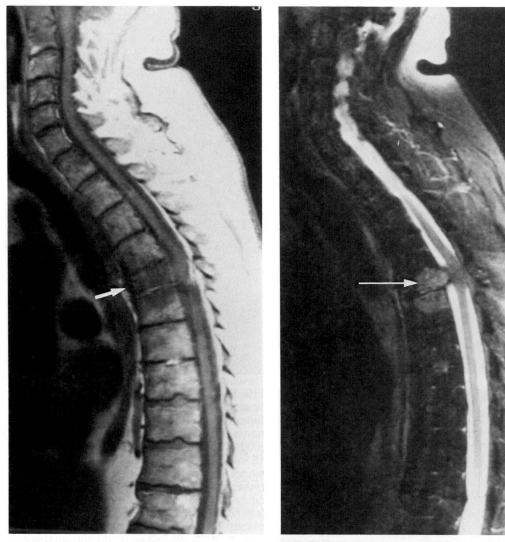

A

B

FIG. 14-8. Metastasis to the thoracic spine, with epidural extension seen with MR imaging using phased array coil. The patient has a known carcinoma of the lung. **A**: Sagittal T1-weighted SE MR image (600/12) shows partial compression of the T5 vertebral body (*arrow*) and low-signal metastasis to the T5 and T6 vertebrae. Epidural extension of tumor is suggested. The phased array coil provides visualization of the spine from C2 to T12 in this patient and is very useful in surveying for metastatic disease. These images were reconstructed in order to present the cervical and thoracic cord in the same plane. **B**: Sagittal T2-weighted FSE MR image (3000/108) of the cervical and thoracic spine obtained with fat-suppression technique. With this pulse sequence the metastatic lesions (*arrow*) are hyperintense relative to the normal vertebrae which have low signal because of the fat-suppression technique. Epidural extension of tumor and spinal cord compression can be seen. The use of the phased array coil provides images of the entire cervical and thoracic spine at the same time, thus markedly reducing imaging time. T1-weighted images may be sufficient when a shortened examination time is required; however, if a T2-weighted image is needed, FSE imaging is useful. This T2-weighted FSE study was performed in 6 minutes and 30 seconds.

Gadopentetate dimeglumine has been used to assess the effectiveness of therapy for spinal metastasis (21). Prior to irradiation or chemotherapy, spinal metastases enhance significantly more than normal vertebrae. After therapy, 70 percent of lesions that respond to treatment and remain clinically asymptomatic for 2–6 months do not show enhancement. Of those lesions that do not respond to therapy and remain clinically symptomatic, 88 percent remain enhanced after contrast injection (21). Some investigators have recommended the use of combined gadopentetate dimeglumine enhancement and fat-suppression techniques for improved lesion detection in the evaluation of metastatic disease (23). Similar combined techniques have

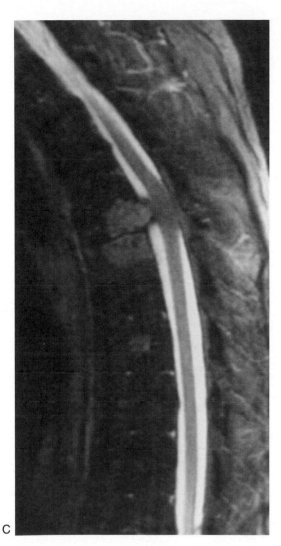

C

FIG. 14-8. (*Continued*). **C:** Magnified view of Fig. 14-8B. Using a phased array coil with a 512 × 512 matrix, high-resolution magnified images can be obtained of the cervical and thoracic spine.

been used for the study of osteomyelitis and postoperative scar.

The early detection of spinal metastasis is important clinically since it can lead to appropriate therapy and may thereby prevent vertebral fracture and/or epidural extension of tumor with subsequent spinal cord or cauda equina compression (17). Magnetic resonance imaging and CTM are particularly well suited for evaluation of epidural tumor extension. Isolated metastasis to the epidural space is found in 5 percent of patients with spinal metastasis presenting with signs of spinal cord or cauda equina compression (6). Much more frequently, epidural metastasis develops from direct extension of osseous vertebral metastasis, usually secondary to carcinoma of the breast, lung, or prostate gland (6,18). Occasionally, tumor from a paraspinal

mass extends into the spinal canal. The effect of the invading tumor on the subarachnoid space and spinal cord can be determined by MR imaging or CTM. Patients with known or suspected primary carcinoma who have back pain and a myelopathy, a radiculopathy, or radiographic evidence of metastasis at the appropriate clinical level need further evaluation for possible epidural metastasis (18). In one study (11), 36 percent of oncological patients with back pain as their only complaint and no signs of neurological dysfunction had MR demonstration of compression of the subarachnoid space or spinal cord.

Myelography, CTM, and MR have been utilized in the evaluation of patients with primary malignancy and clinical suspicion of spinal cord or nerve root compression. Myelography permits the demonstration of a partial or complete block and allows examination of the entire spinal canal, which may reveal other subclinical intraspinal metastases. Magnetic resonance imaging and CTM can better delineate osseous metastatic disease, as well as paravertebral and retroperitoneal extension of tumor. The cortical margins of bone are destroyed and soft-tissue extension of tumor causes obliteration of epidural fat. An epidural tumor causes compression of the subarachnoid space and displacement of the spinal cord or cauda equina (Figs. 14-4, 14-5). Computed tomographic myelography (Fig. 14-6) and MR imaging (Fig. 14-7) can show the soft-tissue epidural mass and spinal cord compression. If a myelogram is performed with water-soluble contrast and a block is seen, CTM can be used to determine the extent of tumor beyond the block, thus providing information that is vitally important if radiation therapy is needed (10).

Magnetic resonance imaging has compared favorably to myelography in the evaluation of epidural metastasis. In one study (3), the MR evaluation of extradural masses causing spinal cord compression had sensitivity of 92 percent and specificity of 90 percent compared to 95 percent and 88 percent, respectively, for myelography. For extradural masses without cord compression, MR imaging had sensitivity of 73 percent and specificity of 90 percent compared to 49 percent and 88 percent, respectively, for myelography. In addition, MR imaging can show multiple metastatic lesions not seen with myelography, such as when a second lesion is present beyond a myelographic block (11). Magnetic resonance imaging is also noninvasive, better tolerated by patients, and is the imaging modality of choice for the initial evaluation of epidural metastasis (11,22). In general, gadopentetate-dimeglumine-enhanced MR imaging is not required in the routine examination for epidural metastasis, although in some cases it may improve the delineation and characterization of certain lesions when combined with precontrast T1-weighted images (22).

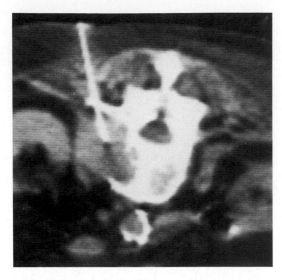

FIG. 14-9. Closed needle biopsy performed under CT guidance. The patient is in the prone position. There is destruction of the left side of the L3 vertebral body with paravertebral extension of tumor. A needle biopsy revealed the presence of metastatic adenocarcinoma. The use of CT for closed needle biopsy guidance represents another important application of CT.

Recent advances in MR imaging with phased array coils provide a method in which multiple surface coils are used in a configuration that produces simultaneous collection of data. The use of phased array coils provides the ability to scan the entire spinal column, which is useful when surveying for pathology such as metastatic disease. Patients being examined for spinal cord compression are often in great distress and cannot tolerate a lengthy study. With the use of phased array coils, diagnostic images with superior lesion localization can be obtained with marked reduction in the examination time (24). A patient with symptoms of spinal cord compression and clinical suspicion of metastatic disease had an MR examination shown in Fig. 14-8. With the use of phased array coils and FSE imaging with fat suppression, the diagnosis of metastasis to the thoracic spine with epidural extension and spinal cord compression was made in a relatively short time. The T2-weighted FSE images shown were obtained in 6 minutes and 30 seconds, and the use of phased array coils eliminated the need to study the cervical and thoracic spine as two separate studies. Appendix 1 provides MR imaging protocols that can be used to evaluate a region of the spine for metastatic disease or to survey the entire spine.

Computerized tomography can be used to guide closed needle biopsy of vertebral and paravertebral tumor, thus diminishing the risk of complications associated with closed needle biopsy performed with conventional radiographic guidance (Fig. 14-9).

REFERENCES

1. Avrahami E, Tadmor R, Dally O, et al. Early MR demonstration of spinal metastases in patients with normal radiographs and CT and radionuclide bone scans. *J Comput Assist Tomogr* 1989;13:598–602.
2. Beltran J, Noto AM, Chakeres DW, et al. Tumors of the osseous spine: staging with MR imaging versus CT. *Radiology* 1987;162:565–9.
3. Carmody RF, Yang PJ, Seeley GW, et al. Spinal cord compression due to metastatic disease: diagnosis with MR imaging versus myelography. *Radiology* 1989;173:225–9.
4. Castillo M, Malko JA, Hoffman JC Jr. The bright intervertebral disk: an indirect sign of abnormal spinal bone marrow on T1-weighted MR images. *AJNR* 1990;11:23–6.
5. Colman LK, Porter BA, Redmond J III, et al. Early diagnosis of spinal metastases by CT and MR studies. *J Comput Assist Tomogr* 1988;12:423–6.
6. Constans JP, DeDivitiis E, Donzelli R, et al. Spinal metastases with neurological manifestations: review of 600 cases. *J Neurosurg* 1983;59:111–8.
7. Dietrich RB, Kangarloo H, Lenarsky C, et al. Neuroblastoma: the role of MR imaging. *AJR* 1987;148:937–42.
8. Dwyer AJ, Frank JA, Sank VJ, et al. Short-TI inversion-recovery pulse sequence: analysis and initial experience in cancer imaging. *Radiology* 1988;168:827–36.
9. Edelstyn GA, Gillespie PJ, Grebbell FS. The radiological demonstration of osseous metastases: experimental observations. *Clin Radiol* 1967;18:158–62.
10. Fink IJ, Garra BS, Zabell A, et al. Computed tomography with metrizamide myelography to define the extent of spinal canal block due to tumor. *J Comput Assist Tomogr* 1984;8:1072–5.
11. Godersky JC, Smoker WRK, Knutzon R. Use of magnetic resonance imaging in the evaluation of metastatic spinal disease. *Neurosurgery* 1987;21:676–80.
12. Jones KM, Mulkern RV, Schwartz RB, et al. Fast spin-echo MR imaging of the brain and spine: current concepts. *AJR* 1992;158:1313–20.
13. Kricun ME. Radiographic evaluation of solitary bone lesions. *Orthop Clin North Am* 1983;14:39–63.
14. Krol G, Haimes A, Sze G. Spinal metastases: difficulties in MR diagnosis. In: *Proceedings of the American Society of Neuroradiology*. Orlando, Florida: American Society of Neuroradiology, 1989.
15. McNeil BJ. Value of bone scanning in neoplastic disease. *Semin Nucl Med* 1984;14:277–86.
16. Muindi J, Coombes RC, Golding S, et al. The role of computerized tomography in the detection of bone metastases in breast cancer patients. *Brit J Radiol* 1983;56:233–6.
17. Redmond J III, Spring DB, Munderloh SH, et al. Spinal computed tomography scanning in the evaluation of metastatic disease. *Cancer* 1984;54:253–8.
18. Rodichok LD, Harper GR, Ruckdeschel JC, et al. Early diagnosis of spinal epidural metastases. *Am J Med* 1981;70:1181–8.
19. Sarpel S, Sarpel G, Yu E, et al. Early diagnosis of spinal-epidural metastasis by magnetic resonance imaging. *Cancer* 1987;59:1112–6.
20. Stimac GK, Porter BA, Olson DO, et al. Gadolinium-DTPA-enhanced MR imaging of spinal neoplasms: preliminary investigation and comparison with unenhanced spin-echo and STIR sequences. *AJNR* 1988;9:839–46, *AJR* 1988;151:1185–92.
21. Sugimura K, Kajitani A, Okizuka H, et al. Assessing response to therapy of spinal metastases with gadolinium-enhanced MR imaging. *JMRI* 1991;1:481–4.
22. Sze G, Krol G, Zimmerman RD, et al. Malignant extradural spinal tumors: MR imaging with Gd-DTPA. *Radiology* 1988;167:217–23.
23. Tien RD. Fat-suppression MR imaging in neuroradiology: techniques and clinical application. *AJR* 1992;158:369–79.
24. Yousem DM, Schnall MD. MR examination for spinal cord compression: impact of a multicoil system on length of study. *J Comput Assist Tomogr* 1991;15:598–604.

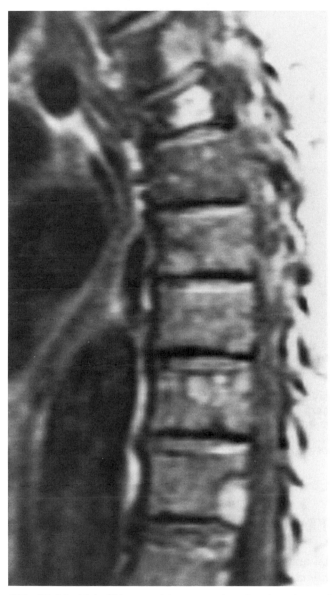

FIG. 15-1A. This 75-year-old woman has back pain and a significant past medical history that is being withheld. Sagittal T1-weighted SE MR image (800/20) of the thoracic spine obtained 6 mm left of the midline.

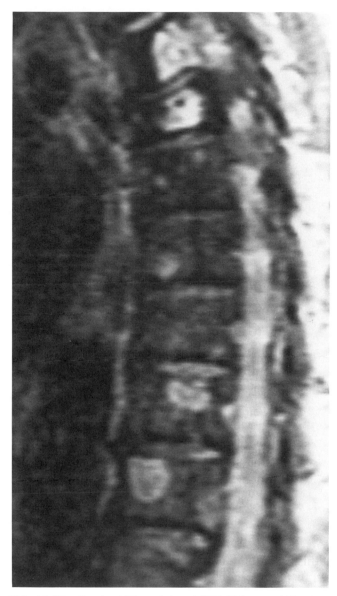

FIG. 15-1B. Sagittal T2-weighted SE MR image (2000/70).

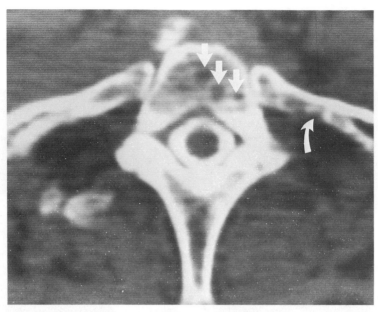

FIG. 16-1. Multiple myeloma. There are multiple small lytic lesions of the T1 vertebral body (*straight arrows*). Additional destruction is seen in the spinous process and the left rib (*curved arrow*). The "punched out" appearance is typical of myeloma. There is no epidural extension of tumor at this level.

MYELOMA

There are small round lytic lesions within the vertebral body, spinous process, and rib (Fig. 16-1). These are caused by multiple myeloma, a malignant proliferation of plasma cells. Multiple myeloma usually develops in individuals over the age of 40 years and is most common in the spine. After metastasis, it is the second most frequent malignancy of the spine and usually involves the vertebral bodies which are rich in red marrow (5). Myeloma does not affect the pedicles early in the disease as there is little red marrow in pedicles. However, the pedicles are involved late in the disease as fat marrow is converted to red marrow (5). Myeloma usually invades marrow with focal, well-defined destructive lesions. Destruction is sometimes so extensive that vertebral collapse occurs and tumor or hemorrhage extends into the paravertebral and epidural spaces, causing spinal cord or cauda equina compression (Fig. 16-2). Myeloma may produce an expansile lesion which encroaches on the spinal canal and neural elements. Rarely, myeloma presents with osteosclerotic bone lesions which may occur in untreated patients or may develop following radiation therapy or chemotherapy. Osteosclerotic myeloma may also be associated with a syndrome of polyneuropathy, organomegally, endocrinopathy, M-protein and skin changes—the so-called POEMS syndrome (8).

Early in its course, myeloma is not readily detected with conventional radiography since it takes approxi-

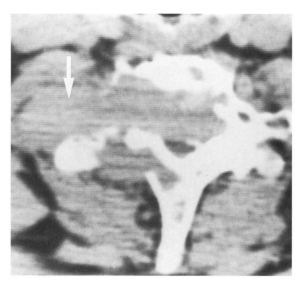

FIG. 16-2. Multiple myeloma. Same patient as in Fig. 16-1. There is extensive destruction of the C7 vertebral body, right pedicle, lamina, and transverse process. A soft-tissue mass extends into the epidural space, causing complete CTM block. A large right paravertebral mass is also present (*arrow*). The extensive osseous, epidural, and paravertebral involvement is the cause of the patient's symptoms of arm pain and leg weakness.

mately 50 percent destruction of cancellous bone before a lesion is radiographically visible (2). Nevertheless, conventional radiography is still more sensitive in detecting myeloma than is the radionuclide scan (12). Radionuclide scanning, which is extremely sensitive to the presence of metastasis, is normal in 27 percent of patients with radiographically proven myeloma (12).

Magnetic resonance imaging is often helpful in detecting the presence and extent of spinal myeloma (1,3, 6,7). The MR characteristics of untreated multiple myeloma may be similar to other infiltrating disorders of marrow in that there may be focal or diffuse decrease in signal intensity on T1-weighted images (1,3). Since myeloma occurs in adults who usually have extensive fat marrow in the spine, T1-weighted images show excellent contrast between the high signal intensity fat and low signal intensity myeloma lesions that replace the fat marrow. However, the MR appearance of my-

eloma is variable and myelomatous lesions may be isointense with hematopoietic marrow on T1-weighted images, making diagnosis difficult. In one series (6), patients with newly diagnosed multiple myeloma were evaluated with MR imaging of the lumbar spine with the following results: 53 percent had focal abnormalities in the bone marrow, 19 percent had diffuse abnormality, and in 28 percent myelomatous involvement could not be suspected. Only 25 percent of patients with myeloma had focal areas of decreased signal intensity on T1-weighted images, whereas 53 percent had focal areas of increased signal intensity on T2-weighted images. In 28 percent of patients, focal lesions were observed only on T2-weighted images, and in no patients were they observed only on T1-weighted images, suggesting that T2-weighted images may be more sensitive to the presence of focal myelomatous nodules (6). When diffuse abnormality of the marrow was identi-

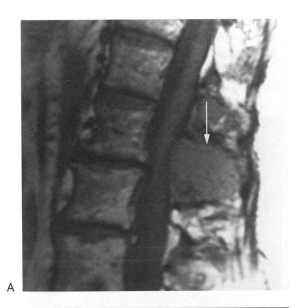

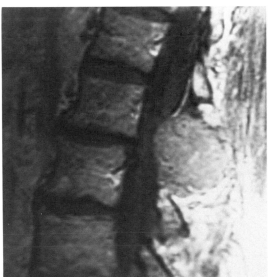

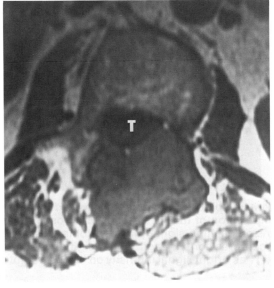

FIG. 16-3. Myeloma. **A**: Sagittal T1-weighted SE MR image (800/23). There is a large mass (*arrow*) of intermediate signal intensity that arises from the lamina of L2 and is compressing the conus. **B**: Sagittal T1-weighted SE MR image (800/23) following the administration of gadopentetate dimeglumine. There is enhancement of the mass. **C**: Axial T1-weighted SE MR image (600/12) shows a large mass of intermediate signal intensity that arises from the lamina of L2 and is encroaching upon the thecal sac (*T*).

of high signal intensity, thus showing reciprocal changes to those seen on T1-weighted images (5).

Patients who have had radiation treatment may have an MR study to evaluate for possible metastatic disease to bone. Metastatic lesions typically produce hypointense alterations in the bone marrow on T1-weighted images and are therefore readily separable from postradiation changes. Cortical destruction and paravertebral soft-tissue mass are other features of metastatic disease not seen in the postradiation patient who lacks tumor involvement.

In addition to the normal diffuse progressive conversion from hematopoietic marrow to fatty marrow, there is a second type of marrow replacement that has a more localized pattern. This focal fatty replacement is common and is seen as isolated or multifocal rounded areas of high signal intensity on T1-weighted images which measure 0.5–1.5 cm in diameter (2). The prevalence of this focal fatty deposition increases with age and is found in 13 percent of those in the first 10 years of life, 52 percent of those 31–40 years of age, and 93 percent of those 50–60 years of age (2). The focal nature of this common appearance should not be confused with changes of radiation therapy which cause uniform involvement of multiple adjacent vertebral bodies.

A serious complication of radiation therapy is radiation myelopathy. Typically, these patients present with paresthesias and inability to perceive pain and temperature, which begins 9–15 months after completion of radiotherapy to the spine (8). Progressive spinal cord symptoms occur over a 6-month period (8). Magnetic resonance imaging can show changes of radiation myelopathy. The spinal cord may be enlarged, of normal size, or atrophic. Performed less than 8 months after the onset of symptoms, MR imaging shows a long segment of abnormal signal intensity within the spinal cord (6). The cord has low signal intensity on T1-weighted images and high signal intensity on T2*-weighted SE images and on T2-weighted GRE images. Swelling of the spinal cord may be present (6). T1-weighted images obtained after the intravenous injection of gadopentetate dimeglumine may show enhancement of the cord that appears more focal than the area of increased signal intensity seen on the T2-weighted preinjection study (8). Performed more than 3 years after the onset of symptoms, MR imaging shows spinal cord atrophy without abnormal signal intensity on unenhanced images (6). The MR appearance of radiation myelopathy is nonspecific and may be seen with neoplasm, demyelination, cord ischemia, or infarction (8).

REFERENCES

1. Dooms GC, Fisher MR, Hricak H, et al. Bone marrow imaging: magnetic resonance studies related to age and sex. *Radiology* 1985;155:429–32.
2. Hajek PC, Baker LL, Goobar JE, et al. Focal fat deposition in axial bone marrow: MR characteristics. *Radiology* 1987;162:245–9.
3. Ramsey RG, Zacharias CE. MR imaging of the spine after radiation therapy: easily recognizable effects. *AJNR* 1985;6:247–51, *AJR* 1985;144:1131–5.
4. Rosenthal DI, Hayes CW, Rosen B, et al. Fatty replacement of spinal bone marrow due to radiation: demonstration by dual energy quantitative CT and MR imaging. *J Comput Assist Tomogr* 1989;13:463–5.
5. Stevens SK, Moore SG, Kaplan ID. Early and late bone-marrow changes after irradiation: MR evaluation. *AJR* 1990;154:745–50.
6. Wang P-Y, Shen W-C, Jan J-S. MR imaging in radiation myelopathy. *AJNR* 1992;13:1049–55.
7. Wismer GL, Rosen BR, Buxton R, et al. Chemical shift imaging of bone marrow: preliminary experience. *AJR* 1985;145:1031–7.
8. Zweig G, Russell EJ. Radiation myelopathy of the cervical spinal cord: MR findings. *AJNR* 1990:11:1188–90.

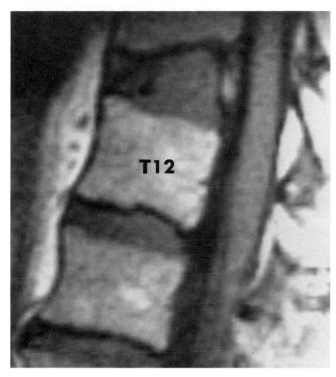

FIG. 18-1A. A 66-year-old woman was examined because of low back pain. Sagittal T1-weighted SE MR image (600/20) of the thoracolumbar spine obtained in the midline.

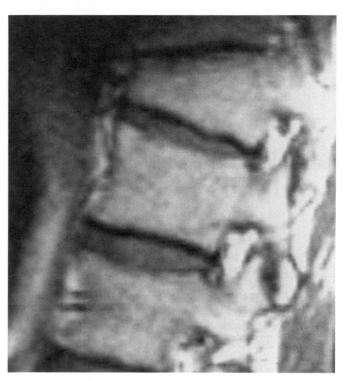

FIG. 18-1B. Parasagittal T1-weighted image obtained 10 mm to the right of the midline. Images obtained to the left of the midline had a similar appearance.

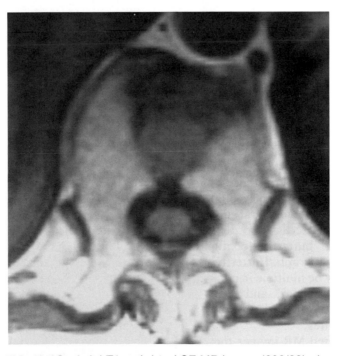

FIG. 18-1C. Axial T1-weighted SE MR image (600/20) obtained at the mid-T11 level.

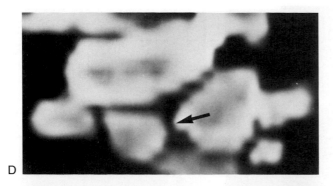

D

FIG. 18-2. *Continued*. **D**: Coronal reconstruction of axial CT images shows the butterfly vertebra of T1 with a midline cleft (*arrow*). Congenital abnormalities such as this may appear somewhat confusing on axial CT. Reconstruction of axial images and conventional radiography are helpful in understanding the complex axial images.

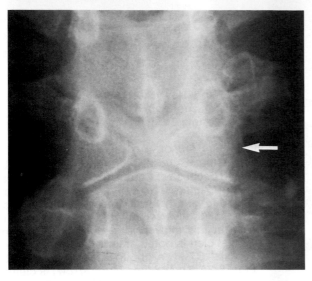

FIG. 18-3. Butterfly vertebra. Conventional AP radiograph of another patient shows butterfly vertebra of T4 (*arrow*).

REFERENCE

1. Schmorl G, Junghanns H. *The human spine in health and disease*. 2nd ed. New York: Grune and Stratton; 1971.

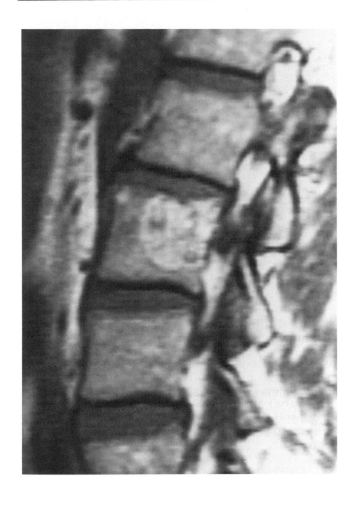

FIG. 19-1A. Magnetic resonance imaging of the lower lumbar spine was performed for a 67-year-old man with back and left leg pain. Sagittal T1-weighted SE image (400/16) obtained to the right of the midline.

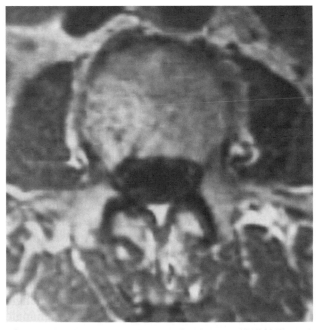

FIG. 19-1B. Axial T1-weighted SE image (600/15) at the level of the L3 vertebral body.

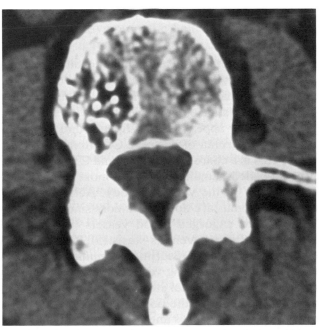

FIG. 19-1C. Axial CT scan at the level of the L3 vertebral body.

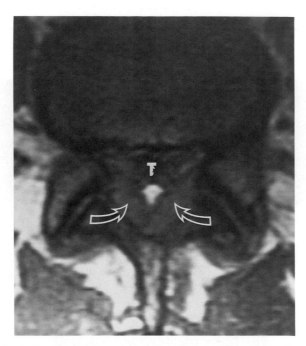

FIG. 20-1. Central spinal stenosis. There is marked thickening of the ligamenta flava (*arrows*) causing compression of the thecal sac (*T*). Disc bulging is also present.

CENTRAL SPINAL STENOSIS

There is degenerative central spinal stenosis secondary to marked thickening of the ligamenta flava (Fig. 20-1). Anatomic classification divides spinal stenosis into central stenosis with impingement on the cauda equina (or the spinal cord at the cervical, thoracic, and upper lumbar levels) and lateral stenosis with impingement on the nerve root. Lateral stenosis can be further subdivided into lateral recess stenosis (subarticular) and neural foraminal stenosis (intervertebral canal) (10).

Another classification of spinal stenosis is congenital-developmental stenosis versus acquired stenosis. Congenital-developmental stenosis includes both idiopathic and achondroplastic stenosis, whereas acquired stenosis includes degenerative (both central and lateral), spondylolisthetic, iatrogenic (postsurgical fibrosis, fusion, chemonucleolysis), and posttraumatic stenosis (1). Other causes such as Paget's disease and fluorosis are included among the acquired forms. Patients with congenital stenosis may develop degenerative changes and are then classified as having a combined form of stenosis.

Developmental and degenerative forms of spinal stenosis can be differentiated. Patients with developmental stenosis typically have uniform narrowing over several or all lumbar segments (9). Examination at the level of the pedicles shows a decreased AP diameter of the spinal canal. There is a decreased interpedicular distance in approximately 20 percent of the vertebrae studied (14). The pedicles may be short and the pedicles and laminae thickened in patients with developmental stenosis (Figs. 20-2, 20-3).

Degenerative spinal stenosis is typically segmental rather than uniform, with stenosis occurring at the level of the disc spaces and articular processes. Between these stenotic segments, the spinal canal and thecal sac may be normal in size (9). Hypertrophic spurs derived from the inferior articular processes and less frequently from the superior articular processes may cause central spinal stenosis of the degenerative form (Figs. 20-4, 20-5). In many cases, marked thickening and buckling of the ligamentum flavum is the major cause of central stenosis (see Fig. 20-1). Frequently, generalized bulging of the disc, thickening of the ligamentum flavum, and hypertrophy of the articular processes act in combination to cause stenosis. Thus, central spinal stenosis may find its etiology in bony and/or soft tissue components.

Patients with developmental spinal stenosis may be asymptomatic for years, their thecal sac just barely accommodated by the small canal. As minor degenerative changes occur, these compromised patients may develop symptoms. This combined form of spinal stenosis has features of both developmental and degenerative stenosis. The entire canal may be narrowed with

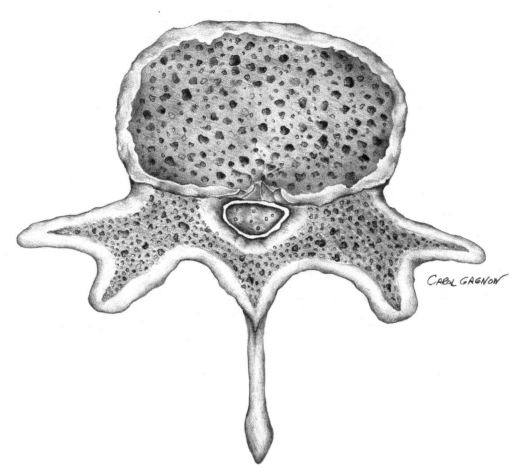

FIG. 20-2. Developmental spinal stenosis. Axial view of a lumbar vertebra at the level of the pedicles. Note the short broad pedicles and thickened laminae, which lead to a decreased AP diameter of the canal.

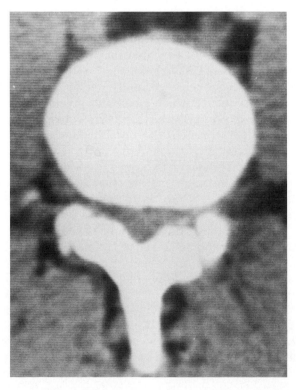

FIG. 20-3. Developmental central spinal stenosis. Axial CT scan just cephalad to the L4-L5 disc. The AP diameter of the canal is narrowed. Bilateral thickening of the laminae is seen.

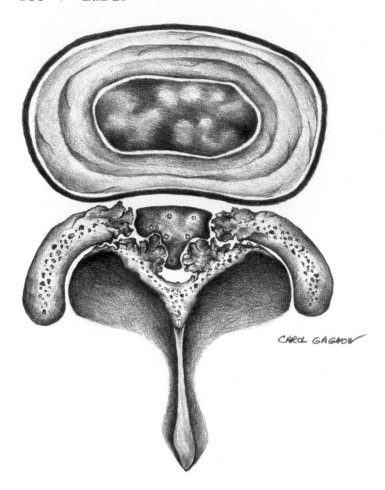

FIG. 20-4. Degenerative central spinal stenosis. Axial view of a lumbar vertebra at level of the disc. Note the osteophytes derived from the articular processes, which lead to compression of the thecal sac.

additional segmental narrowing occurring at the level of the disc spaces and articular processes secondary to disc bulging and facet joint hypertrophy.

Achondroplasia is a classic example of congenital spinal stenosis (Fig. 20-6). It is a congenital disorder of endochondral bone formation that leads to the development of short thick pedicles, which is more pronounced in the lower lumbar spine. This, along with early fusion of the neurocentral synchondroses, causes spinal stenosis that is most severe in the AP dimension. The interpedicular distance is also diminished and narrows progressively from L1 to L5. Thus, the intrinsically normal spinal cord and nerve roots are contained within a small bony canal.

Both MR imaging and CT can be used to evaluate patients suspected of having central spinal stenosis. Magnetic resonance imaging has been shown to be equivalent to CT and myelography in the diagnosis of lumbar canal stenosis and may be used along with CT as an alternative to myelography (12). In examining the images for central stenosis one must study the bony canal, the thecal sac (or cord), the ligamentum flavum, and the epidural fat.

In the MR evaluation of lumbar central spinal stenosis, sagittal T1- and T2-weighted images and axial T1-weighted images are useful for evaluating the level and degree of spinal stenosis. One can evaluate the bony and soft-tissue components of central stenosis, that is, disc bulging, osteophytes, and thickening of the ligamentum flavum. T2-weighted images show the bony central canal and its relationship to the thecal sac. Some investigators are currently utilizing an FSE T2-weighted sequence which creates a "myelographic effect" in a shorter period of time than conventional SE T2-weighted sequences. There is increased signal intensity of cerebrospinal fluid; however, with this pulse sequence, fat tissue is also hyperintense unless a fat-suppression technique is used (Fig. 20-7). A GRE sequence with a low flip angle also creates a myelographic effect.

Osteophytes are bony protrusions arising from the endplates in response to aging and mechanical stress. When small, they are usually composed of cortical bone and sometimes a minimal amount of cancellous bone, making them difficult to differentiate from adjacent hypointense posterior longitudinal ligament or cerebrospinal fluid on T1-weighted images. Large osteophytes contain more cancellous bone (fat marrow), and therefore have easily recognized bright signal on T1-weighted images. In general, osteophytes are easier

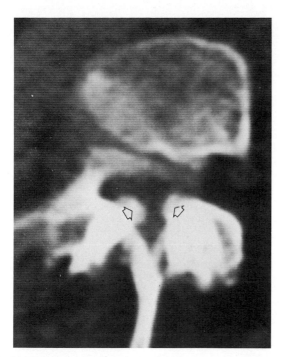

FIG. 20-5. Degenerative central spinal stenosis. Axial CT scan photographed at bone window settings shows large osteophytes (*arrows*) derived from the articular processes. The osteophytes are causing severe spinal stenosis with narrowing of the transverse diameter of the canal. The asymmetry of the scanning plane is caused by severe scoliosis and has led to asymmetric visualization of the pedicles and vertebral body.

to depict and differentiate from soft tissue on proton density-weighted images (5). Osteophytes can be recognized on conventional SE T2-weighted or FSE T2-weighted images as the hypointense cortical margin is contrasted very well with the high signal of cerebrospinal fluid. Large osteophytes containing cancellous bone and fat marrow have high signal intensity surrounded by the low signal intensity of cortical bone.

The ligamentum flavum (yellow ligament) is a yellowish fibro-elastic ligament that joins adjacent laminae. It extends from the anterocaudad surface of the lamina above to the posterocraniad surface of the lamina below. This ligament is thinnest in the cervical spine and becomes progressively thicker in the thoracic and lumbar regions. Normally, the ligamentum flavum is composed of 80 percent elastin and 20 percent type I collagen (5,19). With aging and scarring, collagen replaces the elastin and the collagen content may rise to more than 50 percent. Also, with aging, there is disc and facet joint degeneration and narrowing of the disc space. This leads to buckling of the ligamentum flavum which may encroach upon the spinal canal or intervertebral foramen. Isolated thickening without buckling of the ligamentum flavum is rare (19).

The ligamentum flavum can be observed on T1-weighted parasagittal MR images. It is located between two adjacent laminae and is separated from cerebrospinal fluid by posterior epidural fat. The ligamentum flavum is thicker and more triangular in shape near the midline. Intervening fat separates the two ligamenta flava in the midline (7).

The ligamentum flavum has intermediate signal intensity on both T1- and proton density-weighted MR images. The signal of the ligamentum flavum may not be separated from that of cerebrospinal fluid on proton density-weighted images. The relatively higher signal intensity of the ligamentum flavum compared to other body ligaments is most likely related to its high elastin content (5). On T2-weighted images, the ligamentum flavum has low signal intensity and may not be separated from that of bone. T1-weighted parasagittal images are helpful in delineating the posteromedial fat window. As the ligamentum flavum buckles and thickens, it encroaches on this fat window, contrasting with the surrounding high-signal fat tissue. Similarly, on the axial SE T1-weighted image, thickening of the ligamentum flavum is readily evident, encroaching on the thecal sac. Measurements of thickness of the ligamentum flavum are similar to those obtained with CT, the mean thickness being about 4.58 mm $\pm$ 0.97 mm (5). Occasionally, thickening of the ligamentum flavum is asymmetric or unilateral. Although buckling of the ligamentum flavum is usually associated with other signs of degenerative disease, particularly in the facet joints, it may appear slightly thickened in otherwise normal individuals. In axial images, a chemical shift artifact may cause a medial zone of the right ligamentum flavum to appear hypointense. Occasionally, fatty infiltration or calcification can be identified within the ligamentum flavum (3,5), although CT is more sensitive in detecting ligamentous calcification. With MR imaging, calcifications appear hypointense (signal void) on all pulse sequences (3). The calcifications which are composed of calcium pyrophosphate crystals are associated with either focal or diffuse enlargement of the ligamentum flavum (3) and occasionally with associated ossification of the posterior longitudinal ligament (18).

Computed tomography is an excellent method for detecting spinal canal stenosis in the axial plane. Determination of spinal canal size varies with the window width, window levels, and the density of the intrathecal contents (15). The most consistent measurements are obtained using a wide window width (1,000–4,000 HU). The window level is ideally set at the average between the CT numbers of the object being measured and the surrounding structures as determined in Hounsfield units (15). The use of intrathecal water-soluble contrast permits more reproducible canal size measurements (15). The gantry angle does not have a significant effect on spinal canal measurement as long as scan slice thickness is 5 mm or less (4). When scan slice thickness is 10 mm, gantry angulation that ex-

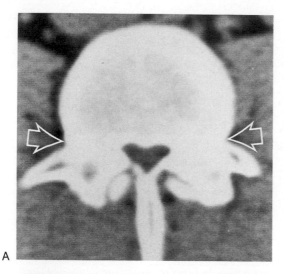

A

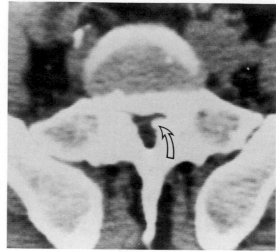

B

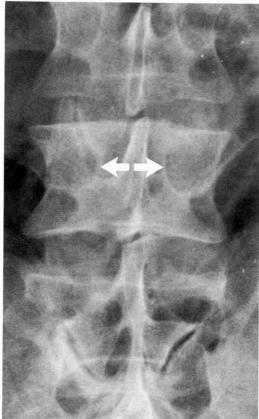

C

FIG. 20-6. Achondroplasia with spinal stenosis. **A**: Axial CT scan at L4 shows spinal stenosis that is typical of the congenital/developmental type. The spinal canal is small, especially in the anterior-posterior dimension. Short, broad pedicles (*arrows*) are typical of this type of stenosis. **B**: Axial CT scan at L5-S1 shows combined developmental and degenerative stenosis. In addition to the findings of developmental stenosis, there are degenerative changes making this a combined form of spinal stenosis. A large osteophyte (*arrow*) derived from an articular process on the left is present and causes additional stenosis. **C**: An AP radiograph shows that the interpedicular distance is diminished (*arrows*) and decreases progressively at the more caudal levels. This abnormality is typical of achondroplasia. Normally the interpedicular distance increases as successive lower lumbar levels are measured.

ceeds 15 degrees from the transverse plane of the canal may result in underestimation of canal size (4).

In the examination of patients with congenital-developmental lumbar stenosis, CT studies have suggested that a midsagittal diameter of 10 mm or less indicates absolute stenosis that may cause compression of the cauda equina (16). Patients with AP diameters measuring 10–12 mm are considered to have relative stenosis. This group may develop symptoms when minimal degenerative changes occur. Although measurements may be useful, it is often helpful to compare the size of the spinal canal to that of the thecal sac, since a small bony canal may not cause symptoms when the thecal sac is also small.

Degenerative central stenosis may be caused by soft-tissue encroachment upon the thecal sac (thickened ligamentum flavum, bulging disc) as well as bony compression (hypertrophy of articular processes). A patient with central stenosis due to ligamentous hypertrophy may have a normal AP diameter of the osseous canal. Therefore, measurement of this diameter is not reliable in determining the presence of degenerative

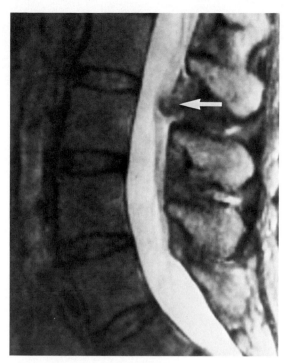

FIG. 20-7. Spinal stenosis. Sagittal T2-weighted FSE MR image (4000/80) with fat suppression shows spinal stenosis of the lumbar spine caused by hypertrophy and buckling of the ligamentum flavum (*arrow*).

stenosis. Only 20 percent of patients with degenerative central stenosis have a decreased AP diameter of the spinal canal (less than 13 mm) as measured by CT (2). Measurement of cross-sectional area of the thecal sac is a more reliable method of evaluating stenosis. In one study, the cross-sectional area of the thecal sac was determined by CT, and the following conclusions were drawn: (a) if the area is 100 mm^2 or less, central lumbar stenosis is present; (b) if the area measures between 100 and 130 mm^2, it is likely that there is early stenosis; (c) an area of 180 mm^2 $\pm$ 50 mm^2 is considered normal (2). These data highlight the importance of studying the size of the thecal sac; however, the diagnosis of central stenosis can be made without these absolute measurements. The demonstration of thickened ligamentum flavum, bulging disc, and/or hypertrophied articular processes compressing the thecal sac is sufficient to make the diagnosis of degenerative spinal stenosis. In evaluating patients who have not had previous surgery, some authors have noted the absence of epidural fat as another sign of stenosis signifying a decrease in effective space (6,11).

Most authors attribute the symptoms of spinal stenosis to pressure on nerve roots within the cauda equina or outside the dura. Other authors suggest the possibility of vascular as well as neural entrapment within the spinal canal or nerve root canal as a cause of symptoms (8). The classic symptoms of spinal stenosis include back pain with either claudication or sciatic pain in the legs (17). The pain is typically present when the patient stands or walks and is relieved by lying down or sitting. Activities that require flexion of the torso such as walking uphill or riding a bike are performed without symptoms, whereas hyperextension leads to severe pain. Compared to patients with disc herniation, patients with spinal stenosis tend to have chronic back pain prior to development of radiating leg pain. Symptoms are more frequently bilateral, and reduced straight leg raising is a less frequent finding (13).

REFERENCES

1. Arnoldi CC, Brodsky AE, Cauchoix J, et al. Lumbar spinal stenosis and nerve root entrapment syndromes: definition and classification. *Clin Orthop* 1976;115:4–5.
2. Bolender NF, Schönström NSR, Spengler DM. Role of computed tomography and myelography in the diagnosis of central spinal stenosis. *J Bone Joint Surg (Am)* 1985;67A:240–6.
3. Brown TR, Quinn SF, D'Agostino AN: Deposition of calcium pyrophosphate dihydrate crystals in the ligamentum flavum: evaluation with MR imaging and CT. *Radiology* 1991;178:871–3.
4. Eubanks BA, Cann CE, Brant-Zawadzki M. CT measurement of the diameter of spinal and other bony canals: effects of section angle and thickness. *Radiology* 1985;157:243–6.
5. Grenier N, Kressel HY, Schiebler ML, et al. Normal and degenerative posterior spinal structures: MR imaging. *Radiology* 1987; 165:517–25.
6. Helms CA, Vogler JB. Computed tomography of spinal stenosis and arthroses. *Clin Rheum Dis* 1983;9:417–41.
7. Ho PSP, Yu S, Sether LA, et al. Ligamentum flavum: appearance on sagittal and coronal MR images. *Radiology* 1988;168: 469–72.
8. Kirkaldy-Willis WH, McIvor GWD. Editorial comment: lumbar spinal stenosis. *Clin Orthop* 1976;115:2–3.
9. Kirkaldy-Willis WH, Paine KWE, Cauchoix J, et al. Lumbar spinal stenosis. *Clin Orthop* 1974;99:30–50.
10. Mall JC, Kaiser JA, Heithoff KB. Postoperative spine. In: Newton TH, Potts DG, eds. *Computed tomography of the spine and spinal cord.* San Anselmo, Calif: Clavadel Press; 1983:187–204.
11. McAfee PC, Ullrich CG, Yuan HA, et al. Computed tomography in degenerative spinal stenosis. *Clin Orthop* 1981;161:221–34.
12. Modic MT, Masaryk T, Boumphrey F, et al. Lumbar herniated disk disease and canal stenosis: prospective evaluation by surface coil MR, CT, and myelography. *AJR* 1986;147:757–65.
13. Paine KWE. Clinical features of lumbar spinal stenosis. *Clin Orthop* 1976;115:77–82.
14. Postacchini F, Pezzeri G, Montanaro A, et al. Computerized tomography in lumbar stenosis: a preliminary report. *J Bone Joint Surg (Br)* 1980;62B:78–82.
15. Rosenbloom S, Cohen WA, Marshall C, et al. Imaging factors influencing spine and cord measurements by CT: a phantom study. *AJNR* 1983;4:646–9.
16. Verbiest H. The significance and principles of computerized axial tomography in idiopathic developmental stenosis of the bony lumbar vertebral canal. *Spine* 1979;4:369–78.
17. Wiltse LL, Kirkaldy-Willis WH, McIvor GWD. The treatment of spinal stenosis. *Clin Orthop* 1976;115:83–91.
18. Yamashita Y, Takahashi M, Matsuno Y, et al. Spinal cord compression due to ossification of ligaments: MR imaging. *Radiology* 1990;175:843–8.
19. Yong-Hing K, Reilly J, Kirkaldy-Willis WH. The ligamentum flavum. *Spine* 1976;1:226–34.

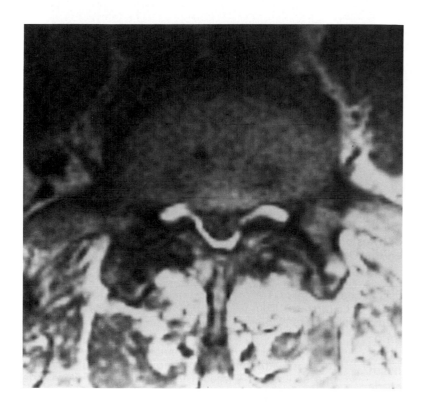

FIG. 21-1A. This 48-year-old man was evaluated because of pain in both legs. Axial T1-weighted SE MR image (800/15) obtained 5 mm caudad to the L4-L5 disc space.

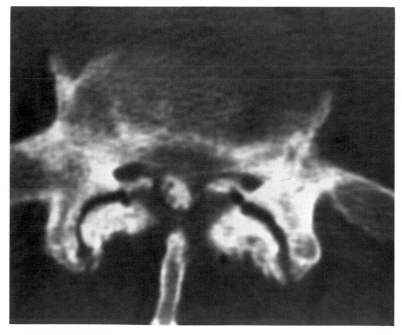

FIG. 21-1B. Axial CTM obtained caudad to the L4-L5 disc space.

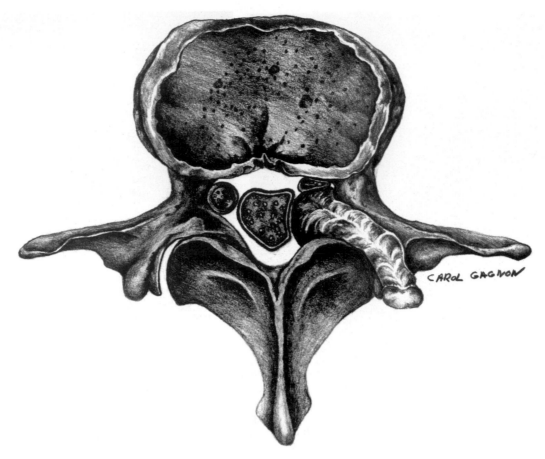

FIG. 21-5. Lateral recess stenosis and central spinal stenosis. Hypertrophy of the superior articular process causes narrowing of lateral recess and compression of the nerve root within the recess. These hypertrophic changes may also compress the thecal sac, causing central stenosis.

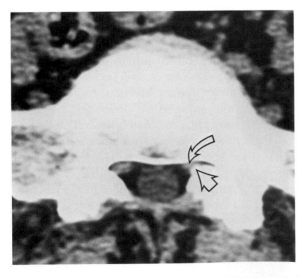

FIG. 21-6. Lateral recess stenosis. Axial CT scan caudad to the L5-S1 disc level in a patient with left hip and buttock pain. Hypertrophy of the superior articular process of S1 on the left (*straight arrow*) has caused severe lateral recess stenosis with compression of the left S1 nerve root (*curved arrow*). Compare with the opposite side where the uncompromised nerve root is seen within a normal lateral recess.

REFERENCES

1. Burton CV, Kirkaldy-Willis WH, Yong-Hing K, et al. Causes of failure of surgery on the lumbar spine. *Clin Orthop* 1981;157: 191–9.
2. Ciric I, Mikhael MA, Tarkington JA, et al. The lateral recess syndrome: a variant of spinal stenosis. *J Neurosurg* 1980;53: 433–43.
3. Eisenstein S. The trefoil configuration of the lumbar vertebral canal: a study of South African skeletal material. *J Bone Joint Surg (Br)* 1980;62B:73–7.
4. Heithoff KB. High-resolution computed tomography of the lumbar spine. *Postgrad Med* 1981;70:193–213.
5. Kirkaldy-Willis WH, Wedge JH, Yong-Hing K, et al. Lumbar spinal nerve lateral entrapment. *Clin Orthop* 1982;169:171–8.
6. Macnab I. Negative disc exploration: an analysis of the causes of nerve-root involvement in sixty-eight patients. *J Bone Joint Surg (Am)* 1971;53A:891–903.
7. McAfee PC, Ullrich CG, Yuan HA, et al. Computed tomography in degenerative spinal stenosis. *Clin Orthop* 1981;161:221–34.
8. Mikhael MA, Ciric I, Tarkington JA, et al. Neuroradiological evaluation of lateral recess syndrome. *Radiology* 1981;140: 97–107.
9. Quencer RM, Murtagh FR, Post MJD, et al. Postoperative bony stenosis of the lumbar spinal canal: evaluation of 164 symptomatic patients with axial radiography. *AJR* 1978;131:1059–64.
10. Risius B, Modic MT, Hardy RW Jr, et al. Sector computed tomographic spine scanning in the diagnosis of lumbar nerve root entrapment. *Radiology* 1982;143:109–14.

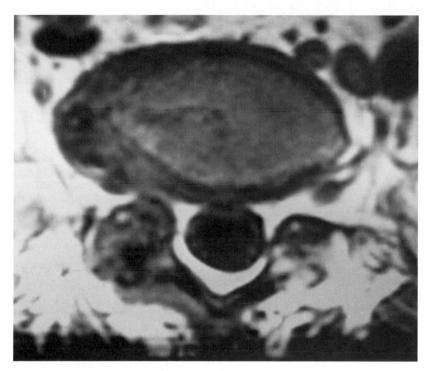

FIG. 22-1. This 68-year-old woman has low back pain and polyneuropathy. Axial T1-weighted (600/14) SE MR image at L5-S1.

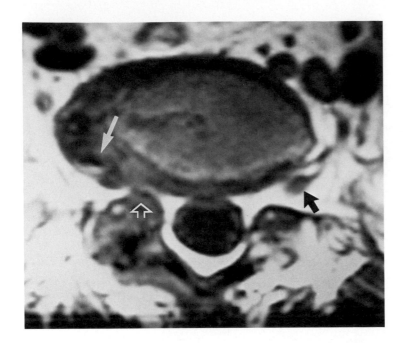

FIG. 22-1. Stenosis of the neural foramen. On the right side there is a large lateral vertebral body osteophyte (*closed white arrow*) and hypertrophy of the articular processes (*open arrow*) causing stenosis of the neural foramen and compression of the right L5 nerve root. Note the normal appearance of the left L5 nerve root (*black arrow*) and neural foramen.

STENOSIS OF THE NEURAL FORAMEN

This patient has neural foraminal stenosis caused by large osteophytes derived from the articular process and the vertebral body margin (Fig. 22-1).

Stenosis of the lumbar neural foramen (intervertebral canal) is best identified by CT and MR imaging. The neural foramen is bordered superiorly by the pedicle of the vertebra above, inferiorly by the pedicle of the vertebra below, and anteriorly by the posterior aspect of the vertebral bodies and the intervertebral disc (5) (Fig. 22-2). The posterior boundary is formed by the pars interarticularis and the apex of the superior articular process of the inferior vertebral body (Figs. 22-3, 22-4). Any bony or soft-tissue encroachment of the neural foramen leads to foraminal stenosis. However, because the nerve root exits through the upper portion of the foramen (approximately 1.0–1.5 cm cephalad to the intervertebral disc) (see Fig. 22-2), stenosis involving the inferior portion of the foramen may be asymptomatic.

The process which results in osseous stenosis of the neural foramen may begin with degenerative changes leading to degradation of the nucleus pulposus and annulus fibrosus with resultant loss of disc height (2,6). This causes additional stress on the facet joints, eventually leading to osteoarthritis and subsequent subluxation of these joints. The superior articular process then moves cephalad and anteriorly, causing narrowing of the neural foramen (2,6). Bony overgrowth of superior and inferior articular processes as well as thickening of the joint capsule and ligamentum flavum also account for foraminal narrowing.

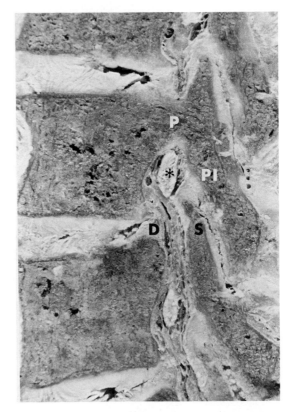

FIG. 22-2. Gross anatomic specimen of the lower lumbar vertebrae in the parasagittal plane showing the nerve root (*asterisk*) exiting the superior portion of the neural foramen just beneath the pedicle (*P*). Note the relationship of the nerve root to the pars interarticularis (*PI*) of the same vertebral level, the superior articular process of the vertebra below (*S*) and the intervertebral disc (*D*).

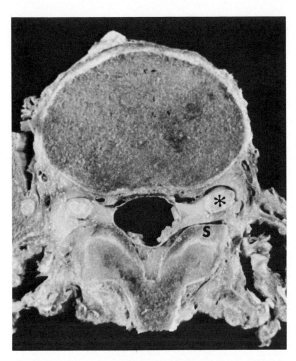

FIG. 22-3. Gross anatomic specimen of L4 vertebra in the axial plane through the level of the neural foramen. The dorsal root ganglion (*asterisk*) is surrounded by fat and has a close relationship to the superior articular process of L5 (*S*).

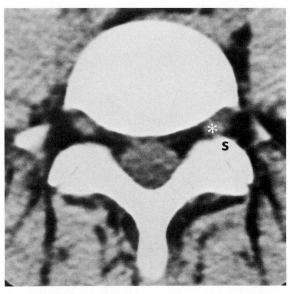

FIG. 22-4. Axial CT scan through the L5 vertebra at the level of the neural foramen. The dorsal root ganglion (*asterisk*) exits the neural foramen bordered anteriorly by the posterior margin of the vertebral body and posteriorly by the superior articular process of S1 (*S*). Fat surrounds the dorsal root ganglion.

Conventional radiography is inadequate for evaluation of intervertebral canal stenosis of the lumbar spine, whereas CT and MR imaging are capable of showing this abnormality (8,10,11). MR imaging can adequately evaluate the neural foramen in both the axial and sagittal planes. Coronal images are not obtained routinely. There is abundant fat within the neural foramen that appears as increased signal intensity on T1-weighted images. This contrasts superbly with the very low signal of the cortex of the articular processes, and the intermediate signal intensity of the nerves, vessels, and dorsal root ganglion within the canal (7). The differentiation between an enlarged, thickened capsule and sclerotic osteophytes may be difficult because of low signal intensity of the capsule found at the posteroinferior aspect of the joint.

In the MR evaluation of lumbar foraminal stenosis, T1- and proton density-weighted SE images are useful. T1-weighted images allow contrast between the increased signal intensity of fat tissue and that of the ligamentum flavum and nerve roots. Proton density-weighted images allow for better contrast between articular (hyalin) cartilage and bone as well as between cortex and marrow. However, with this pulse sequence, the ligamentum flavum and cerebrospinal fluid may be isointense.

The axial MR images are helpful as they allow for better evaluation of the facet joints, articular cartilage, presence and degree of osteophyte formation, and thickness of the joint capsule. One limitation of the T1-weighted axial image is difficulty in differentiating bone from enlarged capsule in some cases of advanced degenerative change. The parasagittal views are helpful for evaluation of displacement of fat tissue and displacement of nerve roots in the region of the intervertebral canal.

Computed tomography can better delineate the bony alterations about the intervertebral canal. CT may reveal hypertrophic changes derived from the superior articular process, or a hard disc representing either posterior vertebral body osteophyte or calcified disc material (Fig. 22-5A). The dorsal nerve root ganglion may appear flattened or enlarged, and the perineural fat within the foramen may be obliterated (3). The grading of stenosis involving the intervertebral canal is based on the amount of narrowing of the canal and the degree of obliteration of perineural fat (11). One word of caution: actual measurements of neural foraminal width from axial CT scans is influenced by several factors (e.g., CT window settings and reference points for measurement) which may lead to interobserver discrepancies (1). Sagittal and oblique reformation of axial CT images may lead to increased diagnostic accuracy of osseous stenosis of the neural foramen (3) (Fig. 22-

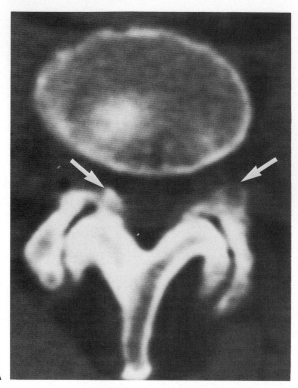

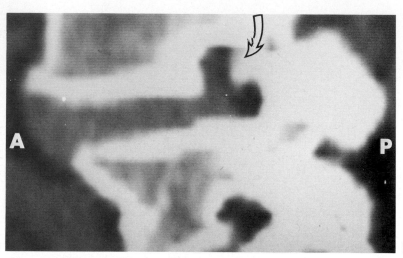

A   B

FIG. 22-5. Stenosis of the neural foramen and degenerative arthritis of the facet joints in patient with degenerative spondylolisthesis at L4-L5. **A**: Computed tomography cephalad to L4-L5 disc at level of neural foramen. There are bilateral hypertrophic changes of the superior articular processes of L5 (*arrows*) and narrowing of the facet joints. Note the somewhat sagittal orientation of the facet joints. The degree of neural foraminal stenosis was better evaluated by the reconstruction technique shown in Fig. 22-5B. **B**: Oblique reconstruction of axial CT images through the plane of the left neural foramen. Encroachment upon the superior portion of the neural foramen is caused by osseous hypertrophy derived from superior articular process of L5 (*arrow*). *A*, anterior; *P*, posterior.

5B). Other causes of foraminal nerve root entrapment may similarly be associated with radiculopathy and a negative myelogram; they include lateral disc herniation, postoperative fibrotic scarring, spondylolisthesis, and tumor (4,10).

As was the case with lateral recess stenosis (see Case 21), patients with FBSS may have stenosis of the neural foramen that was either inaccurately diagnosed preoperatively or inadequately decompressed (Fig. 22-6). It is not certain whether the lateral stenosis is present prior to surgery or is the result of surgery in patients with the FBSS. Some authors, however, believe that in most cases the stenosis precedes the surgery (3). With the advent of CT and the increased ability to diagnose lateral stenosis preoperatively, a decrease in the incidence of the FBSS has been noted by some (3).

Patients with cervical radiculopathy may have compression of a nerve root within the neural foramen caused by a lateral disc herniation or an osteophyte. Evaluation of the cervical neural foramen can be accomplished with conventional SE two-dimensional

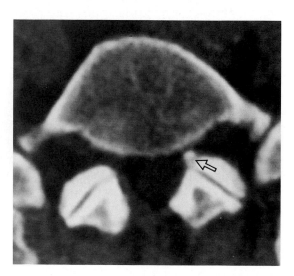

FIG. 22-6. Stenosis of the neural foramen. This patient had previous surgery for central spinal stenosis; however, decompression did not extend to the neural foramen. Hypertrophy of the superior articular process (*arrow*) is causing narrowing of the left neural foramen that was subsequently unroofed at reoperation.

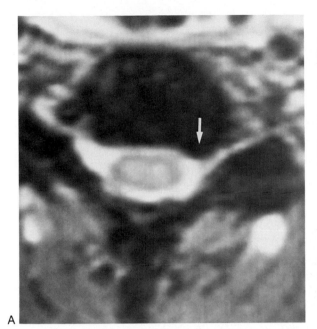
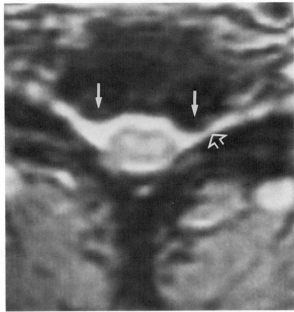

FIG. 22-7. Cervical neural foraminal stenosis. This 60-year-old woman has neural foraminal stenosis at two levels shown by MR imaging. **A**: Axial GRE MR image (MPGR, 600/20 with 20-degree flip angle) at C5-C6. There is spondylosis on the left (*arrow*) causing stenosis of the left neural foramen. **B**: Axial GRE MR image (MPGR, 600/20 with 20-degree flip angle) at C6-C7. At this level there is bilateral spondylosis (*closed arrows*) causing neural foraminal stenosis that is more severe on the left side (*open arrow*).

Fourier transform (2DFT) MR imaging; however this is limited by section thickness, suboptimal signal-to-noise ratio within sections, and cerebrospinal fluid flow artifacts (12). Improved MR techniques to evaluate the cervical neural foramen include: GRE imaging (Fig. 22-7), oblique imaging (9), and thin-section high-resolution gradient-refocussed three-dimensional Fourier transform (3DFT) (12). With the latter technique, contiguous 1.5-mm axial 3DFT images can be obtained and provide high contrast between disc, cord, osteophyte, and cerebrospinal fluid, making it a useful method of evaluating foraminal stenosis. The use of a low flip angle (e.g., 5 degrees) coupled with TR/TE of 50/15 provides excellent visualization of foraminal anatomy and pathology (12). With 3DFT GRE techniques, 60 contiguous 1.5-mm sections can be obtained within a reasonable time frame. The evaluation of these images, however, appears to be strongly interpreter dependent and presumably improves with experience. Computed tomographic myelography remains an excellent method of evaluating pathology of the cervical neural foramen. Using CTM as the "gold standard," 3DFT MR imaging agrees with CTM in detecting cervical neural foraminal narrowing and determining the cause of narrowing in approximately 76 percent of neural foramina studied (12). Osteophytes account for most abnormalities seen on CTM and missed with MR imaging.

REFERENCES

1. Beers GJ, Carter AP, Leiter BE, et al. Interobserver discrepancies in distance measurements from lumbar spine: CT scans. *AJR* 1985;144:395–8.
2. Burton CV, Kirkaldy-Willis WH, Yong-Hing K, et al. Causes of failure of surgery on the lumbar spine. *Clin Orthop* 1981;157:191–9.
3. Heithoff KB. High-resolution computed tomography and stenosis: an evaluation of the causes and cures of the failed back surgery syndrome. In: Post MJD, ed. *Computed tomography of the spine*. Baltimore: Williams and Wilkins; 1984: 506–45.
4. Helms CA, Vogler JB. Computed tomography of spinal stenoses and arthroses. *Clin Rheum Dis* 1983;9:417–41.
5. Kirkaldy-Willis WH, McIvor GWD. Editorial comment: lumbar spinal stenosis. *Clin Orthop* 1976;115:2–3.
6. Kirkaldy-Willis WH, Wedge JH, Yong-Hing K, et al. Lumbar spinal nerve lateral entrapment. *Clin Orthop* 1982;169:171–8.
7. Kostelic JK, Haughton VM, Sether LA. Lumbar spinal nerves in the neural foramen: MR appearance. *Radiology* 1991;178:837–9.
8. McAfee PC, Ullrich CG, Yuan HA, et al. Computed tomography in degenerative spinal stenosis. *Clin Orthop* 1981;161:221–34.
9. Modic MT, Masaryk TJ, Ross JS, et al. Cervical radiculopathy: value of oblique MR imaging. *Radiology* 1987;163:227–31.
10. Osborne DR, Heinz ER, Bullard D, et al. Role of computed tomography in the radiological evaluation of painful radiculopathy after negative myelography: foraminal neural entrapment. *Neurosurgery* 1984;14:147–53.
11. Risius B, Modic MT, Hardy RW Jr, et al. Sector computed tomographic spine scanning in the diagnosis of lumbar nerve root entrapment. *Radiology* 1982;143:109–14.
12. Yousem DM, Atlas SW, Goldberg HI, et al. Degenerative narrowing of the cervical spine neural foramina: evaluation with high-resolution 3DFT gradient-echo MR imaging. *AJNR* 1991;12:229–36, *AJR* 1991;156:1229–36.

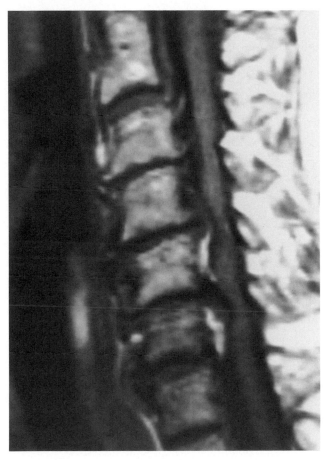

FIG. 23-1A. This 81-year-old woman was examined because of left arm numbness. Sagittal T1-weighted SE MR image (700/15) of the cervical spine.

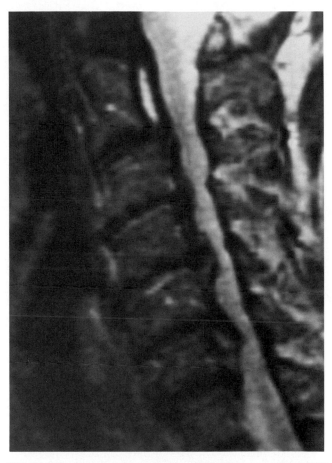

FIG. 23-1B. Sagittal T2-weighted SE MR image (2045/70).

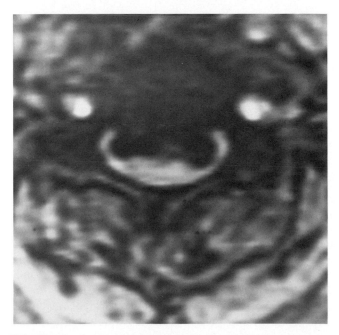

FIG. 23-1C. Axial GRE MR image (GRASS, 24/13 with 8-degree flip angle).

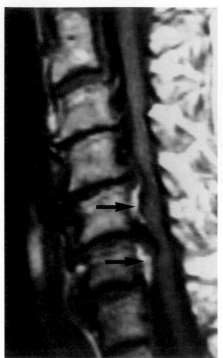
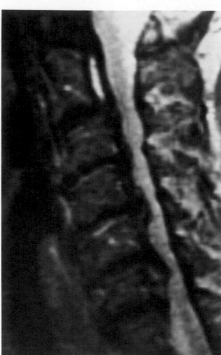
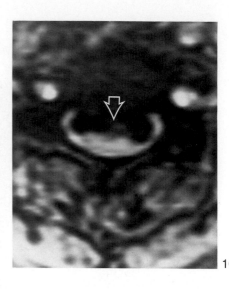

1A

1B

1C

FIG. 23-1A. Ossification of the posterior longitudinal ligament (OPLL). OPLL (*arrows*) is seen posterior to the C5 and C6 vertebrae, and has high signal intensity of fatty marrow. In some cases, ligamentous ossification may have low signal intensity on T1-weighted images and may be difficult to identify because of the similar signal of cerebrospinal fluid. Spinal stenosis is evident.

FIG. 23-1B. The extent of OPLL and the severity of the spinal stenosis is well seen on the T2-weighted image. Bright signal anterior to the ossified posterior longitudinal ligament at C2 is the epidural venous plexus.

FIG. 23-1C. The broad, globular-shaped ossification of the posterior longitudinal ligament (*arrow*) is seen as very low signal intensity on this GRE image. Severe compression of the spinal cord is evident.

OSSIFICATION OF THE POSTERIOR LONGITUDINAL LIGAMENT

In addition to degenerative changes, there is ossification of the posterior longitudinal ligament (OPLL) with severe spinal cord compression shown by MR imaging (Fig. 23-1). This is a clinical disorder that is more prevalent in Japan and eastern Asian countries where it occurs in 1–3 percent of the population with cervical symptoms (6,9). The incidence among Caucasians is only 0.2 percent (6,9). The cervical spine is much more frequently involved than the thoracic or lumbar spine and accounted for 88 percent of cases in one MR study (10). Within the cervical spine, OPLL may occur at any level; however, the most frequent site of ossification is C5 (9). Usually, more than one cervical level is involved. This disorder causes compression of the spinal cord leading to myelopathy and radiculopathy. The most common symptoms at presentation are numbness of the hands, weakness of the legs, difficulty walking

(spastic gait), pain in the neck and arms, and urinary or intestinal symptoms (1,3). Compression of the anterior spinal arteries may also be a cause of symptoms (3). Some individuals are asymptomatic.

The lateral radiograph of the spine shows a bony density having a longitudinal orientation posterior to the vertebral bodies (Fig. 23-2). Several types of ossification have been described: segmental (behind each vertebral body), continuous (involving multiple vertebrae without interruption), mixed segmental and continuous, and localized (limited to the intervertebral disc level) (9). In the cervical spine, the segmental type occurs in 47 percent of cases and the continuous or mixed types of OPLL are found in 53 percent (10). The degree of cord compression and the extent of clinical symptoms are more severe with the continuous than the segmental type of OPLL. In the lumbar spine most cases

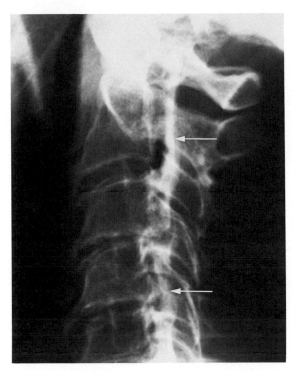

FIG. 23-2. OPLL. Same patient in Fig. 23-1. Lateral radiograph of the cervical spine shows ossification of the posterior longitudinal ligament at several levels (*arrows*).

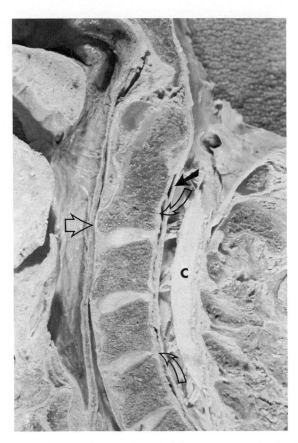

FIG. 23-3. Anatomic specimen of the upper cervical spine in the near-sagittal plane showing the close relationship of the posterior (*curved arrows*) and anterior longitudinal (*open straight arrow*) ligaments to the vertebrae and discs. *C,* spinal cord; *closed arrow,* thecal sac.

are limited to the disc level and may be difficult to differentiate from spondylosis (10).

The methods of CT and MR may be utilized to determine the configuration of the ossified mass, the degree of canal compromise, and the longitudinal extent of ossification. Because OPLL occurs much less frequently than degenerative spondylosis in the cervical spine, the later diagnosis may be made incorrectly in patients with OPLL evaluated by conventional radiography and myelography. Typically, however, CT and MR show that the ossified mass extends posterior to the entire longitudinal extent of the vertebral body rather than being limited to the disc level as typically seen with degenerative spondylosis.

Anatomically, the posterior longitudinal ligament extends from the skull to the sacrum along the posterior aspect of the intervertebral discs and vertebral bodies (Fig. 23-3). It is present in the midline and attaches to the posterior aspect of the discs and vertebral body margins and is separated from the midportion of the vertebral bodies by retrovertebral veins. Ossification of the posterior longitudinal ligament most frequently occurs in the midline and typically has an ovoid or oblong shape on axial images (6). The ossification may appear attached to the vertebral body at some levels and unattached at others (3,6) (Fig. 23-4). The gap between the vertebral body and the ossified ligament is thought to represent an unossified deep layer of the

posterior longitudinal ligament (3,7) or may be due to interposed venous structures. Some authors have described tandem type of ossification with two layers of ossification seen on axial CT (6). This may represent the mixed continuous and segmental type of ossification, with a continuous layer of ossification extending posterior to a separate segmental layer of ossification (6).

The posterior longitudinal ligament normally appears hypointense on all MR SE images. The diagnosis of OPLL can be suggested when there is broad low signal intensity on T1- and T2-weighted images in the distribution of the posterior longitudinal ligament. The low signal intensity is caused by cortical bone which lacks mobile protons. However, on T1-weighted images, intermediate or high signal intensity is seen within the area of ossification in 56 percent of continuous OPLL and 11 percent of segmental OPLL and is thought to represent fatty marrow (10). The differential diagnosis of a low signal abnormality in the anterior subarachnoid space on both T1- and T2-weighted images includes calcified meningioma and arteriovenous malformation (5). However, the extent of the lesion

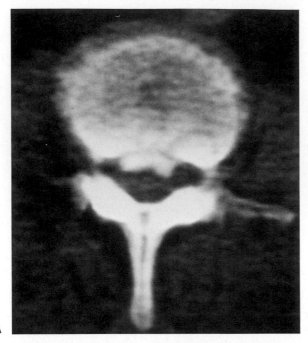
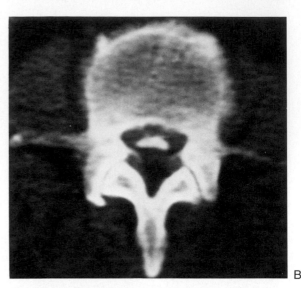

A

B

FIG. 23-4. OPLL of the lumbar spine. **A**: Axial CT scan at vertebral endplate level. The ossified ligament appears attached to the posterior vertebral body. **B**: Axial CT scan at midvertebral level. Ossified ligament is obviously separate from the posterior vertebral body. The unossified area between the vertebral body and the ossified ligament may be caused by an unossified deep layer of the ligament or by interposed venous structures.

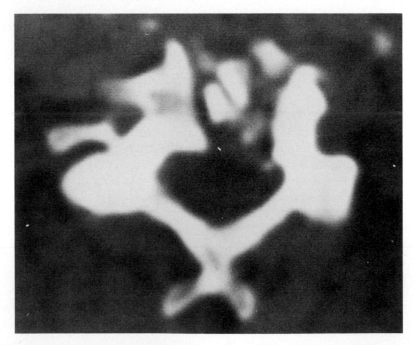

FIG. 23-5. Postoperative status of a patient treated for OPLL. There has been partial resection of the vertebral body, removal of the ossified mass, and insertion of an iliac bone graft.

FIG. 23-6. OPLL and ossification of the ligamentum flavum. **A**: Sagittal T1-weighted SE MR image (833/20) of the thoracic spine shows OPLL (*closed arrows*) and ossification of the ligamentum flavum (*open arrow*) having very low signal intensity. Spinal cord compression is present. **B**: Sagittal T2-weighted SE MR image (2500/70) shows very low signal intensity of the ossified ligaments with this pulse sequence. **C**: Axial T1-weighted SE MR image (833/20) shows OPLL and ossification of the ligamentum flavum (*arrows*) extending into the spinal canal and causing compression of the spinal cord. **D**: Axial CTM image at T10-T11 shows bilateral ossification of the ligamentum flavum (*arrows*) causing spinal cord compression. OPLL was seen at other levels.

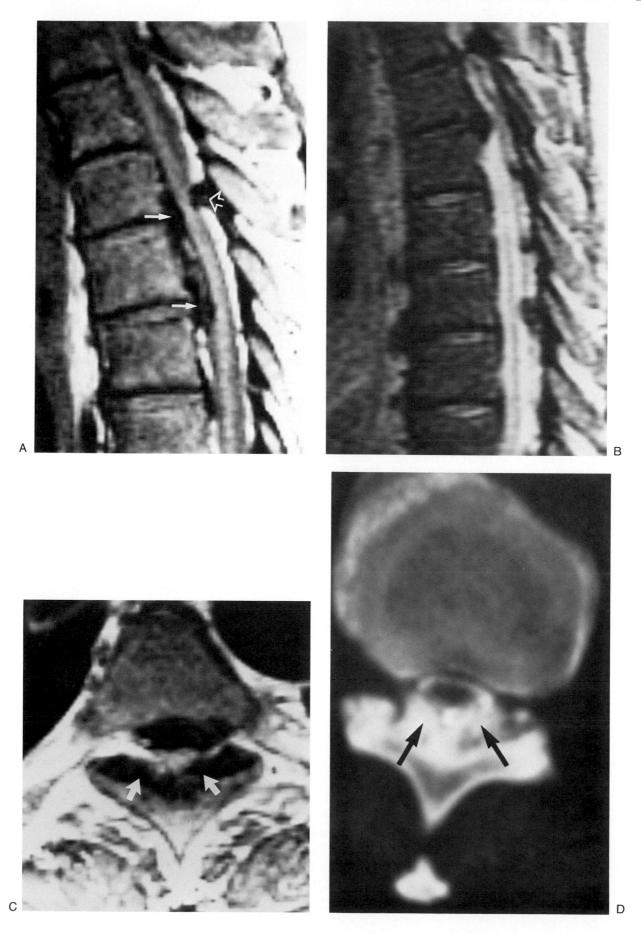

and the possible presence of intermediate or high signal intensity within the areas of ossification on T1-weighted images should enable one to make the correct diagnosis.

Magnetic resonance imaging can also show high signal intensity within the spinal cord on T2- or proton density-weighted images in cases of chronic cord compression. These signal changes may be caused by edema, demyelination, gliosis, or necrosis, and are proportional to the severity of clinical myelopathy and degree of spinal cord compression (8). Spinal cord compression is more severe in the continuous OPLL than in the segmental type. In one series of patients with cervical OPLL, bright signal was found within the cord on T2-weighted images of 34 percent of patients with continuous or mixed OPLL and 16 percent of those with segmental ossification (10). The ligamentous ossification is easier to assess and is thicker with the continuous type. The average thickness of the continuous type is approximately 6 mm while the segmental type is 3 mm (10). Most cervical ossifications greater than 3.2 mm can be detected by MR imaging. Correlation between the degree of spinal canal compromise and clinical symptoms suggest that severe myelopathy is most likely to occur when axial stenosis exceeds 30 percent (1). Sagittal MR imaging or sagittal reconstruction of the axial CT images can further define the longitudinal extent of the ossification as well as the degree of spinal canal compromise. Some patients, however, have a paucity of symptoms despite severe canal stenosis.

Treatment may be conservative or surgical. If surgery is contemplated it becomes important to distinguish OPLL from degenerative spondylosis since the surgical approach differs. OPLL can be surgically treated by a posterior or anterior approach. The anterior approach involves partial resection of the vertebrae, release or removal of the ossified mass, and insertion of an iliac bone graft (2) (Fig. 23-5). The etiology of OPLL is not known; however, certain common characteristics of patients with OPLL have been found. Such patients tend to have abnormal glucose and calcium metabolism and a generalized hyperostotic state with ossification of other paraspinal ligaments (9). Ossification or calcification of the posterior longitudinal ligament has also been seen in 50 percent of patients with DISH (7). Ossification of the ligamentum flavum may occur separately or in association with OPLL. Ossification of the ligamentum flavum is most commonly found in the thoracic spine and may also be a cause of myelopathy with compression of the spinal cord and nerve roots (4) (Fig. 23-6).

REFERENCES

1. Hanai K, Adachi H, Ogasawara H. Axial transverse tomography of the cervical spine narrowed by ossification of the posterior longitudinal ligament. *J Bone Joint Surg (Am)* 1977;59A:481–4.
2. Hanai K, Inouye Y, Kawai K, et al. Anterior decompression for myelopathy resulting from ossification of the posterior longitudinal ligament. *J Bone Joint Surg (Br)* 1982;64B:561–4.
3. Hanna M, Watt I. Posterior longitudinal ligament calcification of the cervical spine. *Brit J Radiol* 1979;52:901–5.
4. Hukuda S, Mochizuki T, Ogata M, et al.: The pattern of spinal and extraspinal hyperostosis in patients with ossification of the posterior longitudinal ligament and the ligamentum flavum causing myelopathy. *Skeletal Radiol* 1983;10:79–85.
5. Luetkehans TJ, Coughlin BF, Weinstein MA. Ossification of the posterior longitudinal ligament diagnosed by MR. *AJNR* 1987; 8:924–5.
6. Murakami J, Russell WJ, Hayabuchi N, et al. Computed tomography of posterior longitudinal ligament ossification: its appearance and diagnostic value with special reference to thoracic lesions. *J Comput Assist Tomogr* 1982;6:41–50.
7. Resnick D, Guerra J Jr, Robinson CA, et al. Association of diffuse idiopathic skeletal hyperostosis (DISH) and calcification and ossification of the posterior longitudinal ligament. *AJR* 1978; 131:1049–53.
8. Takahashi M, Yamashita Y, Sakamoto Y, et al. Chronic cervical cord compression: clinical significance of increased signal intensity on MR images. *Radiology* 1989;173:219–24.
9. Tsuyama N. Ossification of the posterior longitudinal ligament of the spine. *Clin Orthop* 1984;184:71–84.
10. Yamashita Y, Takahashi M, Matsuno Y, et al. Spinal cord compression due to ossification of ligaments: MR imaging. *Radiology* 1990;175:843–8.

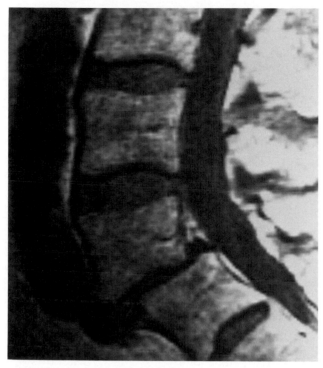

FIG. 24-1A. This 63-year-old man was examined because of pain in the left hip and thigh. Sagittal T1-weighted SE MR image (600/15) of the lumbar spine in the midline.

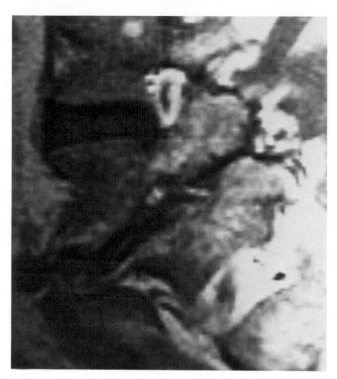

FIG. 24-1B. Sagittal T1-weighted MR image 20 mm left of midline.

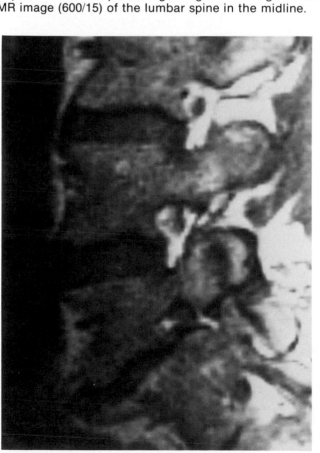

FIG. 24-1C. Sagittal T1-weighted MR image 20 mm right of midline.

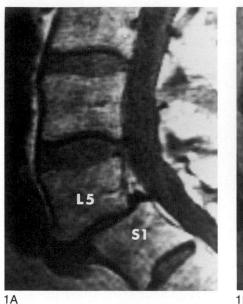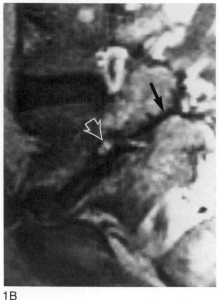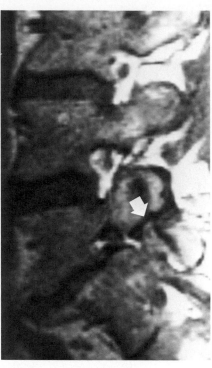

1A

1B

1C

FIG. 24-1A. There is spondylolisthesis at the L5-S1 level with L5 displaced anterior on S1. Narrowing of this disc space is also noted.

FIG. 24-1B. Spondylolysis (*black arrow*) is seen as linear low signal intensity perpendicular to the plane of the pars interarticularis. Neural foraminal stenosis (*white arrow*) is caused by anterior and caudal displacement of L5.

FIG. 24-1C. Similar changes of spondylolysis (*arrow*) and neural foraminal stenosis are seen on the right side. Compare stenotic neural foramen at L5-S1 with normal foramina above this level.

ISTHMIC SPONDYLOLISTHESIS

The midsagittal image shows spondylolisthesis at L5-S1 (Fig. 24-1A). Parasagittal images obtained 20 mm from the midline show linear abnormalities of low signal intensity within the pars interarticularis that lie perpendicular to the plane of the pars and are caused by bilateral spondylolysis (Figs. 24-1B, 1C). The changes of spondylolysis can be readily identified with CT and can also be visualized by careful evaluation of MR images.

The pars interarticularis bridges the superior and inferior articular processes of the same vertebra. It has an oblique course which traverses posteriorly and caudad, as seen on sagittal MR images. On these sagittal MR images, the normal pars has uninterrupted cortex and marrow signal from the superior to inferior articular process. The diagnosis of spondylolysis is suggested when the signal of the marrow and cortical margin of the pars is interrupted by abnormal signal intensity occurring perpendicular to the pars (5,7). In one series, the defect appeared predominantly as low signal intensity on all pulse sequences (7). A gap at the

site of spondylolysis may be present especially if the patient has associated spondylolisthesis. When a gap is present the defect may be of intermediate or increased signal intensity on T1-weighted images because of intervening soft tissue or fat (5,7).

With MR imaging, the sagittal plane is preferred when evaluating for spondylolysis. The sagittal plane provides visualization of the superior and inferior articular processes, the pars, and the pedicle on the same image. The T1-weighted pulse sequences are the SE sequences best suited to image the pars because of superior signal-to-noise ratio and increased contrast between the bone marrow and the signal void of cortical bone (7). In some cases, short TR, short TE, out-of-phase imaging (Dixon technique) may be superior to conventional SE technique in showing spondylolysis (5). With this technique, spondylolysis is seen as a double line of low signal intensity perpendicular to the pars.

MR imaging can also show associated findings such as spondylolisthesis, compression of the sac by hyper-

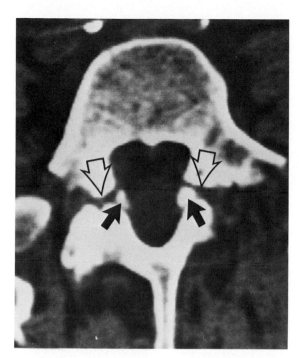

FIG. 24-2. Bilateral spondylolysis. Axial CT scan 10 mm cephalad to the L5-S1 disc. There is bilateral spondylolysis (*open arrows*) which is differentiated from facet joints by the jagged, irregular appearance and the coronal orientation. Osseous fragments adjacent to the medial aspect of the lysis (*closed arrows*) are causing narrowing of the transverse diameter of the canal. These fragments were found to be free at the time of surgery. Note the elongated AP diameter of the canal. This patient had a grade II spondylolisthesis.

trophied tissue about the spondylolysis, foraminal stenosis, and disc herniation. However, MR imaging is less useful than CT in depicting ossified fragments adjacent to the spondylolysis that may compress the sac or nerve roots (5). MR imaging can be used to evaluate for degenerative disc disease at the disc space level below the spondylolysis. Over the age of 25 there is an increase in the incidence of degenerative disc disease below the level of spondylolysis in patients with or without mild spondylolisthesis (12).

Some pitfalls in the MR evaluation of spondylolysis have been described (7). Sclerosis of an intact pars may produce decreased signal of the pars that resembles spondylolysis. Additionally, sagittal MR images slightly lateral to the pars may reveal partial volume imaging of a degenerative spur of the superior articular facet which may simulate spondylolysis (7).

When diagnosing spondylolysis, the CT images are best viewed at bone window settings (e.g., window width 1,000–2,000 HU and window level 200–350 HU) rather than the usual soft-tissue window settings used to visualize the lumbar disc (e.g., window width 500 HU and window level 25–50 HU). With axial scans spondylolysis may have an appearance that resembles

the facet joint; however, several differentiating features have been described (6). The pars defect of spondylolysis is located 10–15 mm above the disc level and has jagged, irregular, noncorticated margins (Fig. 24-2). The facet joint, on the other hand, is located at and adjacent to the disc level and has straight or slightly curved, smooth cortical margins. The pars defect is located anterior to the facet joint and may be in a more coronal plane than the joint (Fig. 24-3). The presence of a complete intact cortical ring outlining the bony spinal canal at the level of the inferior aspect of the pedicle excludes the diagnosis of spondylolysis (9).

Additional CT findings of spondylolysis have been described (6,11). Callus or granulation tissue adjacent to the pars defect is found in 20 percent of cases and may cause compression of the thecal sac or nerve root (11) (Fig. 24-4). Laminal fragmentation has been described in approximately 15 percent of patients with spondylolysis studied by conventional radiography (1) (see Fig. 24-4B). An increased AP diameter of the spinal canal is found with spondylolysis, usually but not always in association with spondylolisthesis. The pars may be narrow or sclerotic. Unilateral spondylolysis may have associated contralateral neural arch sclerosis and hypertrophy (Fig. 24-5). Further delineation of spondylolysis can be obtained by use of sagittal reconstruction (Fig. 24-6).

Both congenital and acquired theories have been offered for the etiology of spondylolysis; however, the most widely accepted theory is that of repeated minor trauma causing a break in the pars interarticularis similar to a stress fracture (11). This may take place in individuals predisposed to spondylolysis because of a congenitally abnormal pars. Spondylolysis occurs in 5 percent of the population. The most frequent site of lysis is L5 (90 percent) followed by L4 (10 percent), with less than 1 percent occurring at L3 (11). Approximately 60 percent of patients with spondylolysis have associated spondylolisthesis (11). Spondylolysis is more commonly bilateral, especially when the lysis is associated with spondylolisthesis.

Isthmic spondylolisthesis is an anterior slippage of one vertebra upon the adjacent caudad vertebra with an associated break in the pars interarticularis of the superior vertebra. This most commonly occurs at L5-S1 and can be readily identified with conventional radiography or MR imaging. When interpreting a CT scan, the lateral digital radiograph should be examined for spondylolisthesis. Spondylolisthesis with pseudoherniation of the disc is shown in Fig. 24-7. The axial CT scan shows a large amount of disc material posterior to the L5 vertebral body (Fig. 24-7A). This is the typical appearance of spondylolisthesis and should not be confused with disc herniation. More caudad, the axial CT scan shows the disc sandwiched between the

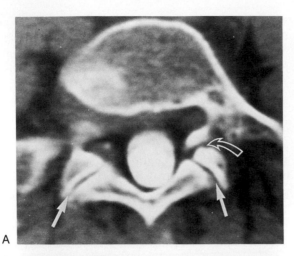

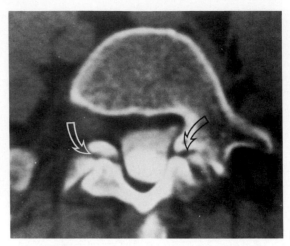

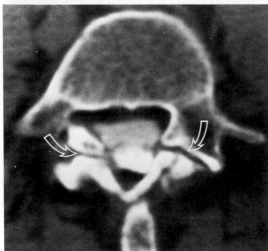

FIG. 24-3. Bilateral spondylolysis. **A**: CTM above the L5-S1 disc level. Slight asymmetry in patient position during scanning accounts for asymmetric visualization of pedicles and disc. The facet joints have an oblique orientation (*straight arrows*). An additional lucent line due to spondylolysis (*curved arrow*) is seen anterior to the left facet joint. This patient also had grade II spondylolisthesis at L5-S1. **B**: CTM 4 mm above Fig. 24-3A. The superior aspect of the facet joints can still be seen. At this level bilateral spondylolysis is noted (*arrows*). The defects of spondylolysis have a more coronal plane than do the facet joints. **C**: Spondylolysis; CTM 8 mm above Fig. 24-3A. The facet joints are no longer seen. The bilateral linear lucencies are due to spondylolysis (*arrows*). Examining the sequence of scans permits CT identification of spondylolysis and prevents mistaking the findings for abnormal facet joints.

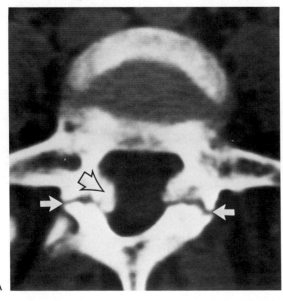

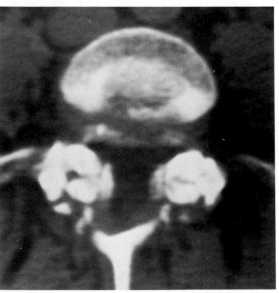

FIG. 24-4. Spondylolysis with callus and fragmentation. **A**: Axial CT scan shows bilateral spondylolysis at L5 as irregular jagged defects having a coronal orientation (*small arrows*). Callus at the site of lysis is more prominent on the right side (*large arrow*). **B**: Axial CT scan 4 mm cephalad to Fig. 24-4A. There is osseous encroachment of the spinal canal, and marked fragmentation is identified.

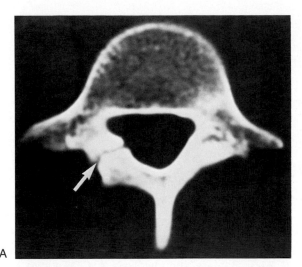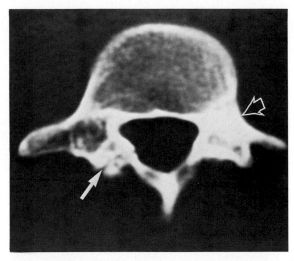

A   B

FIG. 24-5. Unilateral spondylolysis with contralateral sclerosis and hypertrophy of the pedicle shown by CT. **A:** Spondylolysis of L5 is present on the right (*arrow*). **B:** Spondylolysis is again shown on the right (*closed arrow*). This CT scan is through the plane of the pedicles. Note the hypertrophy and sclerosis of the left pedicle (*open arrow*) which develop in response to the unilateral spondylolysis.

vertebral bodies of L5 (anterior) and S1 (posterior) (Fig. 24-7B). Typically, the spinal canal appears elongated in the AP dimension.

The role of MR imaging and CT in evaluating patients with isthmic spondylolisthesis includes the diagnosis of associated central and lateral stenosis and the diagnosis of associated disc disease (4,10). Approximately one-third of symptomatic patients with isthmic spondylolisthesis have spinal stenosis. Commonly there is neural foraminal or lateral recess stenosis at the same interspace level as the spondylolisthesis (4). At the L5-S1 level, anterior and caudal displacement of L5 leads to decreased height of the disc and caudal displacement of the L5 pedicle with subsequent compression of the L5 nerve root in the neural canal (8). Callus and granulation tissue at the site of spondylolysis may encroach on the nerve root at the lateral recess. Central stenosis may occur secondary to thickening of the ligamentum flavum and the laminae at the level of slippage and at the level above the slippage. This may cause compression of the cauda equina.

In those individuals with spondylolisthesis the axial CT scan will reveal disc material posterior to the superior vertebral body and this should not be routinely diagnosed as disc herniation. Disc herniation is unusual at the level of spondylolisthesis and occurs more frequently at the disc level above (4,11). While caution should be exercised in diagnosing disc herniation at the level of spondylolisthesis, this diagnosis may be considered if there is asymmetric compression of the epidural fat, thecal sac, or nerve root (3). Sagittal reconstruction of the axial CT images may be helpful in determining whether the disc extends significantly

beyond the posterior aspect of the sacrum (4,11). Reconstruction views are also helpful in evaluating the previously described stenoses which may accompany isthmic spondylolisthesis.

When severe spondylolisthesis is present, an unusual appearance of the disc may be seen with MR imaging. In one report, the nucleus pulposus appeared to be split into anterior and posterior halves as visualized

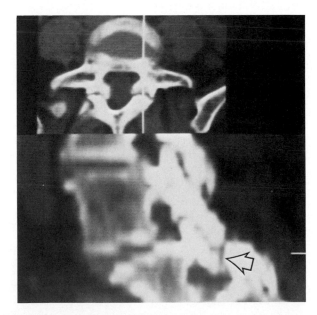

FIG. 24-6. Spondylolysis. Parasagittal reconstruction of axial CT images through the plane of the defect in the left pars interarticularis. The *vertical white line* in the upper insert identifies the plane of scanning. The reconstructed image shows a defect in the pars (*arrow*).

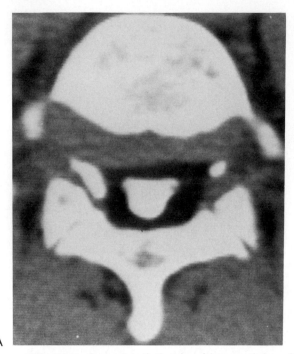
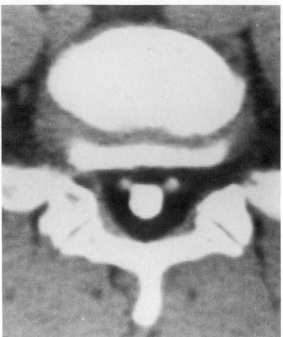

A   B

FIG. 24-7. Spondylolisthesis with pseudoherniation of the disc. **A**: Axial CTM through the plane of the posterior aspect of the L5-S1 disc. The disc is seen extending far posterior to the L5 vertebral body, as a result of grade II spondylolisthesis and the plane of scanning. This finding does not indicate a disc herniation but rather is a form of pseudoherniation of the disc. Note the presence of epidural fat and the lack of thecal sac compression. Bilateral spondylolysis is also present. **B**: This CT scan was obtained 4 mm caudad to Fig. 24-7A. The posterior superior aspect of the sacrum is now visualized in the same relative location as the posterior disc margin seen in Fig. 24-7A. Note the normal appearance of the S1 nerve roots and the epidural fat. A true disc herniation is not present. In patients with isthmic spondylolisthesis, most disc herniations occur at the disc level above the pars defect.

on the sagittal images of patients with grade III spondylolisthesis (2). This was seen on the MR studies of two children who also had decreased signal intensity of the disc, indicating degenerative disc disease thought to be related to the severe spondylolisthesis.

REFERENCES

1. Amato M, Totty WG, Gilula LA. Spondylolysis of the lumbar spine: demonstration of defects and laminal fragmentation. *Radiology* 1984;153:627–9.
2. Birch JG, Herring JA, Maravilla KR. Splitting of the intervertebral disc in spondylolisthesis: a magnetic resonance imaging finding in two cases. *J Pediatric Orthop* 1986;6:609–11.
3. Braun IF, Lin JP, George AE, et al. Pitfalls in the computed tomographic evaluation of the lumbar spine in disc disease. *Neuroradiology* 1984;26:15–20.
4. Elster AD, Jensen KM. Computed tomography of spondylolisthesis: patterns of associated pathology. *J Comput Assist Tomogr* 1985;9:867–74.
5. Grenier N, Kressel HY, Schiebler ML, et al. Isthmic spondylolysis of the lumbar spine: MR imaging at 1.5T. *Radiology* 1989; 170:489–93.
6. Grogan JP, Hemminghytt S, Williams AL, et al. Spondylolysis studied with computed tomography. *Radiology* 1982;145: 737–42.
7. Johnson DW, Farnum GN, Latchaw RE, et al. MR imaging of the pars interarticularis. *AJNR* 1988;9:1215–20, *AJR* 1989;152: 327–32.
8. Kirkaldy-Willis WH, Paine KWE, Cauchoix J, et al. Lumbar spinal stenosis. *Clin Orthop* 1974;99:30–50.
9. Langston JW, Gavant ML. "Incomplete ring" sign: a simple method for CT detection of spondylolysis. *J Comput Assist Tomogr* 1985;9:728–9.
10. McAfee PC, Yuan HA. Computed tomography in spondylolisthesis. *Clin Orthop* 1982;166:62–71.
11. Rothman SLG, Glenn WV Jr. CT multiplanar reconstruction in 253 cases of lumbar spondylolysis. *AJNR* 1984;5:81–90.
12. Szypryt EP, Twining P, Mulholland RC, et al. The prevalence of disc degeneration association with neural arch defects of the lumbar spine assessed by magnetic resonance imaging. *Spine* 1989;14:977–81.

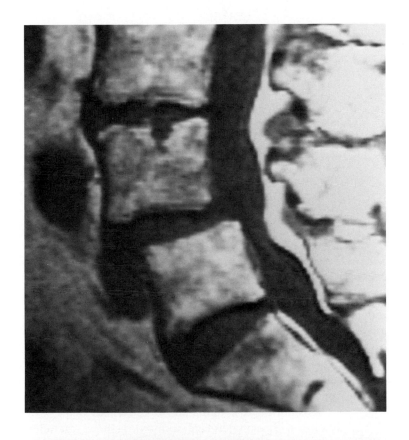

FIG. 25-1A. This 82-year-old woman was examined for possible spinal stenosis. Sagittal T1-weighted SE MR image (600/15) of the lumbar spine.

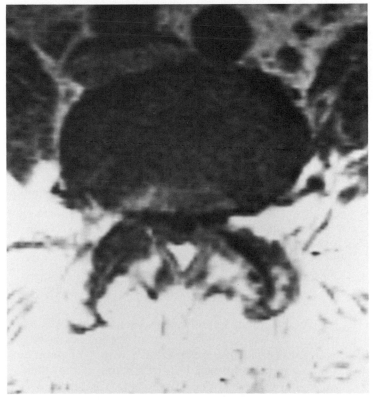

FIG. 25-1B. Axial T1-weighted SE MR image (600/15) at L4-L5.

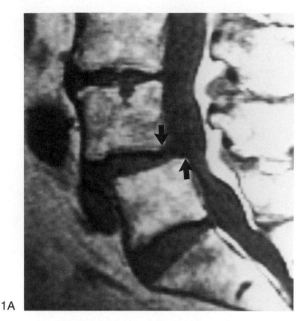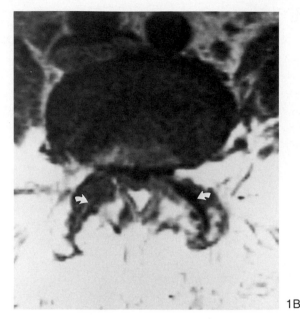

1A
1B

FIG. 25-1A. Degenerative spondylolisthesis. There is grade I spondylolisthesis at L4-L5 (*arrows*) and a decrease in the AP diameter of the thecal sac is noted at this level.

FIG. 25-1B. The axial image shows severe osteoarthritis of the facet joints with joint space narrowing (*arrows*), hypertrophy of the articular processes, and spinal stenosis.

DEGENERATIVE SPONDYLOLISTHESIS

The sagittal image shows anterior subluxation of the L4 vertebra in relation to L5 (Fig. 25-1A). Osteoarthritis of the facet joints is seen on the axial image (Fig. 25-1B). There are changes of central spinal stenosis. This combination of findings is caused by degenerative spondylolisthesis: an anterior slippage of one vertebra on the adjacent caudad vertebra associated with an intact pars interarticularis. This phenomenon occurs secondary to disc degeneration and facet joint instability, which may be related to congenital malalignment of the facets (e.g., sagittal orientation of the facets) (10) (Fig. 25-2). Degenerative changes occur in the facet joints and lead to spinal stenosis.

Degenerative spondylolisthesis most often occurs at L4-L5 (unlike isthmic spondylolisthesis which is usually at L5-S1). The slippage can be seen on the sagittal MR image or on the lateral digital radiograph of the CT study and is usually limited to a grade I/IV. Approximately 30 percent of symptomatic patients with degenerative spondylolisthesis have significant protrusion of the disc at the same level as the spondylolisthesis (4). Magnetic resonance imaging and CT of patients with degenerative spondylolisthesis also reveal degenerative changes of the facet joints such as narrowing, sclerosis, osteophytes, and vacuum phenomenon. Facet joint subluxation may be present, especially if the facet joints have a sagittal orientation.

The role of MR imaging and CT in the evaluation of patients with degenerative spondylolisthesis includes the assessment of central and lateral spinal stenosis (6,7,10). Anterior displacement of the upper vertebra leads to central spinal stenosis with compression of the cauda equina. Lateral stenosis occurs secondary to subluxation of facet joints, osteophyte formation of the articular processes, and bulging of the disc into the intervertebral canal.

Degenerative spondylolisthesis usually occurs after age 50 and affects women four times more frequently than men (9). Patients often have back, buttock, or thigh pain and may have neurogenic claudication or postural symptomatology, the pain occurring with spine extension (5,7). Approximately 10 percent of patients with this disorder have severe symptoms that require decompression laminectomy and excision of the medial portion of the articular processes (9).

Facet Joints

The facet joints can be seen with CT and MR imaging, and pathologic alterations in the joints can be assessed. The facet joints are lined with synovial membrane and are formed by articulation of the inferior articular process of the vertebra above and the superior

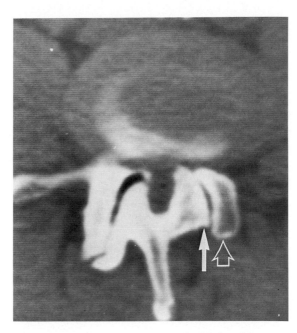

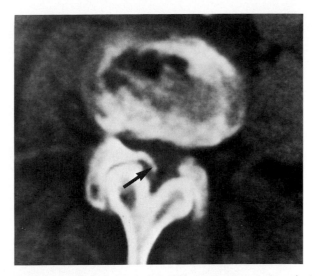

FIG. 25-4. Osteophyte. Axial CT shows an osteophyte (*arrow*) derived from the superior articular process on the right causing spinal stenosis. The facet joints are narrow.

FIG. 25-2. Degenerative spondylolisthesis with stenosis. CT scan at the L4-L5 intervertebral disc level viewed at bone window settings. The facet joints have a somewhat sagittal orientation, and there is anterior subluxation of the inferior articular process of L4 (*long arrow*) in relation to the superior articular process of L5 (*short arrow*). Changes of osteoarthritis of the facet joints are present with joint space narrowing, hypertrophy of articular processes, and vacuum facet phenomenon. The decreased transverse diameter of the spinal canal indicates central spinal stenosis.

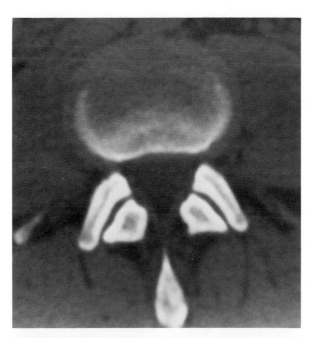

FIG. 25-3. Normal facet joints shown by CT. The normal articular processes have smooth, regular cortical margins. The normal facet joint measures 2–4 mm in width. The facet joints are ideally studied at bone window settings.

articular process of the vertebra below. Computed tomography is an ideal method of evaluating facet joints of the lumbar spine because of the oblique orientation of the joints. The orientation of the lumbar facet joints varies with the level examined. The facet joints tend toward a more sagittal orientation at L3-L4, a more coronal plane at L5-S1, and an intermediate position at L4-L5 (12). Facet joints are best studied at bone window settings.

A normal facet joint has smooth, regular cortical margins with a joint space width of 2.0–4.0 mm (Fig. 25-3). Abnormal facet joints are frequently discovered with CT. In one study, patients with low back pain and/or sciatica were studied by CT, and 43 percent had abnormal facet joints whereas only 18 percent had disc herniation (2). The most frequent abnormality of facet joints is an osteophyte, an outgrowth of cortical bone derived from the articular margin and therefore lacking a medullary space (Fig. 25-4). Articular facet hypertrophy is another common finding and appears as an enlargement of the articular process with normal medullary and cortical proportions (1,2) (Fig. 25-5). Other CT findings of degenerative arthritis of facet joints include: joint space narrowing (<2 mm), subchondral sclerosis, and subchondral erosions and cysts (1,2) (Figs. 25-6, 25-7). Calcifications in the periarticular region and gas within the facet joint (vacuum facet phenomenon) may also be seen. Subluxation of facet joints may be present in association with degenerative spondylolisthesis (anterior subluxation of inferior articular processes) or retrospondylolisthesis (posterior subluxation of inferior articular processes) (Fig. 25-8).

Each facet joint has a dual innervation. The joint capsule of the superior articular process is innervated by branches of the dorsal ramus of the spinal nerve at

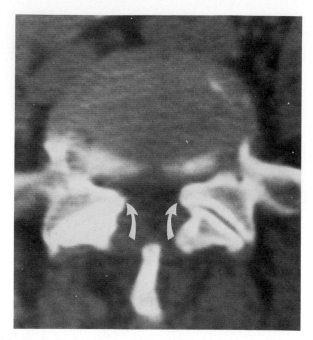

FIG. 25-5. Hypertrophy of articular processes. CT scan at L5-S1 shows bilateral hypertrophy of the superior articular processes of S1 (*arrows*). The right facet joint is narrow.

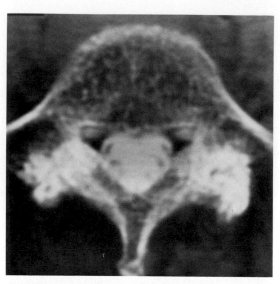

FIG. 25-7. Severe osteoarthritis of the facet joints. CTM at L5 shows extensive subchondral sclerosis, hypertrophy, and posterior osteophyte formation as well as obliteration of the facet joints. Note the lack of stenosis despite severe osteoarthritis.

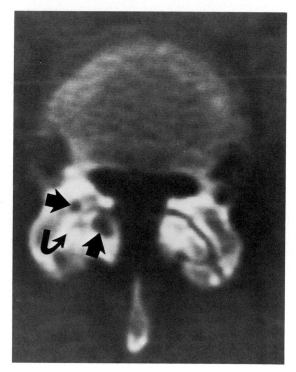

FIG. 25-6. Osteoarthritis of the facet joints. Axial CT at L4-L5 shows severe narrowing of the right facet joint (*curved arrow*) and moderate narrowing of the left facet joint. Subchondral erosions and cysts (*straight arrows*) and sclerosis are present. This image was photographed at bone window settings.

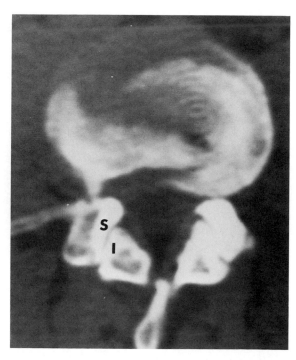

FIG. 25-8. Retrospondylolisthesis at L3-L4. Axial CT shows posterior subluxation of the inferior articular process of L3 (*I*) in relation to the superior articular process of L4 (*S*).

the same level, whereas the joint capsule of the inferior articular process is innervated from branches of the dorsal ramus of the spinal nerve of the next higher vertebral level (3). Pain arising from a facet joint can be referred to the structures innervated by both dorsal root ganglia involved (1,3). Patients with lumbar facet arthropathy may have symptoms of low back pain and sciatica simulating disc herniation. Several methods of treating patients clinically suspected of having the facet joint syndrome have been recommended and include fluoroscopically guided intraarticular injection of a local anesthetic and steroid suspension (2,3), percutaneous radiofrequency facet denervation (11), and surgical fusion (8).

Although presently there is no definite way to identify which facet joints might be responsible for significant low back pain (8), CT may play a role in this evaluation. In a group of patients who had CT examination prior to facet block injection, almost all who obtained relief following the injection had abnormalities of facet joints demonstrated by CT (2). Some patients with abnormal facet joints had no pain relief, suggesting that their pain was either derived from another source or was at least not originating from the capsular innervation (2). Large osteophytes of articular processes, for example, may cause central or lateral stenosis and be responsible for a radiculopathy that would not be relieved by intraarticular injection. Some of these patients might instead be successfully treated by foraminotomy. In the evaluation of patients for possible facet joint syndrome, CT can be used to diagnose other causes of low back pain and sciatica such as herniated nucleus pulposus, spinal stenosis, and metastasis.

REFERENCES

1. Carrera GF, Haughton VM, Syvertsen A, et al. Computed tomography of the lumbar facet joints. *Radiology* 1980;134:145–8.
2. Carrera GF, Williams AL. Current concepts in evaluation of the lumbar facet joints. *Crit Rev Diagn Imaging* 1985;21:85–104.
3. Destouet JM, Gilula LA, Murphy WA, et al. Lumbar facet joint injection, technique, clinical correlation, and preliminary results. *Radiology* 1982;145:321–5.
4. Elster AD, Jensen KM. Computed tomography of spondylolisthesis: patterns of associated pathology. *J Comput Assist Tomogr* 1985;9:867–74.
5. Epstein BS, Epstein JA, Jones MD. Degenerative spondylolisthesis with an intact neural arch. *Radiol Clin North Am* 1977;15:275–87.
6. McAfee PC, Ullrich CG, Yuan HA, et al. Computed tomography in degenerative spinal stenosis. *Clin Orthop* 1981;161:221–34.
7. McAfee PC, Yuan HA. Computed tomography in spondylolisthesis. *Clin Orthop* 1982;166:62–71.
8. Raymond J, Dumas J-M. Intraarticular facet block: diagnostic test or therapeutic procedure? *Radiology* 1984;151:333–6.
9. Rosenberg NJ. Degenerative spondylolisthesis: predisposing factors. *J Bone Joint Surg (Am)* 1975;57A:467–74.
10. Rothman SLG, Glenn WV Jr. Spondylolysis and spondylolisthesis. In: Post MJG, ed. *Computed tomography of the spine.* Baltimore: Williams & Wilkins; 1984:591–615.
11. Shealy CN. Facet denervation in the management of back and sciatic pain. *Clin Orthop* 1976;115:157–64.
12. Van Schaik JPJ, Verbiest H, Van Schaik FDJ. The orientation of the laminae and facet joints in the lower lumbar spine. *Spine* 1985;10:59–63.

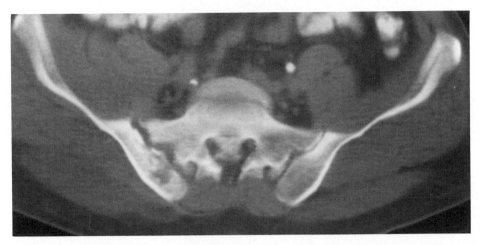

FIG. 26-1A. This 53-year-old man presented with a 2-month history of pain and fever. Axial CT of the sacrum viewed at bone window settings.

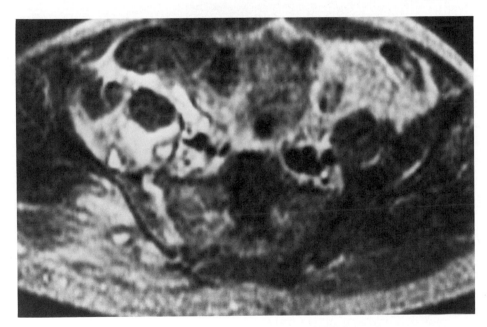

FIG. 26-1B. Axial T2-weighted SE MR image (2800/80) of the sacrum.

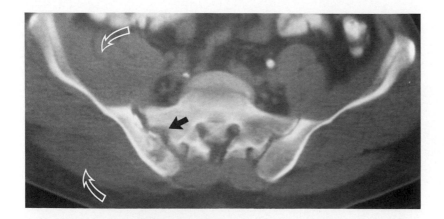

FIG. 26-1A. Pyogenic sacroiliitis. There is widening of the right SI joint and cortical irregularity and erosion of the joint is present (*straight arrow*). Soft tissue thickening of the right iliac and gluteal muscles is seen (*curved arrow*).

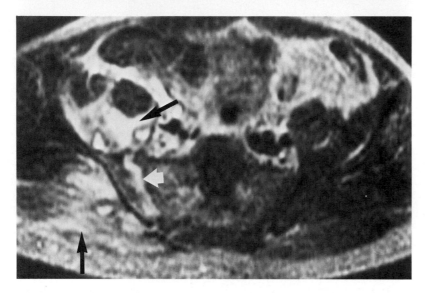

FIG. 26-1B. There is bright signal within a widened right SI joint (*white arrow*) due to infection. Cortical erosion about the joint can be appreciated. Note bright signal in the iliac and gluteal muscles caused by soft tissue extension of the infection (*black arrows*).

PYOGENIC SACROILIITIS

This case illustrates many of the bony and soft-tissue abnormalities of pyogenic sacroiliitis (Fig. 26-1). Pyogenic sacroiliitis may present as a subacute localized process or an acute systemic disorder. The clinical presentation of buttock, hip, or abdominal pain in association with fever may be misleading and may suggest nerve root compression, a hip disorder, or an inflammatory process of the abdomen (7). Septic arthritis of a sacroiliac (SI) joint may occur during pregnancy, immediately postpartum or postabortion; secondary to infection of the skin, bone or urinary tract; or in association with drug abuse (4). The early diagnosis of pyogenic sacroiliitis is important since it is associated with improved therapeutic prognosis. Infectious sacroiliitis (pyogenic or tuberculous) should always be considered in the differential diagnosis of unilateral sacroiliitis.

Generally, radionuclide bone scanning is a useful screening procedure for infectious diseases of the SI joint; however, it is nonspecific. For example, hyper-

emia may result in increased bone activity in patients with cellulitis but without osteomyelitis (1,7). Also, the bone scan may be falsely negative (e.g., normal SI joint activity may obscure appreciation of abnormal activity). Conventional radiographs are usually normal during the first 2–3 weeks following the onset of infection (1,4). Subsequently, radiographs show irregularity of the joint margin, reactive sclerosis, and narrowing of the SI joint, sometimes progressing to fusion.

Computed tomography is more sensitive than conventional radiography in the detection of pyogenic sacroiliitis and can detect widening of the SI joint, cortical irregularity and destruction, and bone fragmentation within the joint (1,7,9) (Fig. 26-2) (see also Fig. 26-1). Soft-tissue extension of infection can be seen as thickening of the iliac and gluteal muscles or as a paraarticular soft-tissue mass. Gas within a soft-tissue abscess is readily seen with CT.

With MR imaging and CT, the synovial and ligamen-

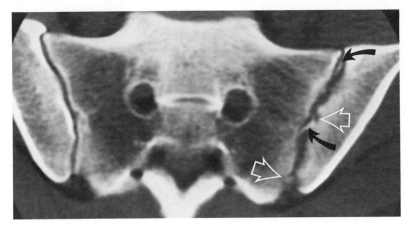

FIG. 26-2. Pyogenic sacroiliitis. Computed tomographic scan of the SI joints. There is unilateral sacroiliitis with cortical irregularity and erosions on both sides of the left SI joint (*straight arrows*). Small bony fragments are noted within the joint (*curved arrows*). This 36-year-old patient is a drug addict who had endocarditis and staphylococcus septicemia, and developed vague back pain and continued fever despite antibiotic therapy.

tous portions of the SI joints can be delineated. The ligamentous portion of the SI joint is posterior, has an oblique course, and is the upper one-third to one-half of the joint. The synovial portion of the SI joint is anterior, is more vertically oriented, and is the lower one-half to two-thirds of the joint. Normally, the ligamentous portion of the joint has increased signal intensity on T1-weighted MR images because of fat, with interposed areas of decreased signal caused by intraosseous sacroiliac ligaments and loose connective tissue (8). The bony margins of the sacrum and innominate bone have low signal intensity. On T2-weighted images, the fat becomes less bright; the ligamentous tissue, connective tissue, and subligamentous bone have low signal intensity. In one-half of normal individuals, there are focal irregularities of the sacrum that represent

sites of ligamentous attachments (8). The adjacent marrow signal varies according to age, with more fat marrow being present in the early adult years compared to childhood.

In the synovial portion of the joint, articular (hyalin) cartilage appears as a thin region of intermediate signal intensity on T1-weighted MR images. Normal cartilage thickness is 2–3 mm anteriorly and 2–5 mm posteriorly (8). In 86 percent of individuals, the opposing cartilage surfaces are separated by a thin zone of low signal intensity (8). The adjacent subchondral bone has low signal intensity. The adjacent marrow is sharply delineated from subchondral bone and, if involved by infection or edema, is of intermediate signal intensity. On T2-weighted MR images the cartilage is not always readily delineated (8). Subchondral bone has low signal

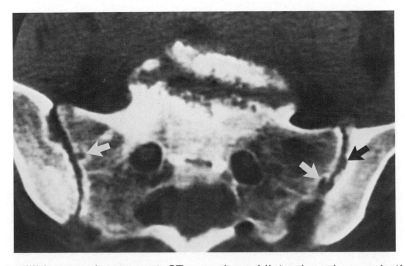

FIG. 26-3. Sacroiliitis secondary to gout. CT scan shows bilateral erosions on both the iliac and sacral sides of the SI joints (*arrows*). This patient had gout involving multiple peripheral joints and presented at this time with a 2-year history of low back and left hip pain.

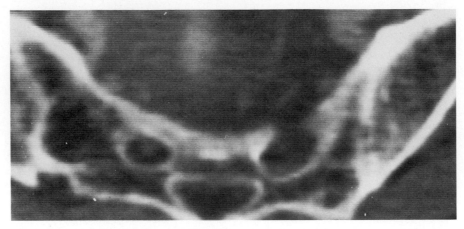

FIG. 26-4. Ankylosing spondylitis. CT shows bilateral fusion of the SI joints secondary to ankylosing spondylitis. At this advanced stage CT does not usually add significant information beyond that obtained from conventional radiographs.

intensity. If the adjacent marrow is involved with infection or edema, it will be hyperintense relative to normal marrow. Reactive sclerosis has low signal intensity.

Magnetic resonance imaging and CT are important for detecting sacroiliitis, particularly when conventional radiography and radionuclide bone scanning are normal or inconclusive. Although CT is superior to MR imaging in evaluating bone production (sclerosis), MR is superior to CT in the evaluation of cartilage and the detection of erosive changes (8). If surgical intervention is required, CT and MR imaging are useful in precisely delineating the location and extent of the infectious process within and around the SI joint (9). In addition, CT can be used as a guide for biopsy of infected paraarticular bone or for joint aspiration.

Noninfectious Sacroiliitis

Occasionally, MR imaging and CT can also be useful in the detection of noninfectious sacroiliitis associated with ankylosing spondylitis, Reiter's syndrome, psoriatic arthritis, intestinal colitides, and gout (Figs. 26-3, 26-4). The radiographic evaluation of the sacroiliac joints plays a key role in the early diagnosis of the spondyloarthropathies. Radionuclide bone scanning is

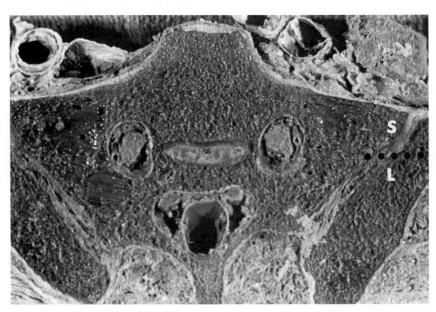

FIG. 26-5. Normal SI joints. Anatomic specimen through the SI joints at the junction of the synovial and ligamentous portions. The synovial portion of the joint (*S, above dotted line*) is more ventral and vertical compared to the more dorsal and oblique ligamentous part of the joint (*L, below dotted line*).

sensitive but nonspecific. Although MR imaging and CT are more sensitive than conventional radiography for the detection of sacroiliitis (3,5), careful examination of good quality radiographs is usually sufficient for proper diagnosis (2,10). In one series, patients with low back pain clinically suspicious for sacroiliitis were examined by conventional radiography and CT (10). The AP radiograph of the pelvis was interpreted unequivocally as either normal or abnormal in approximately 75 percent of cases. Two-thirds of the remaining cases were diagnosed correctly when a complete four-view radiographic series was evaluated. Those patients with equivocal results despite a complete radiographic series (approximately 10 percent) were found to benefit

from CT examination. Both CT and MR imaging are useful in evaluating patients in whom a definitive diagnosis cannot be made by conventional radiography. They may also be used when clinical suspicion is high despite normal radiographic findings (10).

Computed tomography examination of the SI joints can be achieved with contiguous 4- or 5-mm-thick sections obtained from the midportion of the first sacral segment through the entire length of the synovial portion of the SI joint. Optimal scanning is achieved when the gantry is tilted as nearly parallel as possible to the sacrum. This requires maximum angulation of 15–25 degrees. The angulation is opposite the direction normally used for the L5-S1 intervertebral disc space.

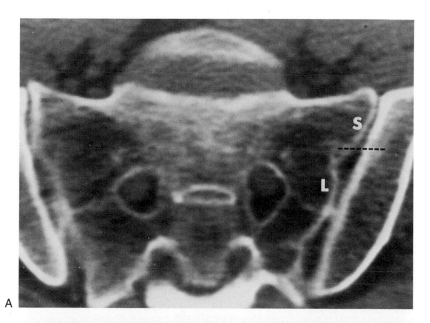

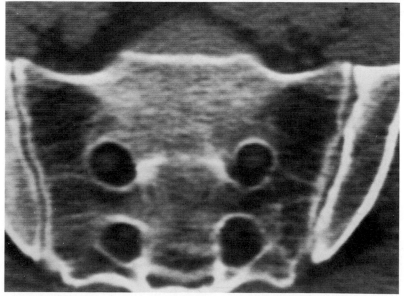

FIG. 26-6. Normal SI joints. CT scans in near-coronal plane. **A:** This CT scan is at the junction of the synovial (S, *above dotted line*) and ligamentous (L, *below dotted line*) portions of the normal SI joints, a similar plane to that shown in Fig. 26-5. The ligamentous portion of the joint is more dorsal, oblique, and irregular than the synovial portion. **B:** This CT scan is obtained caudad to Fig. 26-6A and is through the synovial portion of the normal SI joints, caudad to the ligamentous portion of the joints. Note the uniform symmetric appearance of the joints with no evidence of erosions, joint space narrowing, or other signs of sacroiliitis.

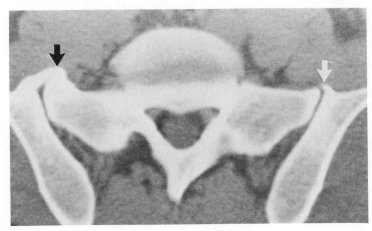

FIG. 26-7. Osteoarthritis of SI joints shown by CT. Anterior paraarticular ankylosis of the right SI joint (*black arrow*) and a small osteophyte of the left ilium (*white arrow*) represent degenerative changes not infrequently encountered in older age groups.

Using this gantry tilt, the synovial portion on the SI joint is differentiated from the ligamentous portion by its more ventral, caudal, and vertical position (6) (Figs. 26-5, 26-6).

The SI joints of asymptomatic patients have been studied by CT and the appearance of the SI joints has been found to vary with age (11). In patients under the age of 30 years, the SI joints are uniform and symmetric. It is not unusual to see iliac sclerosis that is focal and nonuniform. In the older age groups, asymptomatic patients may have focal joint space narrowing, focal iliac and sacral subchondral sclerosis that begins on the iliac side, paraarticular ankylosis, and overall asymmetry of the joints (11) (Fig. 26-7). With these "normal aging" or degenerative findings in mind, diagnostic signs of sacroiliitis at any age would include *uniform* joint space narrowing (<2 mm), *intraarticular* ankylosis, and erosions (3,5,11). Some CT findings that might be seen in asymptomatic older patients are suggestive of sacroiliitis when found in younger age groups. These findings include focal joint space narrowing, focal increased sacral subchondral sclerosis, and overall asymmetry of the joints (11). Isolated iliac sclerosis is not considered a diagnostic finding of sacroiliitis (3).

REFERENCES

1. Bankoff MS, Sarno RC, Carter BL. CT scanning in septic sacroiliac arthritis or periarticular osteomyelitis. *Comput Radiol* 1984; 8:165–70.
2. Borlaza GS, Seigel R, Kuhns LR, et al. Computed tomography in the evaluation of sacroiliac arthritis. *Radiology* 1981;139: 437–40.
3. Carrera GF, Foley WD, Kozin F, et al. CT of sacroiliitis. *AJR* 1981;136:41–6.
4. Gordon G, Kabins SA. Pyogenic sacroiliitis. *Am J Med* 1980; 69:50–6.
5. Kozin F, Carrera GF, Ryan LM, et al. Computed tomography in the diagnosis of sacroiliitis. *Arthritis Rheum* 1981;24:1479–85.
6. Lawson TL, Foley WD, Carrera GF, et al. The sacroiliac joints: anatomic, plain roentgenographic, and computed tomographic analysis. *J Comput Assist Tomogr* 1982;6:307–14.
7. Morgan GJ Jr, Schlegelmilch JG, Spiegel PK. Early diagnosis of septic arthritis of the sacroiliac joint by use of computed tomography. *J Rheumatol* 1981;8:979–82.
8. Murphey MD, Wetzel LH, Bramble JM, et al. Sacroiliitis: MR imaging findings. *Radiology* 1991;180:239–44.
9. Rosenberg D, Baskies AM, Deckers PJ, et al. Pyogenic sacroiliitis: an absolute indication for computerized tomographic scanning. *Clin Orthop* 1984;184:128–32.
10. Ryan LM, Carrera GF, Lightfoot RW Jr, et al. The radiographic diagnosis of sacroiliitis: a comparison of different views with computed tomograms of the sacroiliac joint. *Arthrit Rheum* 1983;26:760–3.
11. Vogler JB III, Brown WH, Helms CA, et al. The normal sacroiliac joint: a CT study of asymptomatic patients. *Radiology* 1984; 151:433–7.

CASE 27

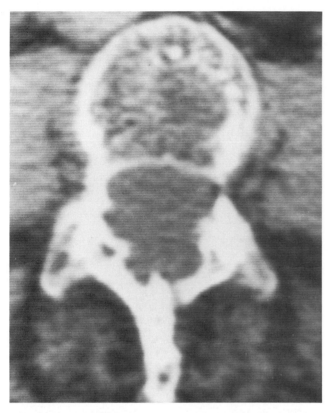

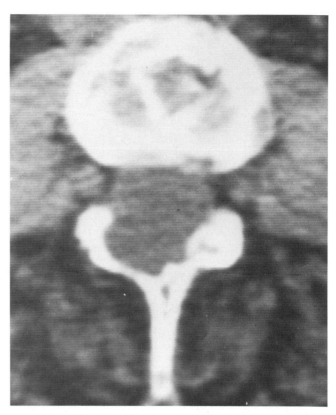

FIG. 27-1A. Axial CT at superior aspect of the L3 vertebra. This 68-year-old woman had slowly progressive right leg weakness of several years' duration associated with atrophy of the right leg. She also had vague chronic back pain and stiffness.

FIG. 27-1B. Axial CT at inferior aspect of the L3 vertebra.

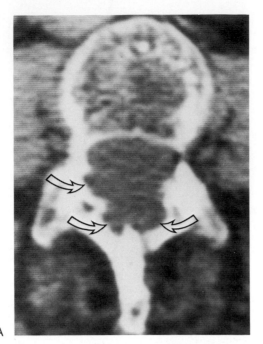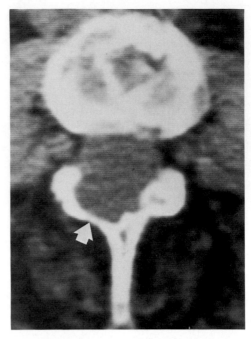

1A   1B

FIG. 27-1A. Ankylosing spondylitis. There are erosions of the inner margin of the laminae bilaterally (*arrows*) due to dorsal diverticula.

FIG. 27-1B. Similar scalloping of the laminae is noted, causing marked thinning of the lamina on the right (*arrow*). Note the moderate fatty replacement of the posterior paraspinal musculature.

ANKYLOSING SPONDYLITIS

In the present case, the CT examination shows findings typical of ankylosing spondylitis with scalloping of the inner margin of the laminae and spinous processes at multiple lumbar levels (Fig. 27-1). Scalloping of the laminae is an uncommon complication of ankylosing spondylitis (1,5,7,9,11,16) caused by pressure erosion from dural ectasia and multiple dorsal diverticulae (13,14).

The imaging diagnosis of ankylosing spondylitis is readily established by conventional radiographs and includes bilateral symmetric sacroiliitis and spondylitis with thin syndesmophytes; squaring of vertebrae and fusion of apophyseal joints. Other less diagnostic features include calcification or ossification of interspinous and supraspinous ligaments; intervertebral disc calcification; and, rarely, atlanto-axial subluxation. Conventional radiographs rarely show erosion of posterior elements (16) such as seen on the present CT study.

The differential diagnosis of spinal canal erosion includes dural ectasia, neurofibromatosis, Marfan's syndrome, Hurler's syndrome, Morquio's disease, achondroplasia, acromegaly, and intraspinal tumors and cysts (12). Typically, patients with dural ectasia secondary to neurofibromatosis, Marfan's syndrome, or other congenital syndromes develop scalloping of the posterior vertebral margin; whereas patients with ankylosing spondylitis in addition develop erosion of the posterior elements (5). An extensive intraspinal tumor may cause scalloping, which is likely to involve both the laminae and posterior vertebral bodies. Magnetic resonance imaging can be used to exclude the possibility of tumor since in patients with ankylosing spondylitis, cerebrospinal fluid fills the posterior diverticula extending into the eroded laminae, and the diverticula appear as decreased signal intensity on T1- and increased signal intensity on T2-weighted images similar to cerebrospinal fluid within the thecal sac.

Some patients with ankylosing spondylitis develop the cauda equina syndrome, with slowly progressive leg or buttock pain, sensory or motor impairment, and bowel or bladder dysfunction (14). Neurologic signs are usually symmetric. Most patients with ankylosing spondylitis and cauda equina syndrome have dural ectasia and dorsal diverticula (16). The etiology of the posterior diverticula is uncertain; however, it has been postulated that inflammation of facet joints induces mild arachnoiditis, causing adhesions with arachnoid pouches formed secondarily into which pulsating cerebrospinal fluid enters (11). In patients with ankylosing spondylitis and the cauda equina syndrome, both CT and MR imaging can show dural ectasia, multiple dorsal diverticulae, and erosion of the laminae, spinous processes, and posterior vertebral bodies. Computed tomography better shows the osseous abnormalities, whereas MR imaging is superior to CT in diagnosing the contents of the dorsal diverticulae as cerebrospinal fluid and not tumor (1,16).

Patients with ankylosing spondylitis are more susceptible to fracture-dislocation secondary to minor trauma than are normal individuals. The spine in patients with ankylosing spondylitis is rigid and tends to fracture as does a long bone, with complete through-and-through fractures rather than the more common vertebral compression fractures. The fractures tend to cross the intervertebral disc spaces to involve adjacent vertebrae, and fractures of the posterior elements are frequent. The fractures are associated with a high morbidity and mortality. In one study (17) 12 percent of patients with ankylosing spondylitis had a spinal fracture and 8 percent of this group had paralytic spinal cord injury. Spinal injuries in patients with ankylosing spondylitis are frequently unstable and have associated dislocation, neural arch displacement or complete transection (4,17) (Fig. 27-2). Computed tomography may show neural arch fractures and ventral displacement of fracture fragments not seen with conventional radiography (17). Three-dimensional CT may be useful in clarifying the nature of the fracture in some cases (Fig. 27-3). The degree of compression of the spinal cord or nerve roots can be evaluated by MR imaging or CT. Spinal cord contusion without evidence of fracture has also been described (17), and can be seen with MR imaging.

Some patients with ankylosing spondylitis have discovertebral destruction that can be evaluated with conventional radiographs, CT, and MR imaging. The abnormalities, referred to as *Andersson lesions,* most frequently affect the lower thoracic and upper lumbar spine, and include: disc space narrowing, destruction of the vertebral endplate, surrounding sclerosis, and kyphosis (8) (Fig. 27-4). Bone destruction, endplate

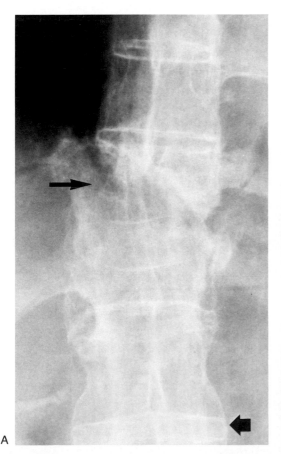
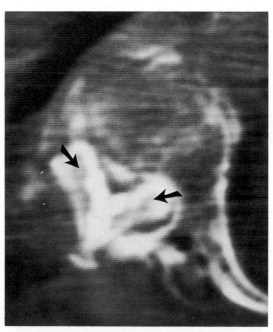

FIG. 27-2. Transection fracture of the thoracic spine in a patient with ankylosing spondylitis. **A**: This patient sustained a severe transection fracture of T11 (*long arrow*) after a fall on stairs. The asymmetry of the spinous processes indicates a rotatory component of the fracture. Note that syndesmophytes (*short arrow*) of ankylosing spondylitis are present. **B**: Axial CT scan dramatically demonstrates the transection fracture through the posterior elements. The laminae (*arrows*) and spinous process are displaced anteriorly with marked narrowing of the spinal canal and compression of the spinal cord.

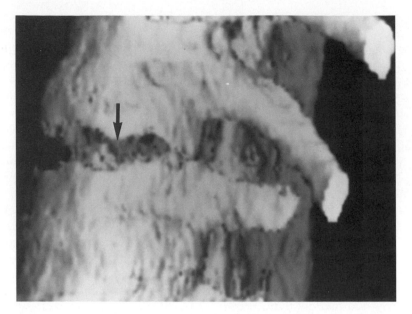

FIG. 27-3. Horizontal fracture through the L1 vertebra in a patient with ankylosing spondylitis. Three-dimensional reconstruction of the axial images in an oblique plane shows the extent of a horizontally oriented fracture (*arrow*). With this technique, the anatomic structures can be viewed in multiple planes for optimal evaluation.

erosions, and adjacent sclerosis are better seen with CT than with conventional radiographs. T2-weighted MR images show decreased signal intensity of most of the disc, although localized areas of increased signal may be seen (8). Focal fatty deposition in the bone marrow adjacent to the destructive lesions may be present. Computed tomography and MR imaging may be useful in differentiating Andersson lesions from osteomyelitis by showing an absence of paravertebral soft-tissue inflammatory mass, often seen with osteomyelitis. In addition, the predominantly low signal intensity of the disc seen on T2-weighted MR images

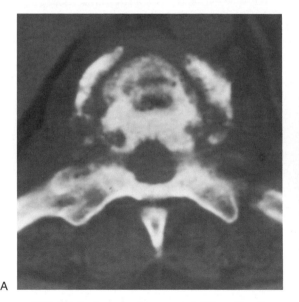
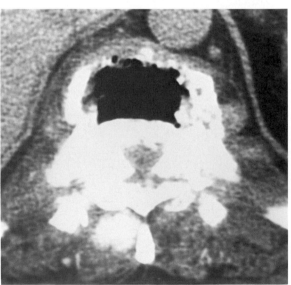

FIG. 27-4. Ankylosing spondylitis with discovertebral destruction. **A**: Axial CT at T10-T11 viewed at bone window settings shows round destructive lesions of the vertebral body. **B**: Axial CT shows bone destruction, vacuum disc phenomenon, and paravertebral soft-tissue mass. This discovertebral destruction, or Andersson lesion, is seen in patients with ankylosing spondylitis and has features that are similar to infection. A vacuum disc phenomenon is usually not seen in patients with acute osteomyelitis.

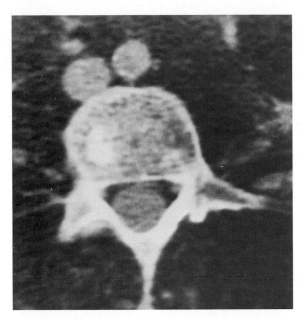

FIG. 27-5. Fatty replacement of the paraspinal musculature. Axial CT shows extensive fatty replacement of the paraspinal musculature in this patient with a 30-year history of paraparesis secondary to poliomyelitis.

differs from the typical high signal intensity of the disc seen in many disc space infections (8).

There is a spectrum of discovertebral destructive lesions in ankylosing spondylitis. The most important biomechanical complication of ankylosing spondylitis is pseudoarthrosis, a state of mobile nonunion that functions as a false joint (2,3). Pseudoarthrosis can be evaluated with CT and MR imaging. Computed tomography shows irregular discovertebral osteolysis with reactive sclerosis and is more sensitive to the detection of a vacuum phenomenon and paraspinal soft-tissue swelling than are conventional radiographs (2); CT is also useful in differentiating a fracture of the posterior elements from mobile facet joints, two abnormalities of pseudoarthrosis. Associated spinal stenosis is also clearly depicted with CT. With T1-weighted MR images, pseudoarthrosis shows decreased signal intensity of the disc and adjacent residual vertebral bodies (3). On T2-weighted images, pseudoarthrosis has heterogeneous signal, with hyperintense edematous granulation tissue and hypointense fibrous tissue. Surrounding the pseudoarthrosis is sclerosis of the vertebral bodies which appears as narrow bands of very low signal on all pulse sequences (3). Paraspinal soft-tissue swelling may be present. Pseudoarthrosis should be considered in the evaluation of a patient with ankylosing spondylitis and discovertebral destruction; however, it may have MR features that are similar to osteomyelitis.

An additional point of interest in the lead case is the fatty replacement of the posterior paraspinal musculature (see Fig. 27-1) which is a nonspecific finding that has been reported to occur in association with ankylosing spondylitis (15). Severe fatty replacement of paraspinal musculature has been reported in patients with neuromuscular disorders such as poliomyelitis and muscular dystrophy (6) (Fig. 27-5). Fatty replacement of the sacrospinal muscle groups may also be seen in varying degrees of severity in patients who have had previous lumbar surgery (10) and in otherwise normal individuals, especially elderly females (6).

REFERENCES

1. Abello R, Rovira M, Sanz MP, et al. MRI and CT of ankylosing spondylitis with vertebral scalloping. *Neuroradiology* 1988;30: 272–5.
2. Chan F-L, Ho EKW, Chau EMT. Spinal pseudarthrosis complicating ankylosing spondylitis: comparison of CT and conventional tomography. *AJR* 1988;150:611–4.
3. Eschelman DJ, Beers GJ, Naimark A, et al. Pseudoarthrosis in ankylosing spondylitis mimicking infectious diskitis: MR appearance. *AJNR* 1991;12:1113–4.
4. Grisolia A, Bell RL, Peltier LF. Fractures and dislocations of the spine complicating ankylosing spondylitis. *J Bone Joint Surg (Am)* 1967;49A:339–44,386.
5. Grosman H, Gray R, St Louis EL. CT of long-standing ankylosing spondylitis with cauda equina syndrome. *AJNR* 1983;4: 1077–80.
6. Hadar H, Gadoth N, Heifetz M. Fatty replacement of lower paraspinal muscles: normal and neuromuscular disorders. *AJNR* 1983;4:1087–90, *AJR* 1983;141:895–8.
7. Helms CA, Vogler JB. Computed tomography of spinal stenoses and arthroses. *Clin Rheum Dis* 1983;9:417–41.
8. Kenny JB, Hughes PL, Whitehouse GH. Discovertebral destruction in ankylosing spondylitis: the role of computed tomography and magnetic resonance imaging. *Br J Radiol* 1990;63: 448–55.
9. Kramer LD, Krouth GJ. Computerized tomography: an adjunct to early diagnosis in the cauda equina syndrome of ankylosing spondylitis. *Arch Neurol* 1978;35:116–8.
10. Laasonen EM. Atrophy of sacrospinal muscle groups in patients with chronic, diffusely radiating lumbar back pain. *Neuroradiology* 1984;26:9–13.
11. Matthews WB. The neurological complications of ankylosing spondylitis. *J Neurol Sci* 1968;6:561–73.
12. Mitchell GE, Lourie H, Berne AS. The various causes of scalloped vertebrae with notes on their pathogenesis. *Radiology* 1967;89:67–74.
13. Rosenkranz W. Ankylosing spondylitis: cauda equina syndrome with multiple spinal arachnoid cysts. *J Neurosurg* 1971;34: 241–3.
14. Russell ML, Gordon DA, Ogryzlo MA, et al. The cauda equina syndrome of ankylosing spondylitis. *Ann Intern Med* 1973;78: 551–4.
15. Sage MR, Gordon TP. Muscle atrophy in ankylosing spondylitis: CT demonstration. *Radiology* 1983;149:780.
16. Sparling MJ, Bartleson JD, McLeod RA, et al. Magnetic resonance imaging of arachnoid diverticula associated with cauda equina syndrome in ankylosing spondylitis. *J Rheumatol* 1989; 16:1335–7.
17. Weinstein PR, Karpman RR, Gall EP, et al. Spinal cord injury, spinal fracture and spinal stenosis in ankylosing spondylitis. *J Neurosurg* 1982;57:609–16.

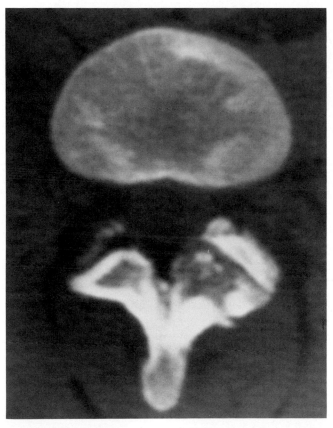

FIG. 28-1A. This 21-year-old man presented with chronic low back pain. Axial CT scan at L3.

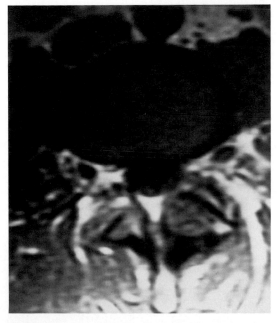

FIG. 28-1B. Axial T1-weighted SE MR image (700/12) obtained at L3.

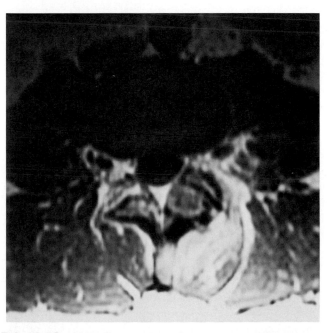

FIG. 28-1C. Axial T1-weighted SE MR image (600/11) obtained after the intravenous injection of gadopentetate dimeglumine.

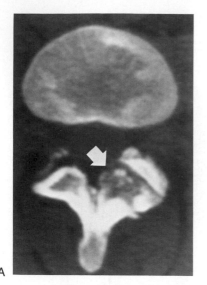 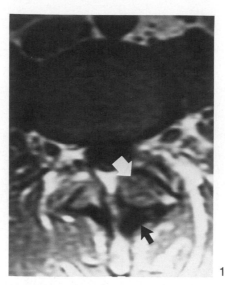 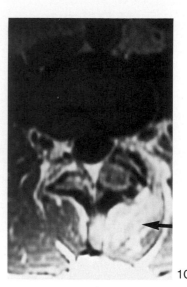

1A 1B 1C

FIG. 28-1A. Osteoid osteoma. There is a slightly expansive osteolytic lesion (nidus), with a partially ossified matrix, involving the left inferior articular process and lamina of L3 (*arrow*). Sclerosis is noted posteriorly.

FIG. 28-1B. The nidus (*white arrow*) has predominantly intermediate signal intensity. Foci of low signal within the lesion are caused by ossification of the matrix. Very low signal intensity posterior to the lesion is caused by sclerosis (*black arrow*).

FIG. 28-1C. After contrast injection there is slight rim enhancement of the nidus. Extensive enhancement of the posterior paraspinal muscles is seen (*arrow*).

OSTEOID OSTEOMA

The axial CT and MR images show the presence of an osteoid osteoma of the lumbar spine (Figs. 28-1A, 1B). The nidus has a partially ossified matrix, and slight enhancement of the rim of the nidus is seen after the injection of gadopentetate dimeglumine (Fig. 28-1C).

Osteoid osteoma is an uncommon tumor. Ten percent occur in the spine (6) with over half of these developing in the lumbar region (8). They usually involve the posterior elements, particularly the lamina, articular process, or pedicle. Osteoid osteoma isolated to the vertebral body occurs in less than 10 percent of cases (8). Most osteoid osteomas develop in individuals under the age of 25 years.

Osteoid osteomas of the spine may be difficult to detect initially by conventional radiography because of their small size and because of overlying bony structures (5,8). When visible, they usually appear as a radiolucent lesion (nidus) 1 cm or less in diameter, surrounded by exuberant sclerosis (8). Ossification which may be present within the nidus is often difficult to detect. Osteoid osteomas of the spine are often entirely sclerotic (Fig. 28-2A). Scoliosis may be present. The tumor is usually located on the concave side of the scoliotic curve. Spinal osteoid osteoma should be considered in young patients who present with painful sco-

liosis. Radionuclide bone scanning is almost always positive in cases of osteoid osteoma (3); however, the radionuclide bone scan, while highly sensitive, lacks specificity.

The CT appearance of osteoid osteoma is characteristic, with a radiolucent nidus usually surrounded by intense reactive sclerosis (5,7) (Fig. 28-2B). In some cases CT may be the only imaging modality to show the nidus (5). Ossification, which may be present within the nidus, is more readily detected by CT than by conventional radiography (8). Osteoid osteoma remains localized and does not progressively destroy or expand surrounding bone or extend into the paravertebral or intraspinal compartments as might osteoblastoma. Mild enlargement of the posterior elements may develop because of cortical thickening from periosteal bone formation rather than marrow expansion (7). The precise anatomic location of the nidus can be shown by CT, which aids the surgeon in determining the best surgical approach and obviates unnecessary resection which otherwise might lead to compromise of spine stability (5,7,8,11,12,14). When osteoid osteoma involves the pedicle, detection of the nidus differentiates osteoid osteoma from other causes of an osteosclerotic pedicle (14) such as osteoblastic metastasis,

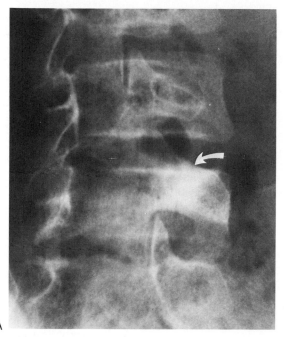
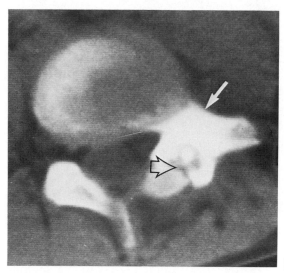

A
B

FIG. 28-2. Osteoid osteoma. **A**: Conventional radiograph of the lower lumbar spine in the left posterior oblique projection. There is osteosclerosis of the left pedicle of L5 (*arrow*). No radiolucent nidus is identified. **B**: Axial CT examination shows a radiolucent nidus (*open arrow*) that was not visible on the conventional radiographic examination. Central ossification of the nidus is identified. There is reactive sclerosis in the pedicle (*closed arrow*) and around the lesion. (Courtesy of Jay Mall, M.D., San Francisco, California.)

Paget's disease, and pedicle sclerosis secondary to a contralateral pars defect or absent pedicle. Occasionally, the nidus of osteoid osteoma is not visible on CT because of partial volume averaging.

Compared to CT, osteoid osteoma is not as well delineated with MR imaging. The MR appearance of osteoid osteoma depends upon the nature of the components of the nidus as well as the tissue surrounding the nidus (6,15). The nidus has decreased signal intensity on T1-weighted images and variable signal on T2-weighted images. Calcification or ossification within the center of the nidus appears either isointense or hypointense relative to the nidus, depending upon the amount of mineralization present. An osteoid osteoma may be surrounded by sclerosis or edema that may be extensive. Sclerosis appears as very low signal intensity on both T1- and T2-weighted images, whereas edema shows decreased signal intensity on T1- and increased signal intensity on T2-weighted images (15).

Osteoblastoma is a rare benign primary bone tumor that is similar to osteoid osteoma histopathologically. Lesions that are 1 cm or less in size are considered osteoid osteoma; those greater than 2 cm are considered osteoblastoma; and those from 1–2 cm may be considered as osteoid osteoma-osteoblastoma complex (10). Osteoblastomas comprise less than 1 percent of all primary tumors of bone (10). Approximately 35 per-

cent of osteoblastomas arise in the spine or sacrum (7), occurring in decreasing frequency in the lumbar, thoracic, and cervical spine and sacrum. Osteoblastoma usually develops within the first three decades of life.

Most cases of osteoblastoma are detected by conventional radiography or radionuclide bone scan. For the delineation of the osseous changes, CT is preferred to MR imaging, although both can be helpful in determining the exact anatomic location and extent of the tumor and its relationship to surrounding structures (4,8,9,12). The CT findings of osteoblastoma are those of an osteolytic, frequently expansive lesion usually involving the posterior elements (pedicle, lamina, articular process) alone or to a lesser extent in combination with the vertebral body. Isolated involvement of the vertebral body is uncommon (10). The margin is usually sharply defined and sclerotic although aggressive margins simulating malignancy may be present. Osteoblastomas are greater than 1 cm and usually larger than 2 cm in diameter when initially discovered (8,10). An ossified matrix is identified by conventional radiography in almost 50 percent of cases (10); however, it is more readily detected by CT because of superior resolution (Fig. 28-3). Ossification of tumor in the spinal canal can be identified (1).

Approximately 25–50 percent of patients with osteo-

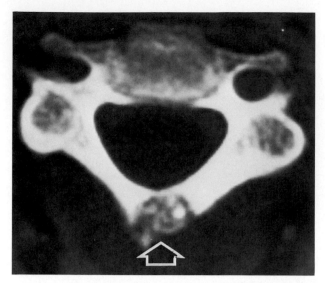

FIG. 28-3. Osteoblastoma. Axial CT of the C4 vertebra in an 11-year-old girl with neck pain. There is an osteolytic lesion involving the junction of the spinous process and both laminae (*arrow*). Ossifications are noted within the matrix.

blastoma present with neurologic signs caused by expansion of tumor into the spinal canal (8,10). In this clinical setting conventional radiographs may show the lesion. To determine the degree of spinal cord compression, MR imaging or CTM is needed (2,13).

The MR signal characteristics of osteoblastoma are variable and may be heterogeneous. On T1-weighted MR images there is intermediate to decreased signal intensity, whereas on T2-weighted images, there may be bright signal (2,3). The presence of an ossified matrix, however, may lead to areas of hypointense signal on all MR pulse sequences. In one case report (3), osteoblastoma was associated with extensive edema and inflammatory tissue, causing increased signal intensity on T2-weighted images that extended to the soft tissues, adjacent vertebra, and ribs. This led to an over-

estimation of the size of the lesion and suspicion for malignancy. All of the involved areas showed enhancement following administration of gadopentetate dimeglumine. In that case, CTM clearly established the diagnosis and the true extent of the lesion. However, in the presence of neurologic signs, MR imaging provides a noninvasive method of evaluating spinal cord compression and may be preferable to CTM, thus obviating the need for intrathecal injection.

REFERENCES

1. Amacher AL, Eltomey A. Spinal osteoblastoma in children and adolescents. *Childs Nerv Syst* 1985;1:29–32.
2. Beltran J, Noto AM, Chakeres DW, et al. Tumors of the osseous spine: staging with MR imaging versus CT. *Radiology* 1987;162:565–9.
3. Crim JR, Mirra JM, Eckardt JJ, et al. Widespread inflammatory response to osteoblastoma: the flare phenomenon. *Radiology* 1990;177:835–6.
4. Epstein N, Benjamin V, Pinto R, et al. Benign osteoblastoma of the thoracic vertebra. *J Neurosurg* 1980;53:710–3.
5. Gamba JL, Martinez S, Apple J, et al. Computed tomography of axial skeletal osteoid osteomas. *AJR* 1984;142:769–72.
6. Glass RBJ, Poznanski AK, Fisher MR, et al. MR imaging of osteoid osteoma. *J Comp Assis Tomogr* 1986;10:1065–7.
7. Jackson RP, Reckling FW, Mantz FA. Osteoid osteoma and osteoblastoma: similar histologic lesions with different natural histories. *Clin Orthop* 1977;128:303–13.
8. Janin Y, Epstein JA, Carras R, et al. Osteoid osteomas and osteoblastomas of the spine. *Neurosurgery* 1981;8:31–8.
9. Kirwan EO'G, Hutton PAN, Pozo JL, et al. Osteoid osteoma and benign osteoblastoma of the spine. *J Bone Joint Surg (Br)* 1984;66B:21–6.
10. McLeod RA, Dahlin DC, Beabout JW. The spectrum of osteoblastoma. *AJR* 1976;126:321–35.
11. Nelson OA, Greer RB III. Localization of osteoid-osteoma of the spine using computerized tomography. *J Bone Joint Surg (Am)* 1983;65A:263–4.
12. Omojola MF, Cockshott WP, Beatty EG. Osteoid osteoma: an evaluation of diagnostic modalities. *Clin Radiol* 1981;32:199–204.
13. Omojola MF, Fox AJ, Viñuela FV. Computed tomographic metrizamide myelography in the evaluation of thoracic spinal osteoblastoma. *AJNR* 1982;3:670–3.
14. Wedge JH, Tchang S, MacFadyen DJ. Computed tomography in localization of spinal osteoid osteoma. *Spine* 1981;6:423–7.
15. Yeager BA, Schiebler ML, Wertheim SB, et al. MR imaging of osteoid osteoma of the talus. *J Comp Assis Tomogr* 1987;11:916–7.

CASE 29

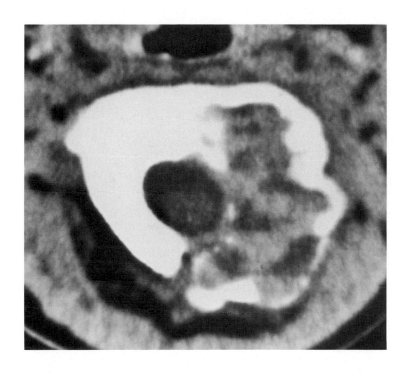

FIG. 29-1A. This 7-year-old boy presented with a 1-year history of neck pain radiating to the occiput. Axial CT at C2.

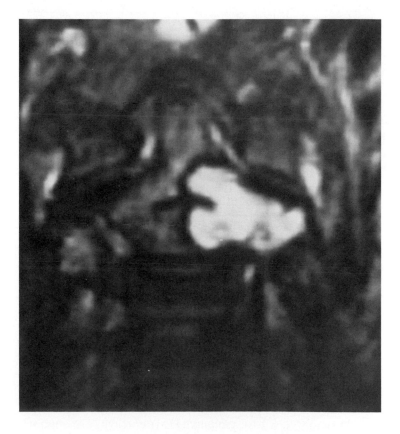

FIG. 29-1B. Coronal T2-weighted SE MR image (2200/90) of the upper cervical spine.

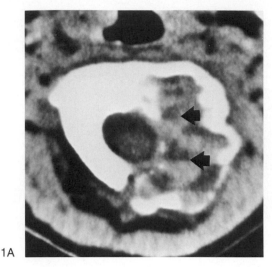

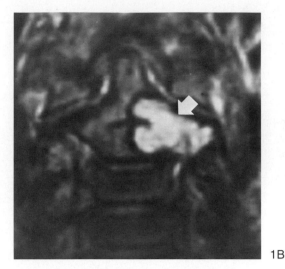

FIG. 29-1A. Aneurysmal bone cyst. There is a large destructive, expansive lesion of the left lamina that extends into the vertebral body and spinal canal. Multiple fluid/fluid levels are seen (*arrows*).

FIG. 29-1B. The aneurysmal bone cyst (*arrow*) shows heterogeneous, predominantly bright signal intensity. The lesion is lobulated and expansive. (Courtesy of Robert Zimmerman, M.D., Philadelphia, Pennsylvania.)

ANEURYSMAL BONE CYST

In this case, the typical features of an aneurysmal bone cyst are seen on the CT and MR images (Fig. 29-1). Aneurysmal bone cyst is a tumor-like lesion that most often occurs during the first three decades of life. Approximately 20 percent of aneurysmal bone cysts develop in the spine and sacrum with a predilection for the cervical and thoracic regions (8). They usually begin in the posterior elements, particularly the lamina or pedicle, or eccentrically in the vertebral body, and then may extend into adjacent bony structures and soft tissues. Aneurysmal bone cyst is an osteolytic lesion that may become highly expansive. A thin rim of bone that surrounds the lesion may not be detected with conventional radiographs. Sometimes the margin of the lesion is poorly defined, giving an aggressive appearance. An aneurysmal bone cyst may extend to involve more than one level, a feature that is unusual for benign and most malignant tumors of the spine.

Pathologically, aneurysmal bone cyst is a highly vascular lesion with areas of blood-filled serous or serosanguinous fluid lined by fibro-osseous tissue (5). Rarely a "solid" aneurysmal bone cyst has been reported and is most common in the spine (7).

Aneurysmal bone cyst may be detected on conventional spine radiographs, whereas CT or MR imaging is able to better evaluate the full extent of the lesion and its relationship to the neural structures. Although CT may better delineate the cortical destruction of the lesion, MR imaging is superior to conventional CT (without intrathecal contrast) in determining the relationship of the lesion to the spinal cord or other neural structures.

With MR imaging, aneurysmal bone cysts are seen as expansive, lobulated lesions with multisignal characteristics and frequent fluid-fluid levels (3,6). A rim of low signal intensity outlines the margin of the lesion and probably represents the intact periosteum (2). The signal characteristics of aneurysmal bone cyst are variable, reflecting the amount and stage of blood products as well as the presence of serous or serosanguinous fluid within the loculations of the lesion (1,2,12). Fluid levels are frequently present and are caused by sedimentation of red blood cells and serum within the loculations (1–3,6,9). Subacute hemorrhage appears as increased signal intensity on T1- and T2-weighted images due to the presence of extracellular methemoglobin. Hemosiderin of chronic hemorrhage is seen as very low signal on T1- and T2-weighted images. Serous fluid appears as decreased signal on T1- and increased signal on T2-weighted images. The signal intensity of an aneurysmal bone cyst may therefore reflect the presence of any or all of these fluids, with the individual loculations showing a variety of signal characteristics because of differing components (6). Fluid levels are best demonstrated if the patient remains motionless for at least 10 minutes prior to scanning (1). The images are obtained in the plane perpendicular to the fluid levels. The presence of fluid levels is a nonspecific finding and has been observed within osteosarcomas, giant cell tumors, malignant fibrous histiocytomas, simple cysts, fibrous dysplasia, and other tumors (9). The presence of a highly expansive, fluid-containing lesion in the posterior elements of the spine of a child or young adult should strongly suggest the diagnosis of aneurysmal bone cyst.

Gadopentetate dimeglumine is not needed routinely in the evaluation of spinal aneurysmal bone cysts, although enhancement of the septations has been observed (2).

Computed tomography is helpful in evaluating not only the osseous extent of aneurysmal bone cyst but also its extent into the paravertebral and intraspinal compartments (10,11). With CT, a faintly calcified thin rim can be seen that often eludes detection on conventional radiographs. Fluid-fluid levels can be observed (3,4).

Patients with aneurysmal bone cyst may present with signs of spinal cord or cauda equina compression. In this clinical setting, MR imaging is preferable to CT and can aid in determining the degree of neural compression. In older patients, slow-growing metastases and myeloma can also appear as osteolytic expansive lesions involving the posterior elements alone or in combination with the vertebral body.

REFERENCES

1. Beltran J, Simon DC, Levy M, et al. Aneurysmal bone cysts: MR imaging at 1.5 T. *Radiology* 1986;158:689–90.
2. Caro PA, Mandell GA, Stanton RP. Aneurysmal bone cysts of the spine in children: MRI imaging at 0.5 tesla. *Pediatr Radiol* 1991;21:114–6.
3. Cory DA, Fritsch SA, Cohen MD, et al. Aneurysmal bone cysts: imaging findings and embolotherapy. *AJR* 1989;153:369–73.
4. Hudson TM. Fluid levels in aneurysmal bone cysts: a CT feature. *AJR* 1984;141:1001–4.
5. Mirra JM. *Bone tumors: diagnosis and treatment*. Philadelphia: JB Lippincott; 1980.
6. Munk PL, Helms CA, Holt RG, et al. MR imaging of aneurysmal bone cysts. *AJR* 1989;153:99–101.
7. Sanerkin NG, Mott MG, Roylance J. An unusual intraosseous lesion with fibroblastic, osteoclastic, osteoblastic, aneurysmal and fibromyxoid elements: "solid" variant of aneurysmal bone cyst. *Cancer* 1983;51:2278–86.
8. Tillman BP, Dahlin DC, Lipscomb PR, et al. Aneurysmal bone cyst: an analysis of ninety-five cases. *Mayo Clin Proc* 1968;43: 478–95.
9. Tsai JC, Dalinka MK, Fallon MD, et al. Fluid-fluid level: a nonspecific finding in tumors of bone and soft tissue. *Radiology* 1990;175:779–82.
10. Volikas Z, Singounas E, Saridakes G, et al. Aneurysmal bone cyst of the spine: report of a case. *Acta Radiolog Diag* 1982;23: 643–6.
11. Wang AM, Lipson SJ, Haykal HA, et al. Computed tomography of aneurysmal bone cyst of the L1 vertebral body: case report. *J Comput Assist Tomogr* 1984;8:1186–9.
12. Zimmer WD, Berquist TH, Sim FH, et al. Magnetic resonance imaging of aneurysmal bone cyst. *Mayo Clin Proc* 1984;59: 633–6.

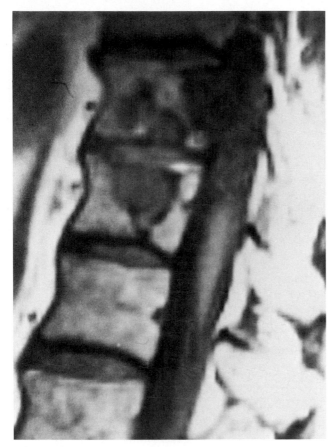

FIG. 30-1A. This 67-year-old man was examined because of weakness in both legs. Sagittal T1-weighted SE MR image (800/20) of the thoracolumbar spine.

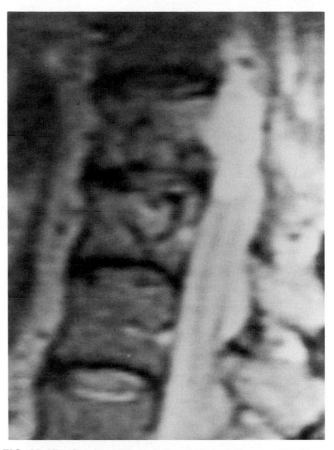

FIG. 30-1B. Sagittal T2-weighted SE MR image (2000/70).

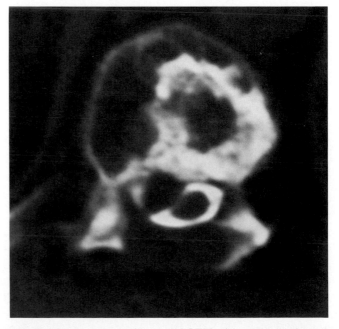

FIG. 30-1C. Postoperative axial CTM with pathologic process still present.

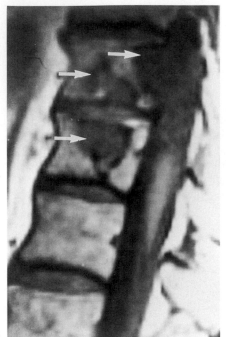

1A

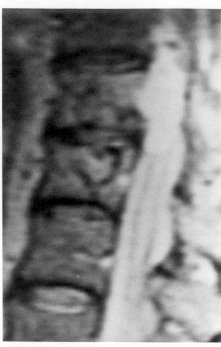

1B

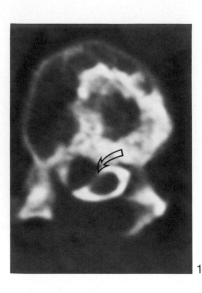

1C

FIG. 30-1A. Chondrosarcoma, low-grade. There are multiple lesions within the T11 and T12 vertebrae (*arrows*) that are hypointense relative to normal bone marrow and display heterogeneous signal. Areas of very low signal intensity are seen in the periphery of the lesions. There is posterior extension of tumor into the spinal canal causing displacement of the spinal cord.

FIG. 30-1B. On the T2-weighted image the lesions are almost isointense relative to normal marrow. The periphery continues to show very low signal intensity that may represent either calcification of the matrix or sclerosis around the lesions. The intraspinal portion of the tumor has very bright signal.

FIG. 30-1C. There is bone destruction with calcification of the osseous and intraspinal components of the tumor that remained following decompressive laminectomy. The presence of bone destruction and a calcified mass is characteristic of chondrosarcoma. Note compression of the anterolateral aspect of the contrast-filled subarachnoid space (*arrow*) caused by the mass.

CHONDROSARCOMA

The MR images show lesions in two adjacent vertebrae with a soft-tissue mass extending posteriorly into the spinal canal (Figs. 30-1A, 1B). The calcified matrix of this tumor is clearly evident on the axial CT image obtained after surgery (Fig. 30-1C). This proved to be a chondrosarcoma. This tumor involved two contiguous vertebral levels, a rare occurrence for most spinal tumors and an unusual feature of chondrosarcoma.

Chondrosarcoma is a malignant tumor of cartilage matrix that is rare in the spine and sacrum. It may arise de novo or from malignant degeneration in Paget's disease or from an osteochondroma, or following radiation to bone. Chondrosarcoma may occur at any level in the spine but is more common in the thoracic spine and sacrum. It develops most often during the fourth through sixth decades, with those tumors developing secondarily in an osteochondroma occurring at an earlier age.

On conventional radiographs there is bone destruction and frequently, extensive punctate or arclike calcifications are seen, indicating a cartilage matrix. The tumor may achieve a large size prior to clinical presentation and frequently extends into the paravertebral and epidural compartments, compressing the spinal cord and nerve roots.

Both MR imaging and CT are important modalities in determining the extent of tumor. In evaluating osseous destruction and in detecting calcifications, CT is preferable to MR imaging (5), whereas MR is preferable for evaluating the extent of tumor in the soft tissues and the degree of spinal cord compression.

The MR signal characteristics of chondrosarcomas are variable and depend upon the presence and degree of hyalin cartilage and the amount of calcification within tumor matrix. Hyalin cartilage contains a cellular portion (chondrocytes) and an acellular portion or matrix composed of collagen and mucopolysaccharides (4). It is the latter which trap water in their interstices. Well-differentiated chondrosarcomas are composed of 95–100 percent hyalin cartilage (4). Enchondromas are composed mainly of hyalin cartilage as well. High-grade chondrosarcomas have a predominantly myxoid to fibrillar matrix with loss of the homogeneity that is seen with pure hyalin cartilage tumors. The high-grade chondrosarcomas contain far less mucopolysaccharides and, therefore, less water than do the low-grade neoplasms. Clear-cell chondrosarcoma is a malignant tumor that behaves as a low-grade lesion (4). These tumors have a cellular stroma with scattered islands of chondroid matrix (2).

Tumors of hyalin cartilage-matrix (including most well-differentiated chondrosarcomas) appear as a mass of low signal intensity on T1-weighted images, and increased homogeneous signal intensity on T2-weighted images because of the high water content of hyalin cartilage (2). They have lobules of varying size, with intervening bands of fibrous tissue or septae of low signal intensity noted on both pulse sequences (2). Calcification of the matrix has very low signal intensity on both T1- and T2-weighted images, but is not as readily detected with MR imaging as with conventional radiography or CT. A sclerotic margin of reactive bone, when present around the tumor, also appears as decreased signal intensity on both pulse sequences. Cortical destruction may be detected as increased signal intensity within the normally low-signal cortical bone on both T1- and T2-weighted images.

The MR signal characteristics of predominantly nonhyalin cartilage chondrosarcomas are intermediate signal intensity on T1-weighted images and intermediate, decreased, and sometimes partially increased signal intensity on T2-weighted images (2). The relative lack of diffuse high signal on T2-weighted images compared with chondrosarcomas containing hyalin cartilage is due to the relative lack of water content in the matrix of the tumor tissue. High-grade chondrosarcomas show a heterogeneous signal intensity (2). The configuration of the tumor is amorphous in appearance compared to the lobular configuration found with tumors composed predominantly of hyalin cartilage. The MR appearance of nonhyalin chondrosarcomas is nonspecific and similar to many primary bone tumors of noncartilage tissue. The MR images of a patient with metastatic clear-cell chondrosarcoma are shown in Fig. 30-2.

On CT, chondrosarcoma appears as an osteolytic lesion, usually with extensive punctate, ring, or arclike calcifications or ossifications (Figs. 30-3, 30-4). Sometimes the calcifications may appear partly amorphous when calcification is extensive or when the tumor is aggressive.

MR imaging and CT can be used in the evaluation of other primary bone tumors of the spine such as osteosarcoma, Ewing's sarcoma, and others.

Osteosarcoma

Osteosarcoma is a rare spinal tumor that usually occurs in the first three decades of life but can be seen in later years. It may develop de novo; however, in the axial skeleton it commonly develops from malignant degeneration from previous radiation, Paget's disease, or other less common lesions. Radiographs of osteosarcoma show bone destruction that is usually associated with production of tumor bone that appears amorphous.

The MR appearance of osteosarcoma is variable, dependent upon the presence of tumor ossification, hemorrhage, and/or tumor necrosis. Osteosarcoma arising from within bone usually has heterogeneous or homogeneous decreased signal intensity on T1-weighted images. On T2-weighted images, either increased and/or decreased signal intensity may be present. Those osteosarcomas with increased signal intensity on T2-weighted images are usually high-grade tumors (5). Very low signal intensity on both pulse sequences can be observed with osteoblastic osteosarcomas. Extraosseous extent of tumor appears isointense or sometimes hyperintense relative to muscle on T1-weighted images (5). Sclerosis appears as very low signal intensity on all pulse sequences. Fluid-fluid levels may also be observed within the lesion and reflect hemorrhage and/or tumor necrosis.

With CT, osteosarcoma appears as an osteolytic, osteosclerotic, or osteolytic-osteosclerotic lesion, depending on the amount of tumor bone formed. Tumor bone appears as an amorphous increase in density and frequently is seen in the paravertebral and even epidural compartments (Fig. 30-5).

Ewing's Sarcoma

Ewing's sarcoma is a highly malignant bone tumor that develops in bone marrow and is extremely rare in the spine. Most cases develop in the first three decades. About 60 percent of axial Ewing's sarcoma develop in the sacrum (6). Metastasis of Ewing's sarcoma to the spine from an extraspinal site is more common than a primary Ewing's sarcoma developing in the spine. Intraspinal metastasis without bone metastasis may occur.

On T1-weighted images, Ewing's sarcoma has decreased signal intensity (1) similar to other marrow-

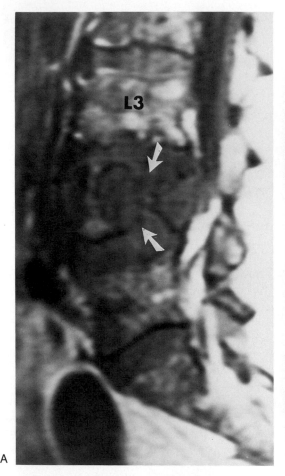

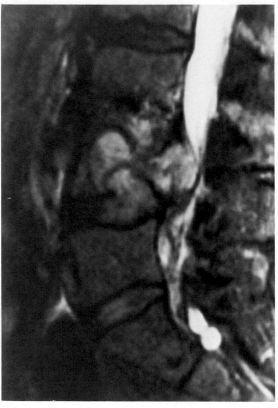

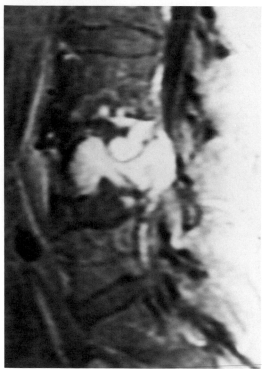

FIG. 30-2. Metastatic clear cell chondrosarcoma. This 74-year-old woman had been treated for chondrosarcoma of the left femur 24 years ago and now presents with discomfort in the right lower extremity in the L4-L5 distribution. **A**: Sagittal T1-weighted SE MR image (600/12) of the lower lumbar spine shows a lesion of low signal intensity of the L4 vertebral body with destruction of the vertebral endplates (*arrows*), vertebral collapse, and posterior extension into the spinal canal. Tumor has crossed the disc and has extended into the adjacent L3 vertebra. **B**: Sagittal T2-weighted FSE MR image (3500/80) with fat suppression shows predominantly bright signal intensity of the chondrosarcoma. Note the increased signal of the tumor that extends into the adjacent disc spaces. **C**: Sagittal T1-weighted SE MR image (600/11) obtained after the intravenous injection of gadopentetate dimeglumine. This image was obtained just parasagittal to Fig. 30-2B and shows marked enhancement of the tumor. Again note extension of tumor into the intervertebral discs.

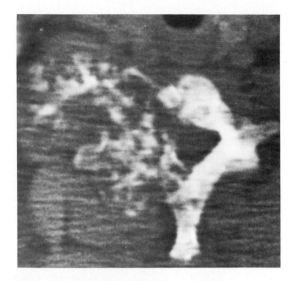

FIG. 30-3. Chondrosarcoma. Computed tomography shows a large, densely calcified osteolytic lesion destroying the right half of the C7 vertebral body, pedicle, and lamina. The punctate nature of the calcifications is characteristic of cartilage matrix. The mass extends deeply into the paravertebral soft tissues and intraspinal compartment. (Courtesy of George Teplick, M.D., Philadelphia, Pennsylvania.)

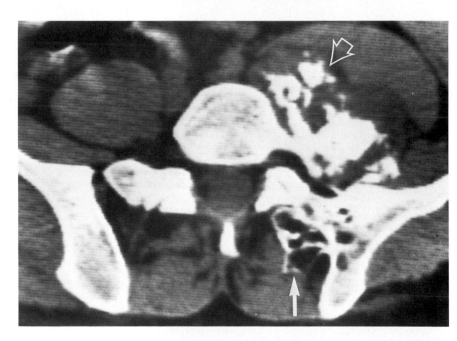

FIG. 30-4. Chondrosarcoma occurring secondary to malignant degeneration of an exostosis. This patient has multiple exostoses. Computed tomography shows a benign exostosis derived from the left ilium (*closed arrow*). This exostosis has corticated margins. A large mass with irregular amorphous clumps of calcification is seen adjacent to the left side of L5 (*open arrow*). This proved to be a chondrosarcoma.

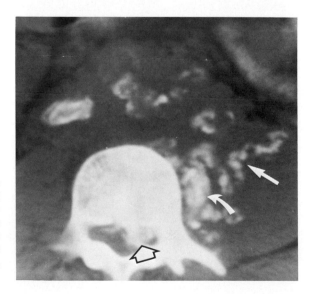

FIG. 30-5. Osteosarcoma. Computed tomography shows an osteosclerotic lesion involving the left half of the L4 vertebral body and pedicle. The tumor extends far anteriorly and laterally into the paravertebral soft tissues. Ossifications of the matrix are both punctate (*straight closed arrow*), resembling cartilage matrix, and amorphous (*curved arrow*), typical of osteosarcoma. Tumor also extends into the epidural space (*open arrow*) (courtesy of Daniel Vanel, M.D., Villejuif, France).

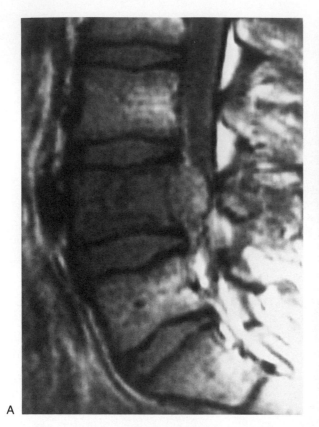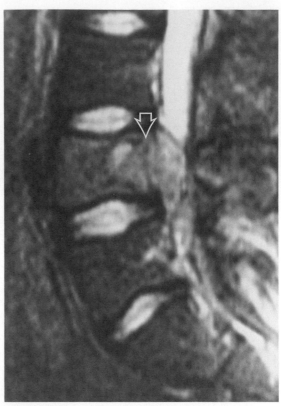

A   B

FIG. 30-6. Ewing's sarcoma of the L4 vertebral body in a 17-year-old male. **A**: Sagittal T1-weighted SE MR image (700/20) shows diffuse decreased signal of the L4 vertebral body and posterior extension of a mass compressing the thecal sac. **B**: Sagittal T2-weighted FSE MR image (3000/90) shows increased signal intensity of the Ewing's sarcoma (*arrow*) and the intraspinal component.

infiltrating lesions (Fig. 30-6A). On T2-weighted images, there is increased signal intensity in most cases due to tumor, necrosis, and inflammatory changes (3) (Fig. 30-6B). Areas of reactive sclerosis (Ewing's sarcoma does not produce tumor bone) appear as very low signal on both T1- and T2-weighted images.

With CT, Ewing's sarcoma appears as an osteolytic lesion often associated with a large soft-tissue mass that extends to the paravertebral or epidural compartments at the time of presentation. Ewing's sarcoma does not produce a mineralized matrix, although sometimes calcific densities are noted in the tumor mass, usually representing islands of bone displaced by tumor mass.

REFERENCES

1. Boyko OB, Cory DA, Cohen MD, et al. MR imaging of osteogenic and Ewing's sarcoma. *AJR* 1987;148:317–22.
2. Cohen EK, Kressel HY, Frank TS, et al. Hyaline cartilage-origin bone and soft-tissue neoplasms: MR appearance and histologic correlation. *Radiology* 1988;167:477–81.
3. Frouge C, Vanel D, Coffre C, et al. The role of magnetic resonance imaging in the evaluation of Ewing's sarcoma. *Skeletal Radiol* 1988;17:387–92.
4. Mirra JM, Gold RH, Marcove RC. *Bone tumors: diagnosis and treatment*. Philadelphia: JB Lippincott Co; 1980.
5. Sundaram M, McGuire MH, Herbold DR. Magnetic resonance imaging of osteosarcoma. *Skeletal Radiol* 1987;16:23–9.
6. Whitehouse GH, Griffiths GS. Roentgenologic aspects of spinal involvement by primary and metastatic Ewing's tumor. *J Can Assoc Radiol* 1976;27:290–7.

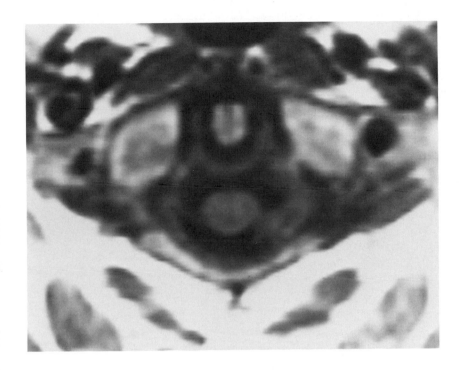

FIG. 31-1A. A 68-year-old woman presented with neck and left arm pain and a previous history of spondylosis and lower cervical spinal fusion. Axial T1-weighted SE MR image (500/12) at the level of C1 and the odontoid process of C2.

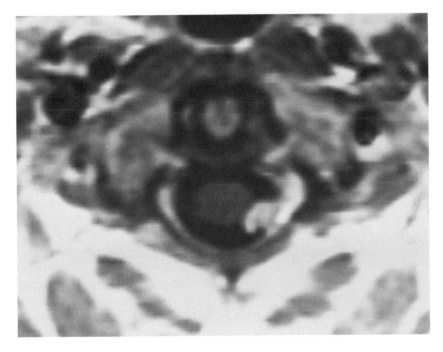

FIG. 31-1B. Axial T1-weighted SE MR image (500/12) obtained after the intravenous injection of gadopentetate dimeglumine.

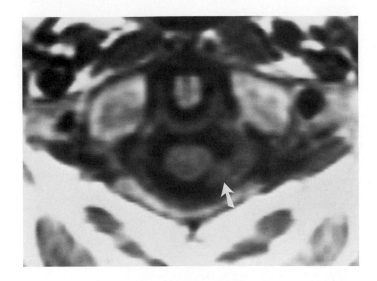

FIG. 31-1A. Meningioma. There is abnormal signal intensity (*arrow*) seen posterior and to the left of the spinal cord. This is of higher signal intensity than the cerebrospinal fluid and is isointense relative to the spinal cord.

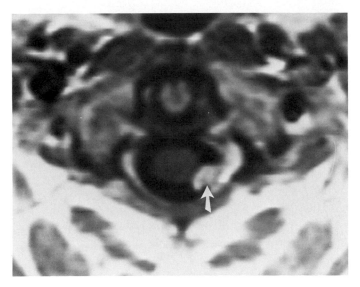

FIG. 31-1B. After the injection of gadopentetate dimeglumine there is marked homogeneous enhancement of this small intradural extramedullary mass (*arrow*) that proved to be a meningioma at surgery.

MENINGIOMA

There is an intradural extramedullary mass at the level of C1 which is isointense to the spinal cord on T1-weighted images (Fig. 31-1A). Marked homogeneous enhancement of the tumor is seen after the intravenous injection of gadopentetate dimeglumine (Fig. 31-1B). Sagittal and coronal images help localize the mass to the intradural extramedullary compartment and show the value of using contrast enhancement in the evaluation of this lesion (Fig. 31-2). This small tumor, which might be difficult to demonstrate with other imaging modalities, is a meningioma.

In adults, meningioma is one of the most frequent primary intraspinal tumors, second only to neurofibroma. Typically, meningiomas occur in the thoracic spine in middle-aged women. Meningiomas are less frequent in the cervical spine and are rare in the lumbar region (19). Predilection for the thoracic spine is not evident in men. They are rare in children (3). Thoracic meningiomas are usually located posteriorly, while cervical meningiomas usually develop anterior to the spinal cord (7). Most meningiomas are purely intradural extramedullary in location, with only about 7 percent involving both the intradural and extradural compartments (7). Meningioma is actually the most frequent tumor confined solely to the intradural extramedullary space, since one-third of neurofibromas involve the extradural compartment. Meningioma is also the most frequent intraspinal tumor that calcifies.

Magnetic resonance imaging is an excellent method of evaluating intraspinal tumors. Tumors can be grouped into compartmental location by dividing them into intramedullary, intradural extramedullary, and extradural lesions. Magnetic resonance imaging can provide accurate assessment of the compartmental loca-

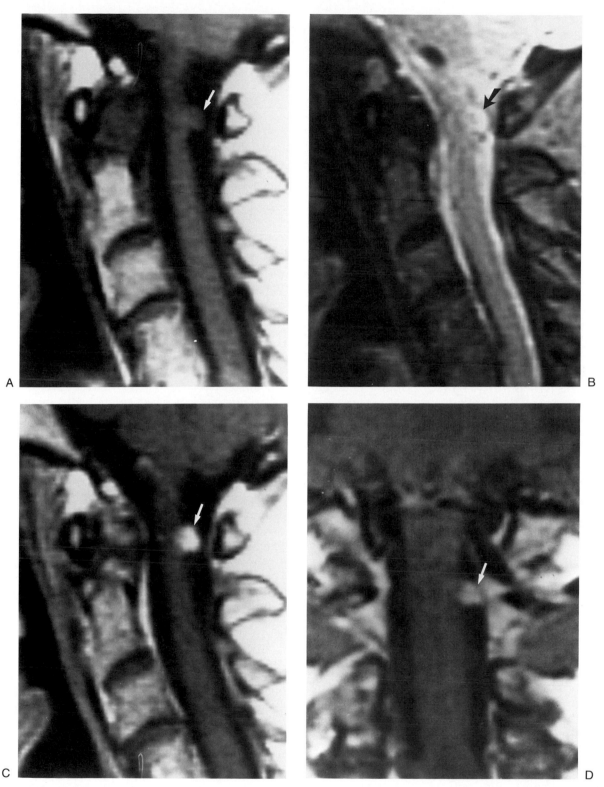

FIG. 31-2. Meningioma. Additional images of the same patient shown in Fig. 31-1. **A**: Sagittal T1-weighted SE MR image shows the meningioma (*arrow*) which is located posteriorly and is isointense relative to the spinal cord. **B**: Sagittal T2-weighted SE MR image (2308/70) does not show the meningioma well (*arrow*) because it has bright signal intensity that is similar to the cerebrospinal fluid with this pulse sequence. **C,D**: After the intravenous injection of gadopentetate dimeglumine, sagittal (C) and coronal (D) T1-weighted SE MR images show marked enhancement of the meningioma (*arrow*) and aid in determining that the tumor has an intradural extramedullary location.

tion of these tumors, with better delineation achieved with the use of gadopentetate dimeglumine. Intramedullary tumors cause spinal cord swelling and enlargement. Intradural extramedullary tumors cause displacement of the spinal cord, widening of the ipsilateral subarachnoid space, and narrowing of the contralateral subarachnoid space (Figs. 31-3, 31-4). Extradural tumors typically displace and compress the ipsilateral subarachnoid space as well as the spinal cord. On occasion, the compartmental location of a meningioma may be in question. Extradural meningiomas may be differentiated from intradural extramedullary lesions in some cases by the presence of a well-defined, low-intensity band seen between the mass and the spinal cord on both T1- and T2-weighted SE images (17). The band is thought to be due to spinal ligaments and dura and is not seen when the mass is located in the intradural extramedullary compartment. Another sign indicating an extradural location of a tumor is the fat cap sign (6). Extradural tumors may splay epidural fat, giving it a capped appearance on sagittal and axial images.

Meningiomas tend to be isointense to the spinal cord on both T1- and T2-weighted images (17). These tumors may be difficult to visualize with conventional

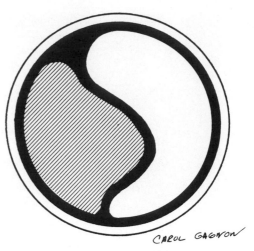

FIG. 31-4. Intradural extramedullary tumor (*shaded area*) and its relationship to the subarachnoid space and spinal cord in the axial plane. The effects of an intradural extramedullary tumor on the spinal cord and subarachnoid space are similar to that seen with axial MR and CTM.

unenhanced MR imaging, but are usually conspicuous after injection of gadopentetate dimeglumine (1,10, 15,18). Meningiomas show immediate and uniform contrast enhancement which improves diagnostic accuracy (Fig. 31-5). These tumors lack a blood-brain (cord) barrier, so contrast enhancement of these lesions is a function of tumor vascularization (10). Meningiomas of the foramen magnum may be difficult to evaluate by other imaging modalities and may be seen with MR imaging, despite a negative myelogram (13). Small meningiomas may sometimes be obscured by cerebrospinal fluid pulsations that cause inhomogeneous decreased signal intensity that is most prominent on T2-weighted images of the upper cervical spine near the foramen magnum (14). These small meningiomas may require contrast enhancement and coronal imaging for accurate diagnosis and compartmental localization (4).

Patients with intradural extramedullary spinal tumors can have associated syringomyelia with cystic cavities extending for considerable distances above and/or below the mass (12). In addition, some patients who have previously undergone surgery for intradural extramedullary tumor such as meningioma or schwannoma may present with new neurologic symptoms caused by syringomyelia that occur after a long symptom-free postoperative period (2). The syrinx cavity may have low signal intensity on both T1- and T2-weighted images. The low signal intensity on T2-weighted images is thought to represent a flow void phenomenon related to fluid motion in clinically enlarging cysts (2). Such patients may benefit most from syrinx decompression. In other cases, the syrinx may

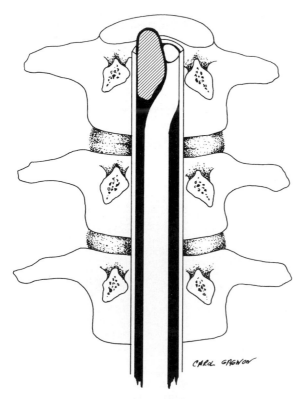

FIG. 31-3. An intradural extramedullary tumor (*shaded area*) and its relationship to the subarachnoid space (*black area*) and spinal cord in the coronal plane. This type of tumor causes displacement of the spinal cord, widening of the ipsilateral subarachnoid space, and narrowing of the contralateral subarachnoid space.

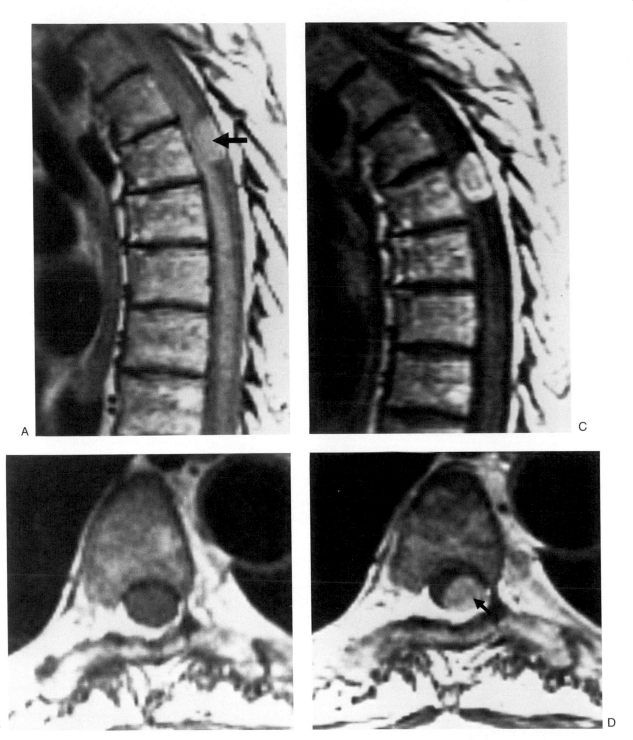

FIG. 31-5. Meningioma of the thoracic spine in a 63-year-old woman with right leg weakness, numbness, and tingling. **A**: Sagittal T1-weighted SE MR image (857/20) of the thoracic spine shows a mass (*arrow*) of moderate increased signal intensity relative to the spinal cord. The mass is causing compression of the spinal cord at the T5 level. **B**: Axial T1-weighted SE MR image (857/20) through the level of the mass fails to separate the mass from the spinal cord. **C,D**: After the intravenous injection of gadopentetate dimeglumine, sagittal (C) and axial (D) T1-weighted SE MR images (600/20) were obtained. There is fairly homogeneous enhancement of the meningioma (*arrow*), although the central portion of the tumor retains some low signal intensity. The tumor has an intradural extramedullary location and is causing spinal cord compression.

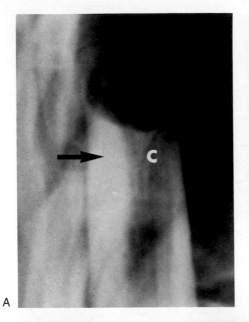

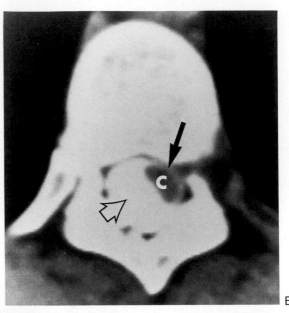

A

B

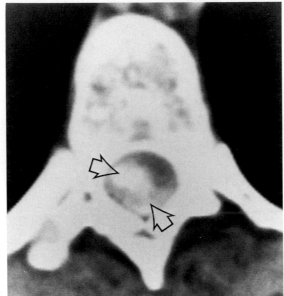

C

FIG. 31-6. Thoracic meningioma in a 46-year-old woman with a history of progressive disturbance of gait and leg weakness. **A**: Lateral radiograph of the lower thoracic spine from a thoracic myelogram performed with water-soluble contrast introduced into the subarachnoid space at a lumbar level. There is a complete myelographic block at the T10-T11 intervertebral disc level. There is widening of the subarachnoid space posteriorly (*arrow*), displacement of the spinal cord anteriorly (*C*), and narrowing of the subarachnoid space anteriorly. This appearance is that of an intradural extramedullary lesion located posteriorly. **B**: Axial CTM just below the level of myelographic block shows widening of the subarachnoid space posteriorly and on the right (*open arrow*), thinning of the subarachnoid space anteriorly on the left (*closed arrow*), and displacement of the spinal cord (*C*). **C**: CTM above the level of the block shows a mass with amorphous calcification filling the posterior and right side of the canal (*arrows*). This mass measured 2.5 × 1.0 cm and proved to be a psammomatous meningioma. Calcifications can be more readily identified with CT than with MR.

have low signal intensity on T1-weighted images and bright signal intensity on T2-weighted images similar to nonpulsatile cerebrospinal fluid. The high signal intensity on T2-weighted images may indicate a syrinx cavity that is not actively expanding. The mechanism for the formation of the syrinx is uncertain, but may be the result of intramedullary edema and microcystic changes that occur from chronic spinal cord compression as well as alterations in cerebrospinal fluid dynamics that occur after surgery (2).

It is not clear whether signal intensity characteristics can be useful in distinguishing meningioma from neural tumor. In one study (17) meningiomas were typically found to be isointense to the spinal cord on both T1- and T2-weighted images, whereas schwannomas had marked hyperintensity on T2-weighted studies. Neurofibromas were found to have signal intensity characteristics similar to meningiomas (17).

Although MR imaging with gadopentetate dimeglumine enhancement is the best method for evaluating intradural extramedullary spinal lesions, some patients may, for various reasons, still be evaluated by myelography followed by CTM, as shown in Fig. 31-6. Conventional myelography can adequately show the presence of tumor and its compartmental location (Fig. 31-6A). When there is a "complete" myelographic block,

CTM may be useful. Small amounts of contrast which pass beyond the block may not be seen with conventional myelography but may be visualized on CTM examination (16). Information gained from CT may be useful in planning the surgical approach (8). For example, a densely calcified or ossified meningioma may occasionally be adherent to the cord and more difficult to remove surgically. This is especially true if the tumor is located anteriorly where it is less accessible to the surgeon (7). Extradural extension of meningioma can also be detected by CT and suggests a more invasive tumor and a more ominous course (7). These tumors may invade bone and resemble metastatic disease.

The differential diagnosis of an intradural extramedullary tumor is usually between neurofibroma or meningioma. Several characteristic findings may be useful in differentiating these two tumors. Meningiomas, for example, may contain globular or punctate calcifications that are more readily visualized by CT than by conventional radiography (9) or MR imaging (Figs. 31-6B, 6C). Reactive sclerosis of the adjacent vertebral body may be seen in association with meningioma on CT examination. Both of these findings are uncommon with neurofibromas. However, other osseous abnormalities are more frequent with neurofibroma than with meningioma and include widening of the neural foramen and vertebral body erosion that are well demonstrated by MR imaging and CT. A "dumbbell" tumor (i.e., an intradural tumor that extends into and beyond the neural foramen) is more likely to represent neurofibroma than meningioma.

Multiple meningiomas are rare and are usually associated with schwannomas or gliomas in patients with neurofibromatosis. They may also develop following radiation therapy (5,11), with the spine having been included in the radiation portal. When multiple meningiomas occur, both intracranial and intraspinal lesions may be present (5). The meningiomas may be so numerous that it may be impossible to differentiate between multiple meningiomas and meningiomatosis (5).

REFERENCES

1. Breger RK, Williams AL, Daniels DL, et al. Contrast enhancement in spinal MR imaging. *AJNR* 1989;10:633–7, *AJR* 1989; 153:387–91.
2. Castillo M, Quencer RM, Green BA, et al. Syringomyelia as a consequence of compressive extramedullary lesions: postoperative clinical and radiological manifestations. *AJNR* 1987;8: 973–8, *AJR* 1988;150:391–6.
3. Desousa AL, Kalsbeck JE, Mealey J Jr, et al. Intraspinal tumors in children. *J Neurosurg* 1979;51:437–45.
4. Dillon WP, Norman D, Newton TH, et al. Intradural spinal cord lesions: Gd-DTPA-enhanced MR imaging. *Radiology* 1989;170: 229–37.
5. Holliday PO III, Davis C Jr, Angelo J. Multiple meningiomas of the cervical spinal cord associated with Klippel-Feil malformation and atlantooccipital assimilation. *Neurosurgery* 1984;14: 353–7.
6. Homer NB, Pinto RS. The fat-cap sign: an aid to MR evaluation of extradural spinal tumors. *AJNR* 1989;10:S93.
7. Levy WJ Jr, Bay J, Dohn D. Spinal cord meningioma. *J Neurosurg* 1982;57:804–12.
8. Memon MY, Schneck L. Ventral spinal tumor: the value of computed tomography in its localization. *Neurosurgery* 1981;8: 108–11.
9. Nakagawa H, Huang YP, Malis LI, et al. Computed tomography of intraspinal and paraspinal neoplasms. *J Comput Assist Tomogr* 1977;1:377–90.
10. Parizel PM, Balériaux D, Rodesch G, et al. Gd-DTPA-enhanced MR imaging of spinal tumors *AJNR* 1989;10:249–58, *AJR* 1989; 152:1087–96.
11. Patronas NJ, Brown F, Duda EE. Multiple meningiomas in the spinal canal. *Surg Neurol* 1980;13:78–80.
12. Quencer RM, El Gammal T, Cohen G. Syringomyelia associated with intradural extra-medullary masses of the spinal canal. *AJNR* 1986;7:143–8.
13. Scotti G, Scialfa G, Colombo N, et al. MR imaging of intradural extramedullary tumors of the cervical spine. *J Comput Assist Tomogr* 1985;9:1037–41.
14. Sherman JL, Citrin CM, Gangarosa RE, et al. The MR appearance of CSF pulsations in the spinal canal. *AJNR* 1986;7:879–84.
15. Sze G, Abramson A, Krol G, et al. Gadolinium-DTPA in the evaluation of intradural extramedullary spinal disease. *AJNR* 1988;9:153–63, *AJR* 1988;150:911–21.
16. Tadmor R, Cacayorin ED, Kieffer SA. Advantages of supplementary CT in myelography of intraspinal masses. *AJNR* 1983; 4:618–21.
17. Takemoto K, Matsumura Y, Hashimoto H, et al. MR imaging of intraspinal tumors—capability in histological differentiation and compartmentalization of extramedullary tumors. *Neuroradiology* 1988;30:303–9.
18. Valk J. Gd-DTPA in MR of spinal lesions. *AJNR* 1988;9:345–50, *AJR* 1988;150:1163–8.
19. Wood JB, Wolpert SM. Lumbosacral meningioma. *AJNR* 1985; 6:450–1.

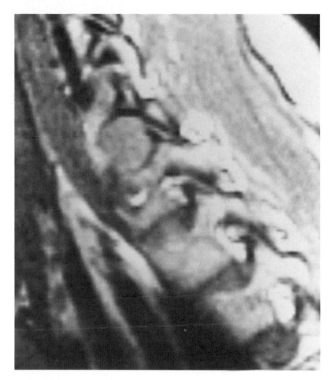

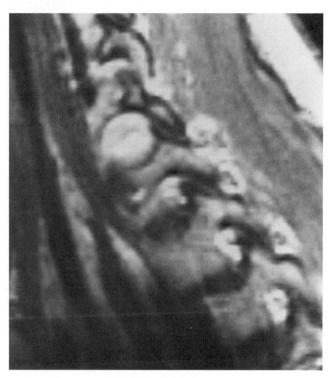

FIG. 32-1A. MR imaging of the cervical and upper thoracic spine was performed in this 22-year-old woman who had neck pain for 2 weeks. Sagittal T1-weighted SE image (700/15) obtained 14 mm left of the midline.

FIG. 32-1B. Sagittal T1-weighted SE image (700/15) obtained 14 mm left of the midline after the intravenous injection of gadopentetate dimeglumine.

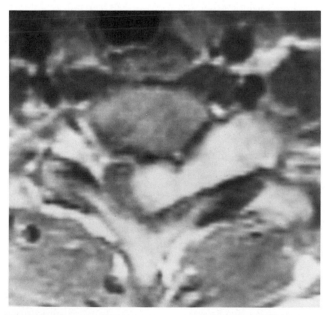

FIG. 32-1C. Axial T1-weighted SE image (600/15) obtained at C7-T1 after the intravenous injection of gadopentetate dimeglumine.

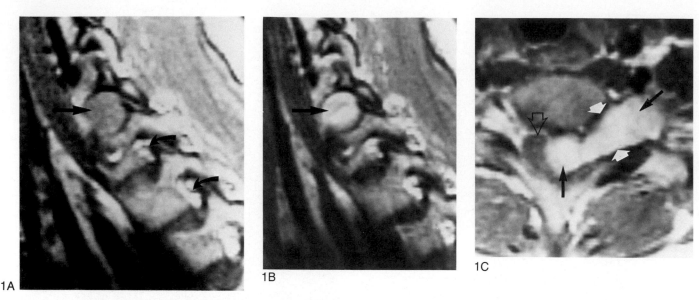

FIG. 32-1A. Dumbbell-shaped schwannoma. There is a mass of slightly low to intermediate signal intensity (*straight arrow*) within the C7-T1 intervertebral foramen. This is causing widening of the foramen compared to normal neural foramina (*curved arrows*).

FIG. 32-1B. There is marked enhancement of the mass (*arrow*) after the intravenous injection of gadopentetate dimeglumine.

FIG. 32-1C. The axial image shows the contrast-enhanced dumbbell-shaped schwannoma (*closed black arrows*). Tumor within the spinal canal is displacing the spinal cord (*open arrow*). The schwannoma is causing marked widening of the left intervertebral foramen (*white arrows*).

DUMBBELL-SHAPED SCHWANNOMA

The T1-weighted parasagittal MR image shows a slightly hypointense mass within the C7-T1 intervertebral foramen (Fig. 32-1A). The mass shows marked enhancement on sagittal and axial T1-weighted images obtained after the intravenous injection of gadopentetate dimeglumine (Figs. 32-1B, 1C). The axial image also reveals that the mass has both an intradural component displacing the spinal cord to the right and an extradural component within the intervertebral foramen. Midsagittal T1-weighted images obtained before and after contrast injection confirm the presence of the mass within the spinal canal and again show marked enhancement (Fig. 32-2). This is a typical appearance of a dumbbell-shaped schwannoma.

A schwannoma is a neural tumor of nerve sheath origin that occurs along nerve roots or peripheral nerves (4). Other names used interchangeably for schwannoma include neuroma, neurilemoma, and peripheral fibroblastoma. These tumors are usually solitary but may be multiple and sometimes occur in patients with neurofibromatosis (4,5). Approximately 67 percent of schwannomas occur in the intradural compartment, while 16 percent have an extradural location, and 16 percent are both intradural and extradural (7).

Extension into the neural foramen creates the typical dumbbell-shaped lesion. Widening of the neural foramen and osseous erosion can be seen (Fig. 32-3). Frequently, two or more vertebral levels are involved.

Neurofibroma is a tumor of nerve root or peripheral nerve origin, usually occurring at multiple sites in association with neurofibromatosis (4). These tumors may also extend into the neural foramen, presenting a similar appearance to our present case (Fig. 32-4). Meningiomas, on the other hand, are less likely to have extradural extension into the neural foramen.

With MR imaging, schwannomas tend to be isointense or hypointense relative to the spinal cord on T1-weighted images, and have mild to marked hyperintensity on T2-weighted images (2). These tumors show enhancement after the intravenous injection of gadopentetate dimeglumine (1,2,6) (Fig. 32-5). The use of contrast enhancement provides high tumor contrast and more clearly delineates compartmentalization of lesions into intramedullary, intradural-extramedullary, and extradural. Schwannomas may have cystic and hemorrhagic components in addition to their solid portion. Correlation between the MR imaging appearance of schwannomas and their gross and histologic charac-

178

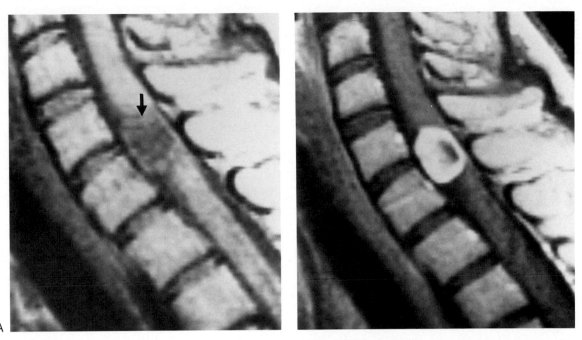

FIG. 32-2. Schwannoma. Same patient as in Fig. 32-1. **A**: Sagittal T1-weighted SE MR image (700/15) obtained in the midline shows the mass (*arrow*) within the spinal canal that is hypointense relative to the spinal cord. **B**: Sagittal T1-weighted SE MR image (700/15) after the intravenous injection of gadopentetate dimeglumine shows marked enhancement of the schwannoma. A small central area lacks enhancement.

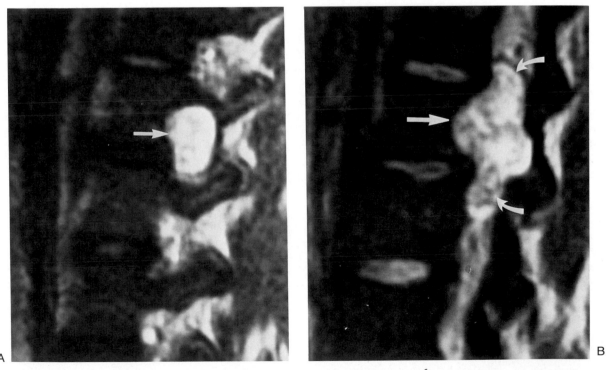

FIG. 32-3. Schwannoma at L1-L2. **A**: Sagittal T2-weighted SE MR image (2000/70) obtained 20 mm to the right of the midline. On the T2-weighted study there is bright signal intensity within the L1-L2 foramen (*arrow*) and widening of the foramen. **B**: Sagittal T2-weighted image obtained 10 mm medial to Fig. 32-3A. There is a large heterogeneous mass (*curved arrows*) causing posterior vertebral body scalloping (*straight arrow*).

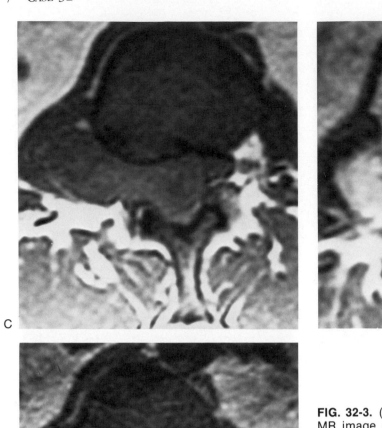

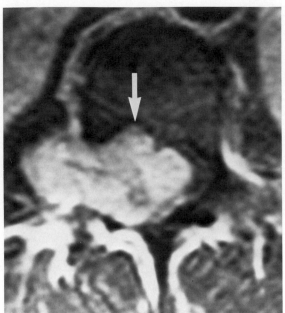

C

E

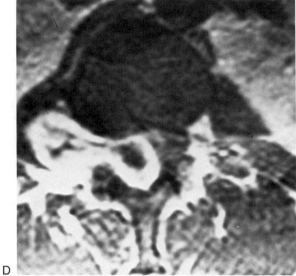

D

FIG. 32-3. (*Continued*). **C**: Axial T1-weighted SE MR image (700/14) shows the dumbbell-shaped configuration of the schwannoma. Widening of the right intervertebral foramen is seen. **D**: Axial T1-weighted SE MR image (700/14) after the intravenous injection of gadopentetate dimeglumine. There is bright enhancement of most of the schwannoma. Central portions of the tumor remain unenhanced. After the injection of contrast, the boundaries of the tumor within the spinal canal are more readily apparent. **E**: Axial T1-weighted image obtained 15 mm cephalad to Fig. 32-3D after intravenous injection of contrast. The heterogeneous, predominantly high-signal intensity schwannoma is seen. Posterior vertebral body scalloping (*arrow*) is noted.

teristics have been studied (1). Areas that are markedly hyperintense on T2-weighted images correspond to areas of cystic degeneration within the tumor, whereas areas of relative hyperintensity represent the solid component. After intravenous injection of gadopentetate dimeglumine, enhancement on T1-weighted images corresponds to the solid component of the tumor, whereas the cystic portions remain unenhanced (1). A peripheral pattern of contrast enhancement has been described and should suggest the diagnosis of schwannoma when seen in an intradural extramedullary tumor (2). In some cases, areas of hyperintensity on T1-weighted images are found and are due to hemorrhage. The MR appearance does not correlate, however, with the histologic classification of schwannomas into Antoni A (cell-rich and composed of compact bundles of fibrillated cells) and Antoni B (loosely textured stroma, often with microcystic degeneration with mucin) (1). Neurofibromas are histologically more uniform solid tumors that usually do not have cystic change but may have central areas of decreased signal intensity on T2-weighted images because of dense collagenous stroma (2).

Although it may not be possible to differentiate between schwannoma and neurofibroma with preoperative imaging, the histologic diagnosis does have clinical importance. One study (3) suggests that a patient with an intraspinal nerve sheath neurofibroma is very likely

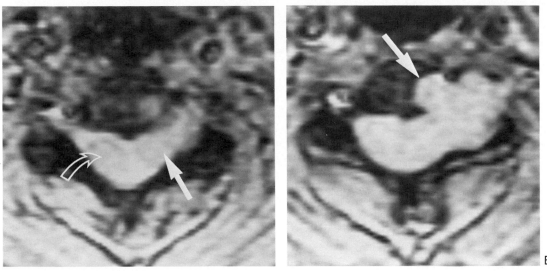

A

B

FIG. 32-4. Neurofibroma of the cervical spine in a 53-year-old woman. **A**: Axial GRE MR image (GRASS, 24/13 with 8-degree flip angle) obtained at C3-C4. There is a neurofibroma on the left (*straight arrow*) that is causing widening of the left intervertebral foramen and displacement of the spinal cord (*curved arrow*). **B**: Axial GRE MR image (GRASS, 24/13 with 8-degree flip angle) shows marked widening of the left intervertebral foramen with erosion and scalloping of the vertebral body margin (*arrow*).

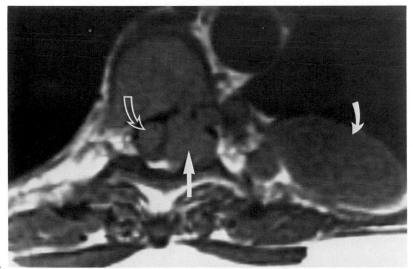

A

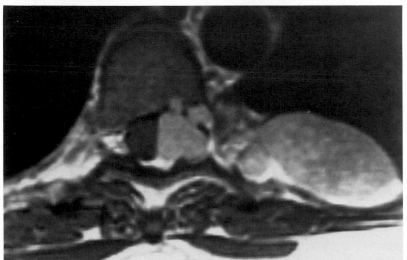

B

FIG. 32-5. Schwannoma. **A**: Axial T1-weighted SE MR image (800/20). There is a large intraspinal mass on the left (*straight arrow*) compressing and displacing the spinal cord (*open arrow*) to the right. The mass is isointense to the spinal cord. Note also a large left paraspinal mass (*closed curved arrow*). **B**: Axial T1-weighted SE MR image (800/20) obtained after the intravenous injection of gadopentetate dimeglumine shows fairly uniform enhancement of both the intraspinal and paraspinal masses. Tumor can be seen extending into the vertebral body and is causing osseous scalloping. Compression of the spinal cord is now more readily apparent after enhancement of the tumor.

to have neurofibromatosis 1, while a patient with a schwannoma is likely to have a sporadic condition or neurofibromatosis 2.

REFERENCES

1. Demachi H, Takashima T, Kadoya M, et al. MR imaging of spinal neurinomas with pathologic correlation. *J Comput Assist Tomogr* 1990;14:250–4
2. Friedman DP, Tartaglino LM, Flanders AE. Intradural schwannomas of the spine: MR findings with emphasis on contrast-enhancement characteristics. *AJR* 1992;158:1347–50.
3. Halliday AL, Sobel RA, Martuza RL. Benign spinal nerve sheath tumors: their occurrence sporadically and in neurofibromatosis 1 and 2. *J Neurosurg* 1991;74:248–53.
4. Lott IT, Richardson EP Jr. Neuropathological findings and the biology of neurofibromatosis. *Adv Neurol* 1981;29:23–32.
5. Russell DS, Rubinstein LJ. *Pathology of tumours of the nervous system*. 4th ed. Baltimore: Williams and Wilkins; 1977.
6. Schroth G, Thron A, Guhl L, et al. Magnetic resonance imaging of spinal meningiomas and neurinomas. *J Neurosurg* 1987;66:695–700.
7. Shapiro R. *Myelography*. 4th ed. Chicago: Year Book Medical Publishers; 1984.

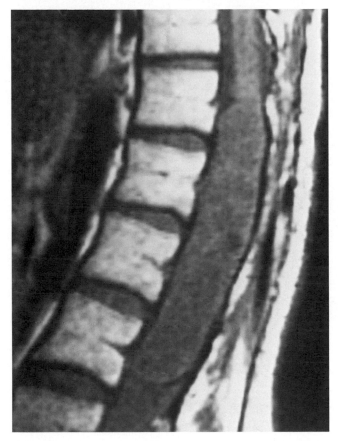

FIG. 33-1A. This 42-year-old woman had been treated previously for a spinal disorder. Sagittal T1-weighted SE MR image (600/20) of the thoracolumbar spine.

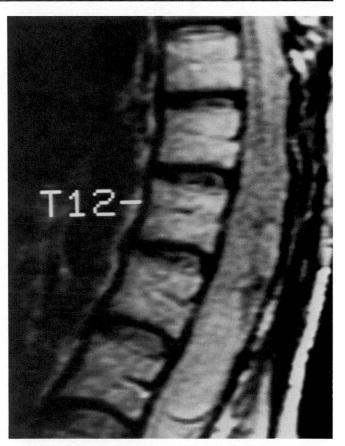

FIG. 33-1B. Sagittal T2-weighted SE MR image (2000/70).

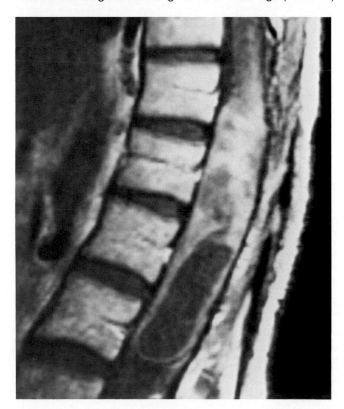

FIG. 33-1C. Sagittal T1-weighted SE MR image (600/20) after intravenous injection of gadopentetate dimeglumine.

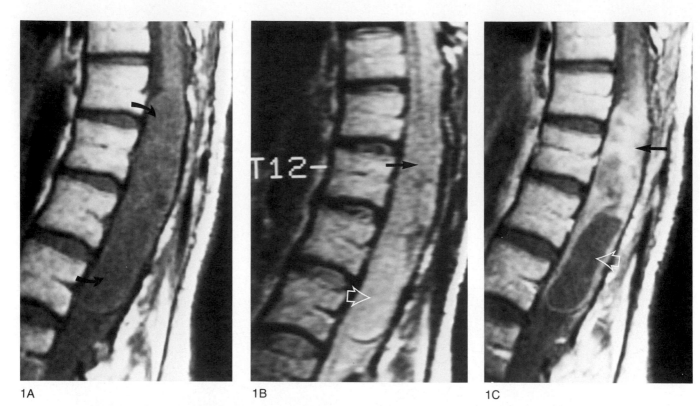

1A   1B   1C

FIG. 33-1A. Intramedullary tumor, astrocytoma. There is marked swelling and enlargement of the spinal cord caused by a large intramedullary mass (*arrows*) that is slightly hypointense relative to the spinal cord.

FIG. 33-1B. On the T2-weighted image the mass appears heterogeneous with intermediate signal seen superiorly (*black arrow*) and brighter signal seen inferiorly (*white arrow*).

FIG. 33-1C. After the injection of gadopentetate dimeglumine, the solid portion of the tumor displays marked enhancement (*black arrow*), whereas the cystic component remains unenhanced (*white arrow*).

INTRAMEDULLARY TUMOR

There is a large intramedullary tumor (Figs. 33-1A, 1B) with cystic cavitation that is best delineated on the contrast-enhanced images (Fig. 33-1C). This is a recurrent astrocytoma.

Gliomas (ependymomas and astrocytomas) comprise the majority of intramedullary tumors. The most frequent intramedullary tumor is ependymoma. Astrocytoma is the second most common and in some series is more frequent than ependymoma in children (5). These tumors may be focal or quite extensive, involving the entire cord (holocord) (1,7); this is a common finding with astrocytomas in children (7). Less frequent intramedullary tumors include hemangioblastoma, metastasis, and lipoma.

Symptoms associated with a spinal cord tumor depend on the spinal level involved. Cervical tumors cause upper extremity weakness and cervical pain. Thoracic tumors present with mild progressive paraparesis and pain over the thoracic spine. These patients may have disturbance of the bowel and bladder sphincters (7). Some patients may present with gait disturbance, whereas others present with scoliosis without neurologic signs (4). Idiopathic scoliosis in a young person is painless and usually not associated with neurologic deficit. Painful scoliosis should raise the question of an underlying pathologic process that should be further evaluated.

Conventional radiography may reveal clues to the presence of an intramedullary tumor. The most frequent radiographic changes are widening of the interpedicular distance over several segments; thinning, flattening, or erosion of the pedicles; and increase in the sagittal diameter of the spinal canal. In the cervical spine, evaluation of the interpedicular distance is not reliable. Thus, an increase in the sagittal diameter of the cervical canal is more meaningful than an apparent increase in the interpedicular distance (1).

Magnetic resonance imaging is the method of choice in the evaluation of patients suspected of having a spinal cord tumor. The location and full extent of an intramedullary tumor can be identified. Images can be obtained in sagittal, axial, and coronal planes as needed for complete evaluation. Sagittal imaging is particularly useful because of the long segments of the spinal cord that may be involved with intramedullary tumors. Paramagnetic contrast enhancement can be used in the evaluation of these patients (Appendix 1).

An intramedullary tumor infiltrates and swells the spinal cord, thus thinning the surrounding subarachnoid space (Figs. 33-2 to 33-4). Edema may be present around the tumor. Inhomogeneous MR signal may be caused by cystic degeneration, necrosis, and hemorrhage. In attempting to differentiate tumor with necrosis or cystic degeneration from syringomyelia, the combination of nonuniform signal, nonisointensity with cerebrospinal fluid, and indistinct margins proved to be a neoplasm in only 60 percent of intramedullary lesions studied, and is therefore not diagnostic of neoplasm (15). Also, intratumoral cysts and cysts located rostral and caudal to tumor may have signal isointense with tumor or spinal cord, making identification difficult (8). This may be related to their contents, which includes proteinaceous fluid and possibly chronic hemorrhage (8,11).

Intramedullary tumors may be difficult to visualize with conventional unenhanced MR imaging. These tumors may be isointense relative to the spinal cord on T1-weighted images (10). On T2-weighted images, a

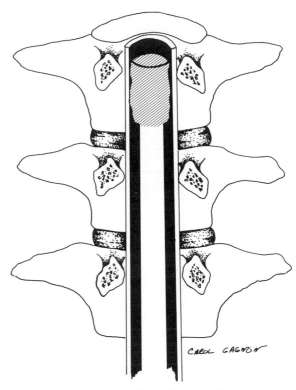

FIG. 33-3. Relationship of an intramedullary tumor to the thecal sac in the coronal plane. *Shaded area* indicates the intramedullary mass. Notice the symmetric thinning of the subarachnoid space (*black area*).

multinodular appearance may be seen that is difficult to distinguish from surrounding edema. Small intramedullary tumors may not be seen because of partial volume averaging. Tumors may also be difficult to differentiate from adjacent isointense gliosis or from

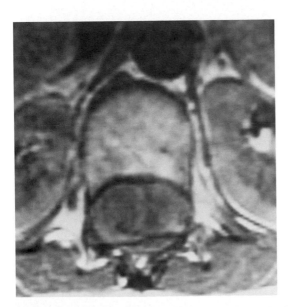

FIG. 33-2. Astrocytoma. Same patient as shown in Fig. 33-1. Axial T1-weighted image shows the tumor filling and expanding the spinal cord.

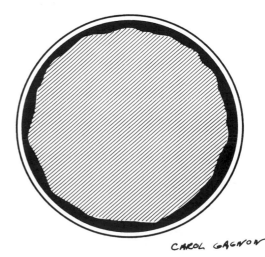

FIG. 33-4. Relationship of an intramedullary tumor to the thecal sac in the axial plane. This representation highlights the features of an intramedullary tumor similar to that seen with axial MR. The intramedullary mass (*shaded area*) compresses the subarachnoid space (*black area*).

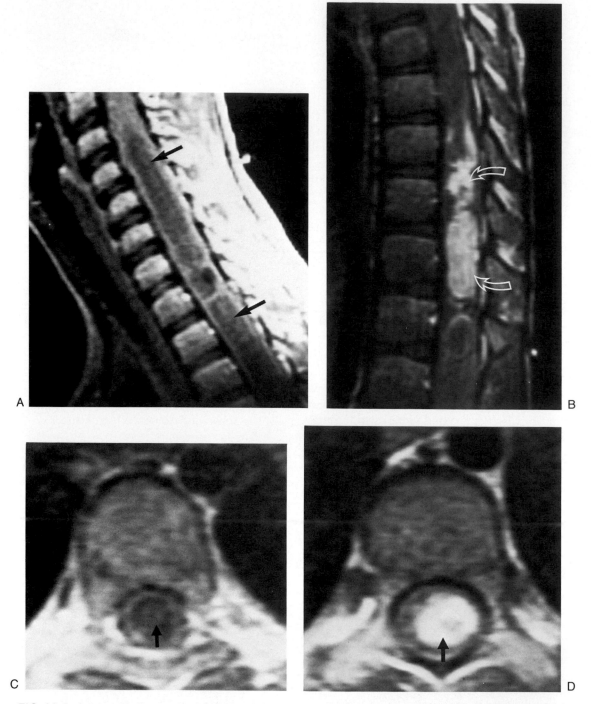

FIG. 33-5. Intramedullary ependymoma of the thoracic spine with extensive cystic cavitation in an 8-year-old girl. **A**: Sagittal T1-weighted SE MR image (800/25) after the injection of gadopentetate dimeglumine shows enlargement of the spinal cord and intramedullary cavitation over multiple cervical and upper thoracic levels (*arrows*). No solid tumor is seen. **B**: Sagittal T1-weighted SE MR image (800/25) after injection of contrast shows enhancement of solid portion of the ependymoma in the lower thoracic spine (*arrows*). **C**: Axial T1-weighted SE MR image (600/20) of lower thoracic spine prior to contrast injection shows low-signal-intensity lesion (*arrow*) within intermediate-signal spinal cord. The surrounding cerebrospinal fluid has been effaced. **D**: Axial T1-weighted SE MR image (600/20) after intravenous injection of gadopentetate dimeglumine shows marked enhancement of the solid portion of the ependymoma (*arrow*).

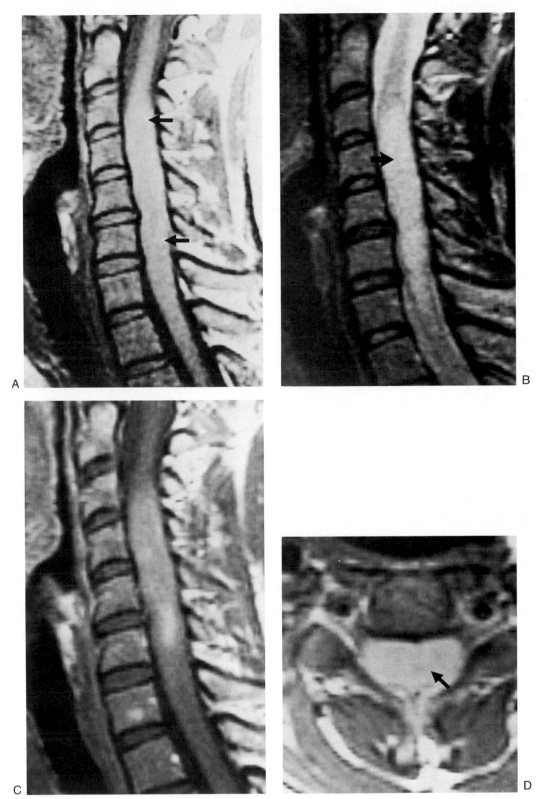

FIG. 33-6. Ependymoma of the cervical spine in a 36-year-old woman who presented with numbness and tingling of the hands. **A**: Sagittal T1-weighted SE MR image (700/20) shows widening of the spinal cord (*arrows*) from C3 to C7. **B**: Sagittal T2-weighted SE MR image (2250/70) shows hyperintensity of intramedullary mass (*arrow*) relative to normal cord. **C**: Sagittal T1-weighted SE MR image (700/20) after the intravenous injection of gadopentetate dimeglumine shows patchy inhomogeneous enhancement of the mass which proved at surgery to be an ependymoma. An astrocytoma could have a similar appearance. **D**: Axial T1-weighted SE MR image (600/20) after injection of contrast shows enhancement of the mass (*arrow*) which fills the canal and compresses the surrounding subarachnoid space.

isointense cysts with exudative fluid (6,11,14). The intravenous injection of gadopentetate dimeglumine can be very useful in the evaluation of patients with intramedullary tumors (Fig. 33-5). The enhancement of intramedullary gliomas depends on a breakdown of the blood-brain (cord) barrier. Ependymomas tend to show intense, homogeneous, sharply marginated enhancement (6,10). This enhancement may be marked on delayed images (14). Cystic degeneration or cavitation which may be present within an ependymoma is best visualized after contrast enhancement of the tumor (6,10). Spinal astrocytomas, including low grade astrocytomas, also show contrast enhancement which tends to be inhomogeneous and patchy with either smooth or irregular margins (6,10). Intratumoral cavitation can be seen. Although there are some enhancement pattern differences between ependymomas and astrocytomas, there is overlap in the appearance of these tumors which prevents accurate differentiation on the basis of postenhancement characteristics (2,3, 6,10) (Fig. 33-6).

In one study, thirteen patients with proved intramedullary spinal cord neoplasm were examined with high-field-strength MR imaging (1.5-T) before and after the intravenous injection of gadopentetate dimeglumine (6). Portions of each neoplasm showed marked enhancement. The diagnosis of an intramedullary tumor could be made on only the postenhancement studies in four of thirteen patients, and in an additional five patients the use of contrast improved diagnostic confidence. In a literature review of 55 cases of spinal cord glioma studied with contrast-enhanced MR, 98 percent showed enhancement (12). Gadopentetate dimeglumine may also be useful in differentiating intramedullary tumors from extramedullary lesions, and residual or recurrent tumor from postsurgical and postradiation changes (6,10,13). Delayed imaging obtained 20 minutes after injection of gadopentetate dimeglumine may show further increase in signal intensity of intramedullary tumors, making them more conspicuous (14).

One other interesting observation should be mentioned. In a study of thirty-five patients with intramedullary spinal tumors, eight (23 percent) had hypointen-

sity on T1- and T2-weighted images caused by hemosiderin deposition, usually at the tumor margin or less frequently within the tumor (9). All of the surgically proved tumors with hypointense areas of hemosiderin were ependymomas, and these accounted for 64 percent (seven of eleven) of the ependymomas in the series. The MR demonstration of an intramedullary tumor with hemosiderin at the tumor margin is believed to be suggestive, but not pathognomonic, of an ependymoma (9).

REFERENCES

1. Banna M, Gryspeerdt GL. Intraspinal tumors in children (excluding dysraphism). *Clin Radiol* 1971;22:17–32.
2. Breger RK, Williams AL, Daniels DL, et al. Contrast enhancement in spinal MR imaging. *AJNR* 1989;10:633–7.
3. Bydder GM, Brown J, Niendorf HP, et al. Enhancement of cervical intraspinal tumors in MR imaging with intravenous gadolinium-DTPA. *J Comput Assist Tomogr* 1985;9:847–51.
4. Citron N, Edgar MA, Sheehy J, et al. Intramedullary spinal cord tumors presenting as scoliosis. *J Bone Joint Surg (Br)* 1984;66B: 513–7.
5. DeSousa AL, Kalsbeck JE, Mealey J Jr, et al. Intraspinal tumors in children. *J Neurosurg* 1979;51:437–45.
6. Dillon WP, Norman D, Newton TH, et al. Intradural spinal cord lesions: Gd-DTPA-enhanced MR imaging. *Radiology* 1989;170: 229–37.
7. Epstein F, Epstein N. Surgical treatment of spinal cord astrocytomas of childhood: a series of 19 patients. *J Neurosurg* 1982; 57:685–9.
8. Goy AMC, Pinto RS, Raghavendra BN. Intramedullary spinal cord tumors: MR imaging, with emphasis on associated cysts. *Radiology* 1986;161:381–6.
9. Nemoto Y, Inoue Y, Tashiro T, et al. Intramedullary spinal cord tumors: significance of associated hemorrhage at MR imaging. *Radiology* 1992;182:793–6.
10. Parizel PM, Balériaux D, Rodesch G, et al. Gd-DTPA-enhanced MR imaging of spinal tumors. *AJNR* 1989;10:249–58, *AJR* 1989; 152:1087–96.
11. Slasky BS, Bydder GM, Niendorf HP, et al. MR imaging with gadolinium-DTPA in the differentiation of tumor, syrinx, and cyst of the spinal cord. *J Comput Assist Tomogr* 1987;11:845–50.
12. Sze G. MR imaging of the spinal cord: current status and future advances. *AJR* 1992;159:149–59.
13. Sze G, Krol G, Zimmerman RD, et al. Intramedullary disease of the spine: diagnosis using gadolinium-DTPA-enhanced MR imaging. *AJNR* 1988;9:847–58, *AJR* 1988;151:1193–204.
14. Valk J. Gd-DTPA in MR of spinal lesions. *AJNR* 1988;9:345–50, *AJR* 1988;150:1163–8.
15. Williams AL, Haughton VM, Pojunas KW, et al. Differentiation of intramedullary neoplasms and cysts by MR. *AJNR* 1987;8: 527–32, *AJR* 1987;149:159–64.

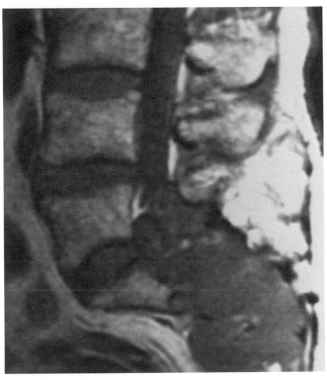

FIG. 34-1A. This 66-year-old man was evaluated because of low back pain. Sagittal T1-weighted SE MR image (600/20) of the lumbosacral spine.

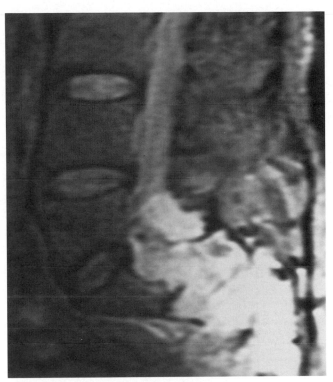

FIG. 34-1B. Sagittal T2-weighted SE MR image (2000/70).

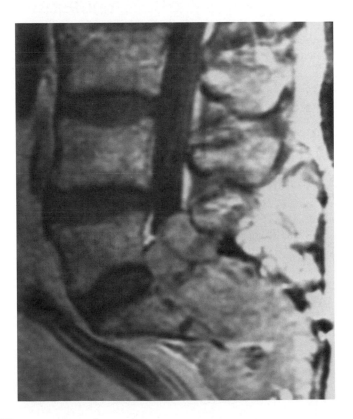

FIG. 34-1C. Sagittal T1-weighted SE MR image (600/20) obtained after the intravenous injection of gadopentetate dimeglumine.

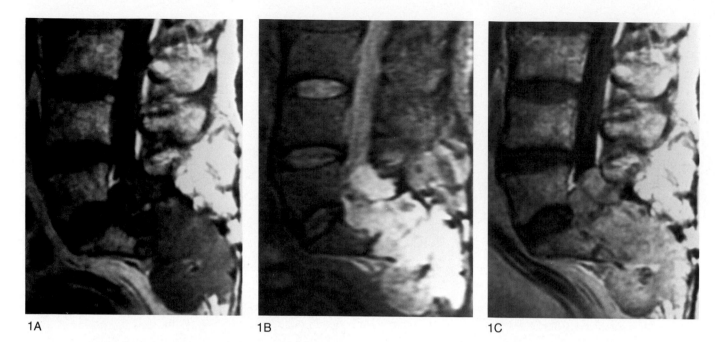

1A　　　　　　　　　　1B　　　　　　　　　　1C

FIG. 34-1A. Chordoma. There is destruction of the sacrum and a large lobulated soft-tissue mass with low signal intensity is seen extending into the sacral and lower spinal canal.

FIG. 34-1B. The mass has heterogeneous increased signal intensity on the T2-weighted image.

FIG. 34-1C. After the injection of contrast there is moderate enhancement compared to the precontrast T1-weighted image shown in Fig. 34-1A.

CHORDOMA OF THE SACRUM

A large destructive mass is well seen on the T1- and T2-weighted MR images and proved to be a chordoma of the sacrum (Figs. 34-1A, 1B). Moderate enhancement of the mass is seen after the intravenous injection of gadopentetate dimeglumine (Fig. 34-1C); CTM shows sacral destruction with soft-tissue extension into the sacral canal and foramina (Fig. 34-2).

Chordoma is a rare primary bone tumor that arises from notochord rests. A review of several large series finds chordoma most prevalent in the sacrococcygeal region (50 percent), followed by the clivus (35 percent), and vertebral column (15 percent) (1,10). It most commonly develops during the fourth through seventh decades. In the sacrum, chordoma usually begins in the midline of the 4th and 5th sacral vertebrae and is typically a progressive, slow growing tumor that reaches large size (5).

There are two types of chordoma: a conventional chordoma which consists of cords of physaliphorous cells varying from a compact tumor mass to strands of tumor within a gelatinous matrix and a chondroid tumor which has varying amounts of cartilage tissue (11).

Chordoma of the sacrum begins centrally and is often symmetric when discovered but may appear asymmetric when large. It may involve the sacral foramina and central sacral canal. Extension of tumor into the presacral soft-tissues or buttocks is common and massive soft tissue involvement may seem out of proportion to the bone destruction (1). Although slow growing, chordomas may metastasize, usually to the lungs or lymph nodes (4). Rarely, chondromas metastasize to the subarachnoid space (4) or spinal cord (2).

The sacrum is a difficult bone to evaluate with conventional radiographs because of its curvature and the presence of overlying bowel gas and feces. Magnetic resonance imaging or CT can be helpful since they allow for excellent evaluation of the bony sacrum, neural foramina, central sacral canal, parasacral soft-tissues, and sacroiliac joints.

With MR, T1- and T2-weighted images are usually sufficient to evaluate the extent of sacral lesions (Fig. 34-3). On T1-weighted images, chordomas appear as lobulated masses and have intermediate signal intensity in 75 percent of cases and low signal intensity in 25 percent (11), typically with a heterogeneous pattern.

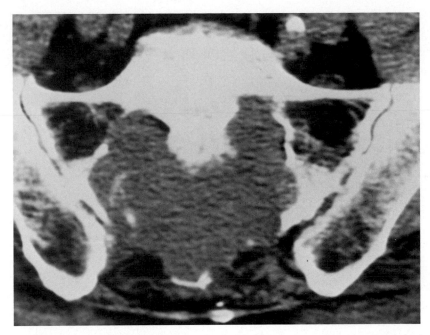

FIG. 34-2. Chordoma of sacrum. Axial CTM of the same patient as Fig. 34-1. There is destruction of the sacrum. The soft-tissue mass fills the sacral canal and foramina and there is blockage to the flow of myelographic contrast.

The amount of calcification present within the tumor may alter the signal characteristics of the tumor since large amounts of calcification appear as flocculent, low signal within the tumor mass. All chordomas have increased signal intensity on T2-weighted images. About 70 percent have low signal fibrous septations within the mass and a pseudocapsule of low signal intensity may be observed as well (11). Conventional chordomas have longer T1 and T2 relaxation times than do chondroid chordomas. This is probably due to the gelati-

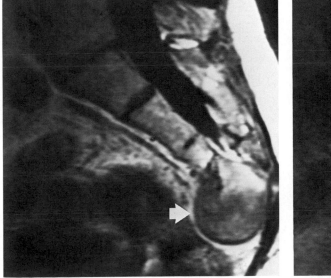
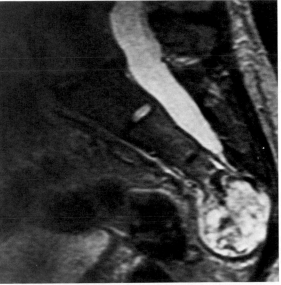

A   B

FIG. 34-3. Recurrent chordoma of the sacrum. There had been partial surgical resection for chordoma 13 years ago. **A**: Sagittal T1-weighted SE MR image (600/25) of the sacrum. There is a destructive, expansive mass in the region of the distal sacrum (*arrow*) that shows heterogeneous intermediate signal intensity as well as a low signal intensity rim (pseudocapsule). **B**: Sagittal T2-weighted SE MR image (2500/80). The tumor appears heterogeneous with predominantly increased signal intensity interspersed with areas of intermediate and decreased signal. Although these signal characteristics are not specific for chordoma, the location of the tumor should suggest the diagnosis. The low signal intensity rim is again seen.

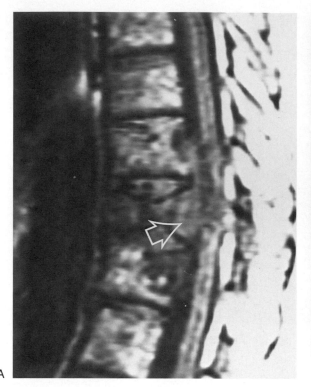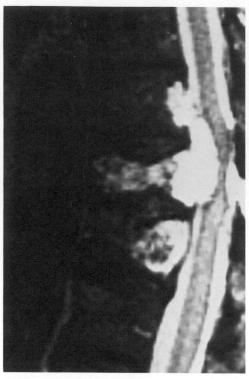

A

B

FIG. 34-4. Chordoma involving three contiguous vertebral bodies. **A**: Sagittal T1-weighted SE MR image (500/23) of the thoracolumbar spine. There is diffuse decreased signal intensity of the T10 vertebral body with a soft-tissue mass extending posteriorly (*arrow*), compressing the spinal cord. Involvement of the posterior aspect of the T9 and T11 vertebral bodies is noted. **B**: Sagittal T2-weighted SE MR image (2400/80). The chordoma involves three contiguous vertebrae and shows heterogeneous, predominantly high signal intensity. The epidural extension of the mass shows homogeneous increased signal intensity and is causing compression and displacement of the spinal cord.

nous watery matrix of conventional chordomas compared to the cartilaginous matrix of chondroid chordomas (11).

Computed tomography shows a mixed osteolytic and osteoblastic pattern although pure osteoblastic or pure osteolytic lesions may develop (3) (see Fig. 34-2). Calcification is frequently detected with CT and is found more commonly in chordomas of the sacrum than in those of other axial sites (3).

Chordoma occurs more frequently in the cervical and lumbar spine than in the thoracic spine (6,7,10). Pain is the most frequent initial complaint of patients with chordoma of the cervical spine. Occasionally these patients present with dysphagia or with respiratory difficulty caused by soft-tissue extension of the mass into the posterior pharynx (9).

Spinal chordoma extending into the posterior elements is not common initially but occurs frequently with recurrent disease (6). Chordoma is usually associated with an anterior or lateral paraspinal mass. There may be involvement of two contiguous vertebral bodies with invasion of the intervertebral disc, a feature

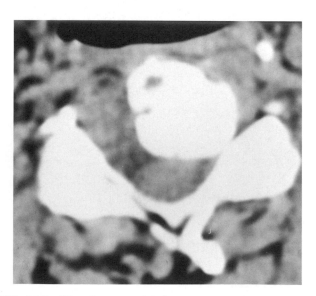

FIG. 34-5. Chordoma. Axial CT through the level of the C4-C5 neural foramina. There is destruction of the right side of the C4 vertebral body and marked widening of the right neural foramen. Tumor extends into the intervertebral canal and spinal canal. Adjacent images showed spinal cord compression. Chordoma is an uncommon cause of widening of the neural foramen.

that is unusual in other tumors of the spine (1,2,7) (Fig. 34-4). Rarely, a chordoma may enlarge the intervertebral foramen and simulate a neurofibroma (12) (Fig. 34-5).

The CT appearance of spinal chordoma is similar to that of sacral chordoma. Amorphous calcification of the tumor mass is found in 40 percent of vertebral chordomas (6). Calcification is more extensive in the periphery of the tumor (3). A sharply defined pseudo-capsule may be evident (6). In over 50 percent of vertebral chordomas, there are single or multiple areas of low attenuation within tumor mass (6), probably representing myxomatous or gelantinous tissue (10).

The MR appearance of spinal chordoma is similar to that of sacral chordoma. Rarely, chordoma may be entirely osteoblastic on the conventional radiograph, resembling an ''ivory'' vertebra (8). Such a lesion appears as very low signal intensity on T1-weighted images because of the sclerosis. Magnetic resonance imaging can delineate the morphology and extent of tumor in the paraspinal and epidural spaces as well as any involvement of the posterior elements and contiguous vertebrae.

REFERENCES

1. Friooznia H, Golimbu C, Rafii M, et al. Computed tomography of spinal chordomas. *CT* 1986;10:45–50.
2. Friooznia H, Pinto RS, Lin JP, et al. Chordoma: radiologic evaluation of 20 cases. *AJR* 1976;127:797–805.
3. Krol G, Sundaresan N, Deck M. Computed tomography of axial chordomas. *J Comput Assist Tomogr* 1983;7:286–9.
4. Krol G, Sze G, Arbit E, et al. Intradural metastases of chordoma. *AJNR* 1989;10:193–5.
5. Levine E, Batnitzky F. Computed tomography of sacral and presacral lesions. *Crit Rev Diag Imaging* 1984;21:307–74.
6. Meyer JE, Lepke RA, Lindfors KK, et al. Chordomas: their CT appearance in the cervical, thoracic and lumbar spine. *Radiology* 1984;153:693–6.
7. Murali R, Rovit RL, Benjamin MV. Chordoma of the cervical spine. *Neurosurgery* 1981;9:253–6.
8. Schwarz SS, Fisher WS III, Pulliam MW et al. Thoracic chordoma in a patient with paraparesis and ivory vertebral body. *Neurosurgery* 1985;16:100–2.
9. Shallat RF, Taekman MS, Nagle RC. Unusual presentation of cervical chordoma with long-term survival. *J Neurosurg* 1982;57:716–8.
10. Sundaresan N, Galicich JH, Chu FCH, et al. Spinal chordomas. *J Neurosurg* 1979;50:312–9.
11. Sze G, Uichanco LS, Brant-Zawadski MN, et al. Chordomas: MR imaging. *Radiology* 1988;166:187–91.
12. Wang A-M, Joachim CL, Shillito J Jr, et al. Cervical chordoma presenting with intervertebral foramen enlargement mimicking neurofibroma: CT findings. *J Comput Assist Tomogr* 1984;8:529–32.

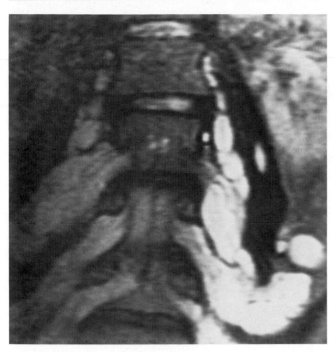

FIG. 35-1A. This 25-year-old woman has a systemic disorder. Coronal T2-weighted SE MR image (2000/70) of lumbar spine.

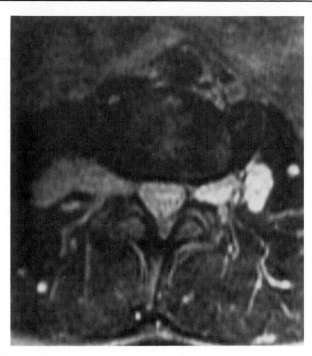

FIG. 35-1B. Axial T2-weighted SE MR image (2000/70) at L3-L4.

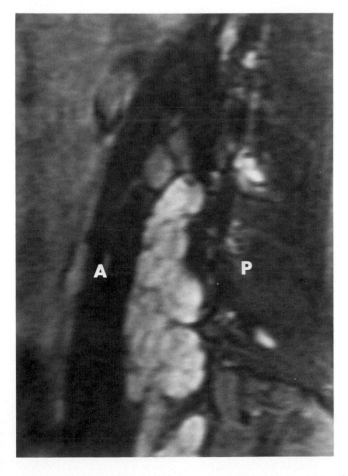

FIG. 35-1C. Sagittal T2-weighted SE MR image (2000/70) obtained 4 cm left of midline. A, anterior; P, posterior.

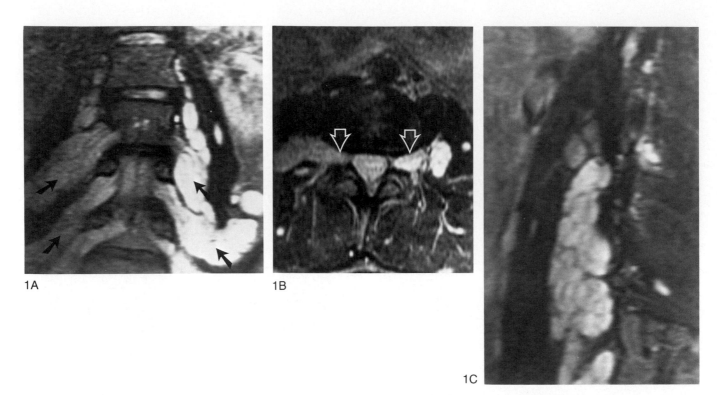

FIG. 35-1A. Neurofibromatosis. Numerous neurofibromas (*arrows*) are present bilaterally extending along the lumbar nerves, and are well seen on the coronal image. These tumors have high signal intensity on T2-weighted images. The lack of high signal of the tumors on the right is caused by asymmetric positioning of the surface coil off of the midline.

FIG. 35-1B. The neurofibromas are seen within the neural foramina (*arrows*) at this L3-L4 level.

FIG. 35-1C. The T2-weighted parasagittal image shows bright signal of the multiple lobulated neurofibromas.

NEUROFIBROMATOSIS

In this case, T2-weighted coronal, axial, and parasagittal MR images show extensive bilateral neurofibromas (Fig. 35-1). High-signal-intensity fusiform masses are seen along all of the spinal nerve roots visualized. A T2-weighted axial image obtained at the sacral level shows neurofibromas within the sacral foramina (Fig. 35-2). Paravertebral neurofibromas are also seen anteriorly.

Neurofibromatosis is a hereditary hamartomatous disorder, probably of neural crest origin, involving neuroectodermal, mesodermal, and endodermal tissues (6). It is classified as one of the phacomatoses (4). There are two major distinct forms of neurofibromatosis which differ in their clinical, biochemical, and genetic manifestations (11,13,14). Neurofibromatosis 1 (NF-1) is characterized by multiple café au lait spots, multiple cutaneous and subcutaneous neurofibromas, freckling in the axillary or inguinal regions, optic glioma and central nervous system tumors such as spinal neurofibroma, plexiform neurofibroma, meningioma,

and other gliomas, as well as iris hamartomas (Lisch nodules) and distinctive osseous lesions such as sphenoid dysplasia and pseudoarthrosis (11,13,14). This is the classical neurofibromatosis as described by von Recklinghausen, an autosomal dominant disorder that affects approximately 1 in 4000 individuals (13). Neurofibromatosis 2 (NF-2) is an autosomal dominant disorder that occurs in about 1 in 50,000 individuals and is characterized by the presence of bilateral acoustic neuromas (11,13). These patients may also have multiple tumors such as neurofibroma, meningioma, glioma, or schwannoma. Cutaneous manifestations are typically less prominent in NF-2 than they are in classic von Recklinghausen neurofibromatosis. There are genetic differences as well, with the gene locus of NF-1 on chromosome 17 and that of NF-2 on chromosome 22. Both forms have autosomal transmission and are highly penetrant. Because NF-1 and NF-2 may have both central and peripheral nervous system manifestations, the previously used terms *peripheral neurofibro-*

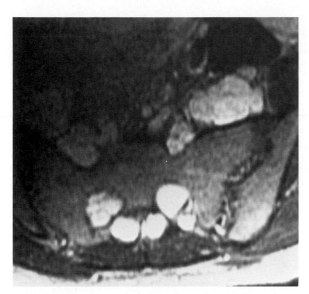

FIG. 35-2. Neurofibromatosis. Axial T2-weighted SE MR image (2000/70) at sacral level in same patient as Fig. 35-1. Multiple neurofibromas fill the sacral canal and foramina and are seen as high signal intensity on the T2-weighted image. Presacral neurofibromas are also seen.

matosis for the classic von Recklinghausen form and *central neurofibromatosis* for the bilateral acoustic neuroma form have been discarded (13).

Multiple neurofibromas are well seen with MR imaging. These tumors have slightly greater signal intensity than muscle on T1-weighted images and markedly increased signal intensity on T2-weighted images (2). This corresponds to the typical CT appearance of low attenuation masses (20–30 HU). In one MR study, 63 percent of patients with neurofibromatosis had central areas of decreased signal intensity in many of the neurofibromas seen on T2-weighted images (2). The low-intensity center is thought to correspond to relatively fibrous components of the neurofibroma, while the bright signal of the surrounding mass on T2-weighted images is due to its myxoid matrix (2). Within large neurofibromas that measure 3–5 cm, several distinct central areas of decreased signal intensity may form a ring pattern (2). In some patients, such as in the present case, numerous neurofibromas are seen as an elaborate network of fusiform and spherical masses depicted by MR imaging. Dumbbell-shaped neurofibromas may be found causing spinal cord compression and enlargement of neural foramina. Occasionally, a neurofibroma degenerates into a neurofibrosarcoma. MR imaging of a neurofibrosarcoma was described in one report as a large, well-circumscribed mass that had a heterogeneous center on T2-weighted images due to necrosis (2).

Patients with neurofibromatosis may develop intramedullary abnormalities such as astrocytoma, ependymoma, syringomyelia, and central schwannoma which can be seen with MR imaging (2,8,12). Asymptomatic hamartomas or heterotopic lesions of the spinal cord may also be present and are seen as increased signal intensity on T2-weighted images without spinal cord enlargement (7). These lesions appear normal on T1-weighted images and do not produce mass effect. Associated hamartomas of the brain may be found in the basal ganglia, thalamus, hypothalamus, cerebral peduncles, and cerebellar white matter (7).

Magnetic resonance imaging permits noninvasive evaluation of patients with neurofibromatosis (Fig. 35-3), including demonstration of the size and location of the masses, compression of the spinal cord, and paravertebral extension. This imaging modality can be very useful in the pediatric population. Multiple planes, including direct coronal imaging, are useful in studying patients with neurofibromatosis. Extensive neurofibromata can be seen, sometimes involving each spinal nerve root with extension into the intercostal region.

In one study, gadopentetate dimeglumine-enhanced T1-weighted images and STIR images were compared and found to be complementary in screening patients with neurofibromatosis (15). Neurofibromas enhance on T1-weighted images obtained after the intravenous injection of gadopentetate dimeglumine. This technique is particularly useful for intradural tumors, since these may be difficult to visualize with conventional unenhanced SE sequences, especially when the tumors are small (Figs. 35-3, 35-4). The STIR sequences may be favored for evaluating extradural lesions, with the neurofibromas appearing bright compared to the intensity of surrounding muscle and suppressed fat (15).

In one study, twenty-eight patients with NF-1 and nine patients with NF-2 were studied with contrast-enhanced spinal MR imaging (5). All patients with NF-2 had intradural extramedullary masses, most often schwannomas or meningiomas. These patients had multiple masses that frequently had more than one histology. Intramedullary masses were found in five of nine patients (55 percent), most often ependymomas. Patients with NF-1 had intradural extramedullary masses consistent with neurofibromas in five of twenty-eight cases (18 percent) and extradural masses in one case (4 percent). Intramedullary tumors occur in a smaller percentage of patients with NF-1 than with NF-2. This study found that intradural tumors occur frequently in both NF-1 and NF-2 in asymptomatic, relatively young patients. This observation has prompted the investigators to recommend routine MR imaging of the entire spine in patients with neurofibromatosis (5).

Spinal alterations are frequent in neurofibromatosis and are most often due to mesodermal dysplasia (bone, dura) but may also be caused by neural tumors and lateral thoracic meningoceles (6,9). In the general population, the most common cause of posterior scalloping of one or more vertebral bodies is neurofibromatosis

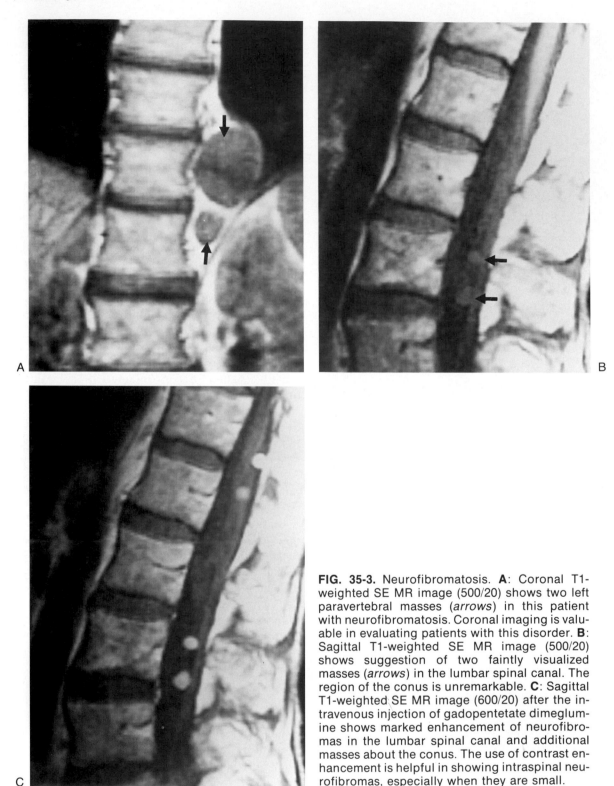

FIG. 35-3. Neurofibromatosis. **A**: Coronal T1-weighted SE MR image (500/20) shows two left paravertebral masses (*arrows*) in this patient with neurofibromatosis. Coronal imaging is valuable in evaluating patients with this disorder. **B**: Sagittal T1-weighted SE MR image (500/20) shows suggestion of two faintly visualized masses (*arrows*) in the lumbar spinal canal. The region of the conus is unremarkable. **C**: Sagittal T1-weighted SE MR image (600/20) after the intravenous injection of gadopentetate dimeglumine shows marked enhancement of neurofibromas in the lumbar spinal canal and additional masses about the conus. The use of contrast enhancement is helpful in showing intraspinal neurofibromas, especially when they are small.

(9). Posterior scalloping is present in approximately 14 percent of patients with neurofibromatosis and is most often due to dural ectasia (4). The dural ectasia occurs secondary to mesenchymal abnormality which allows dilatation of the subarachnoid space (9) (Fig. 35-5A).

Posterior scalloping can also occur secondary to one or more neurofibromas. Although posterior scalloping of the vertebral body can be seen with conventional radiography, CTM and MR imaging are useful modalities capable of determining the cause of the posterior

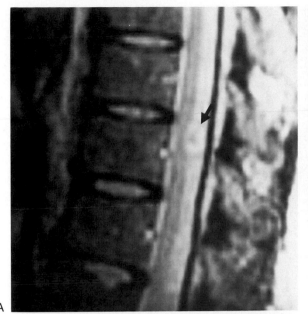

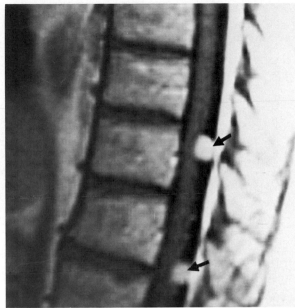

A

B

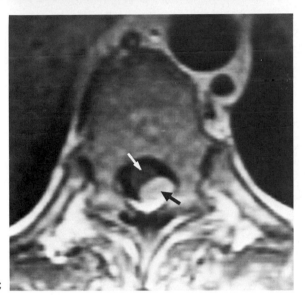

C

FIG. 35-4. Neurofibromatosis. **A**: Sagittal T2-weighted SE MR image (2000/70) shows faint suggestion of small intraspinal mass (*arrow*) at T10 in this patient with neurofibromatosis. **B**: Sagittal T1-weighted SE MR image (600/10) after the intravenous injection of gadopentetate dimeglumine reveals marked enhancement of the tumor at T10, and an additional unsuspected mass at T11-T12 (*arrows*) that proved to be schwannomas at surgery. The demonstration of additional neural tumors is greatly aided by the use of contrast enhancement. **C**: Axial T1-weighted SE MR image (600/20) at T10 after contrast injection shows enhancement of the schwannoma (*black arrow*) compressing the spinal cord (*white arrow*).

vertebral scalloping (i.e., distinguishing between dural ectasia and tumor) (1). Lateral and anterior vertebral body scalloping may occur either secondary to adjacent neural tumor or as a primary mesodermal dysplasia of bone (3).

Kyphoscoliosis is the most frequent skeletal abnormality in neurofibromatosis and occurs in approximately 45 percent of patients (4). Again, this is usually the result of mesodermal dysplasia but in some cases may be related to thoracolumbar spinal tumors (4). The kyphoscoliosis found in patients with neurofibromatosis is classically angular and of a short segment with a predominance of the kyphotic portion. The ky-

phoscoliosis may be rapidly progressive and when severe enough may cause spinal cord or cauda equina compression (Fig. 35-5B). One or more pedicles may be abnormal in patients with neurofibromatosis. Agenesis, hypoplasia, and mesial erosion of the pedicles have been described (4,10) (Fig. 35-5C). Other skeletal manifestations of neurofibromatosis include widening of the neural foramen, widening of the spinal canal, hypoplasia of the transverse process, spina bifida, and thinning of the ribs (4,6,17). Patients with neurofibromatosis may sustain subluxation or dislocation of the spine that may even occur in the absence of significant trauma or preexisting scoliosis or kyphosis (16).

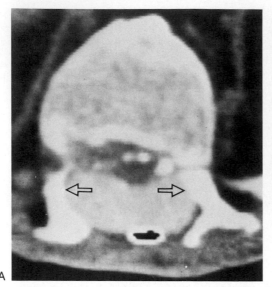

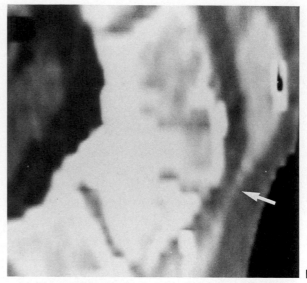

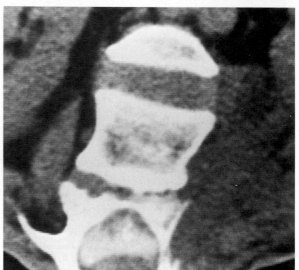

FIG. 35-5. Neurofibromatosis. **A**: Axial CTM of the thoracolumbar spine shows dural ectasia causing mesial scalloping of the pedicles (*arrows*). The pedicles are hypoplastic. In addition there is spina bifida. These abnormalities are due to neurofibromatosis. A droplet of Pantopaque contrast is seen posteriorly and is from a previous myelogram. **B**: Sagittal reconstruction of axial CTM images. Kyphosis, most severe from T11 to L2, is causing marked compression of the subarachnoid space (*arrow*). **C**: This axial CTM is obtained at the level of maximum kyphosis. Because of the severe kyphosis, three vertebrae and two intervertebral disc spaces are examined on the same axial CT section. Posterior scalloping of the vertebral body and mesial scalloping of the pedicles can be appreciated. There is a left paravertebral mass that was better seen on other axial images.

REFERENCES

1. Angtuaco EJC, Binet EF, Flanigan S. Value of computed tomographic myelography in neurofibromatosis. *Neurosurgery* 1983; 13:666–71.
2. Burk DL Jr, Brunberg JA, Kanal E, et al. Spinal and paraspinal neurofibromatosis: surface coil MR imaging at 1.5 T. *Radiology* 1987;162:797–801.
3. Casselman ES, Mandell GA. Vertebral scalloping in neurofibromatosis. *Radiology* 1979;131:89–94.
4. Casselman ES, Miller WT, Lin SR, et al. Von Recklinghausen's disease: incidence of roentgenographic findings with a clinical review of the literature. *Crit Rev Diag Imag* 1977;9:387–419.
5. Egelhoff JC, Bates DJ, Ross JS, et al. Spinal MR findings in neurofibromatosis types 1 and 2. *AJNR* 1992;13:1071–7.
6. Holt JF. Neurofibromatosis in children. *AJR* 1978;130:615–39.
7. Katz BH, Quencer RM. Hamartomatous spinal cord lesion in neurofibromatosis. *AJNR* 1989;10:S101.
8. Kim T, Foust RJ, Mojtahedi S. MR imaging of asymptomatic brainstem and spinal cord lesions in sisters with neurofibromatosis. *AJNR* 1989;10:S71–2.
9. Leeds NE, Jacobson HG. Spinal neurofibromatosis. *AJR* 1976; 126:617–23.
10. Mandell GA. The pedicle in neurofibromatosis. *AJR* 1978;130: 675–8.
11. Martuza RL, Eldridge R. Neurofibromatosis 2-(Bilateral acoustic neurofibromatosis). *N Engl J Med* 1988;318:684–8.
12. Mayer JS, Kulkarni MV, Yeakley JW. Craniocervical manifestations of neurofibromatosis: MR versus CT studies. *J Comput Assist Tomogr* 1987;11:839–44.
13. National Institutes of Health Consensus Development Conference. Neurofibromatosis: conference statement. *Arch Neurol* 1988;45:575–8.
14. Riccardi VM. Von Recklinghausen neurofibromatosis. *N Engl J Med* 1981;305:1617–27.
15. Stimac GK, Porter BA, Olson DO, et al. Gadolinium-DTPA-enhanced MR imaging of spinal neoplasms: preliminary investigation and comparison with unenhanced spin-echo and STIR sequences. *AJNR* 1988;9:839–46, *AJR* 1988;151:1185–92.
16. Stone JW, Bridwell KH, Shackelford GD, et al. Dural ectasia associated with spontaneous dislocation of the upper part of the thoracic spine in neurofibromatosis: a case report and review of the literature. *J Bone Joint Surg* 1987;69A:1079–83.
17. Yaghmai I. Spine changes in neurofibromatosis. *RadioGraphics* 1986;6:261–85.

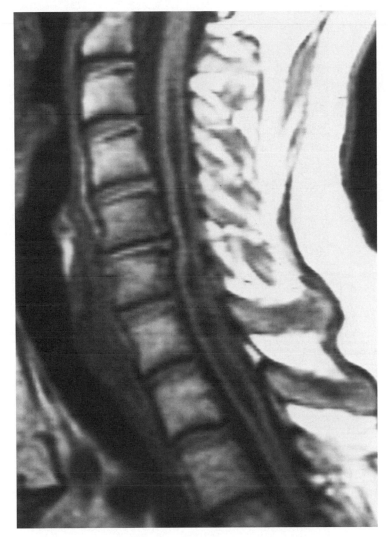

FIG. 36-1. Sagittal T1-weighted SE MR image (500/12) of the cervical spine in a 48-year-old woman.

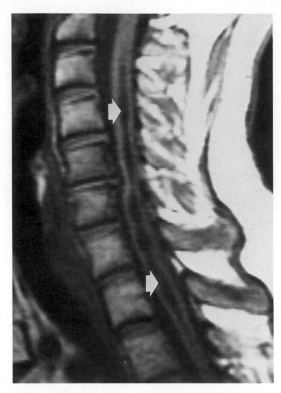

FIG. 36-1. Syringohydromyelia. There is a syrinx of low signal intensity within the central canal (*arrows*) extending from C2-C3 to the upper thoracic spine. Mild disc bulging is seen at C5-C6. A Chiari I malformation was present but is not shown.

SYRINGOHYDROMYELIA

In this case, MR imaging shows an area of low signal intensity within the spinal cord on the T1-weighted image (Fig. 36-1). This patient has syringohydromyelia. The syrinx is seen as low signal intensity on the axial T1-weighted image (Fig. 36-2A) and as high signal on the sagittal GRE image (Fig. 36-2B).

Hydromyelia is an intramedullary cavity lined by ependymal cells. It represents cystic dilatation of the central canal of the spinal cord. Hydromyelia is of congenital origin and is frequently associated with hindbrain abnormalities such as Chiari malformation (8). Some patients with hydromyelia may develop syringomyelia. Syringomyelia is another type of intramedullary cavity that is lined by glial cells and develops extrinsic to the central canal of the spinal cord. Since syringomyelia and hydromyelia are so closely associated developmentally, clinically, and even radiographically, they may be considered together as syringohydromyelia (2). Usually, syringohydromyelia involves the dorsal aspect of the cervical cord. In most cases, the cavity is found in the cervicothoracic junction (13) and, in some cases, may even involve the entire cord.

Patients with syringohydromyelia typically present with diminution of pain and temperature perception in the upper extremities, which progresses to paresis and muscle atrophy (2). Thoracic scoliosis and neurotrophic joints in the upper extremities also occur in this disorder. Rapidly progressive scoliosis in patients with myelomeningocele may be associated with extensive syringohydromyelia and Chiari malformation (12).

Syringohydromyelia is sometimes "acquired," developing secondary to spinal cord tumor (see Case 33, Fig. 5A), extramedullary tumor, trauma with hematomyelia, or arachnoiditis (2–4,6,9,10). Tumor should be considered when the syrinx spares the cervical cord (the typical location of "true" syringomyelia), extends for only a short segment, or has a nodular, irregular wall.

Magnetic resonance imaging is the modality of choice in the evaluation of syringohydromyelia, and may disclose cysts that are not detectable by other imaging modalities. T1- and T2-weighted images (Appendix 1) are used to establish the presence, morphology, and extent of the syrinx; the extent of cord edema, gliosis, or myelomalacia; the presence or absence of an associated tumor, Chiari malformation, or hydro-

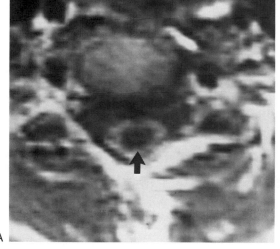
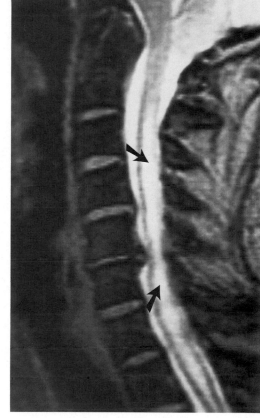

A

B

FIG. 36-2. Syringohydromyelia. Same patient as in Fig. 36-1. **A**: Axial T1-weighted SE MR image (650/14) shows the syrinx as low signal intensity (*arrow*) within the spinal cord of intermediate signal. **B**: Sagittal GRE image (MPGR, 500/15 with 15-degree flip angle) of the cervical spine shows the syrinx with bright signal intensity (*arrows*) within the spinal cord of intermediate signal.

cephalus; and the fluid dynamics within the cyst. The diagnosis of syringohydromyelia is established with the demonstration of a cyst within the spinal cord. A cyst with relatively stationary fluid has decreased signal intensity on T1- and increased signal intensity on T2-weighted images, with greater signal intensity seen on T2-weighted images than on proton density-weighted images (7). A cyst that has fluid in motion may be inhomogeneous with areas of decreased signal intensity on both T1- and T2-weighted images (flow-void) (14) with greater signal intensity seen on proton density-weighted images than on T2-weighted images (7). The flow-void is maximized on ungated, non-motion-compensated T2-weighted images. It may be large at times and is most likely to be seen in larger cysts (13). Flow-void prevents accurate assessment of the exact intensity of the syrinx fluid. Although a cyst with flow-void is usually seen in the congenital form of hydromyelia, it has been noted in cysts associated with other causes (13). The presence of a signal flow-void within a syrinx may have prognostic significance, since shifting of pulsatile fluid may be important in the extension of syrinx

cavities, independent of the factors that caused the syrinx to form initially (13).

Sagittal T1-weighted images are ideal for evaluating the size and extent of the syrinx (Fig. 36-3) and the location of the cerebellar tonsils. Septations may be evident in some large cysts. They consist of fibrous-glial tissue, may reside in a single large cyst or in multiple cysts, and may give an appearance of a "beaded" syrinx (13).

On T1-weighted images hypointense signal intensity within the cord does not always represent fluid within a cyst, as myelomalacia may also have this appearance. Proton-density images may be useful in differentiating cystic fluid from myelomalacia. A cyst shows low signal intensity on the proton-density image, whereas myelomalacia typically has intermediate to high signal intensity (7).

There is a truncation artifact (Gibbs phenomenon) that may be seen on sagittal MR images and should not be mistaken for syringohydromyelia. It appears as linear low signal intensity in the center of the spinal cord (5,11). This artifact can be eliminated by increas-

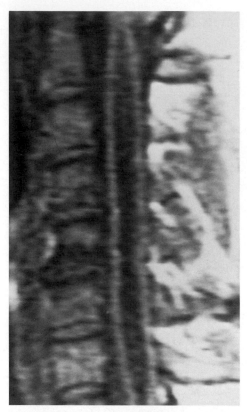

FIG. 36-3. Syringohydromyelia. Sagittal T1-weighted SE MR image (600/20) of the cervical spine shows a syrinx that is causing spinal cord enlargement. Note the decrease in size of the subarachnoid space caused by the widened spinal cord.

ing the number of phase-encoding steps (using an acquisition matrix of 256 × 256 rather than 256 × 128), decreasing the field of view, and switching phase- and frequency-encoding axes (5).

Axial T1-weighted images show the relationship of the syrinx to the spinal cord and can show the presence of multiple cysts not visible on sagittal views. The size of the spinal cord can be determined with axial T1-weighted images as well. In one large series of adults with syringohydromyelia examined by CTM, spinal cord size was most frequently normal (45 percent) or reduced (45 percent); it was enlarged in only 10 percent (1).

Syringohydromyelia may develop following significant spinal cord trauma (3,4), seen in about 3 percent of patients with spinal cord injury (4). It usually presents with new and/or progressively deteriorating neurologic symptoms which begin months to many years

after the injury. Less frequently, there is progressive deterioration in the neurologic status from the onset of injury and in some cases there is a failure of new or progressive symptoms to develop. A cyst is formed by liquefaction of the hemorrhagic necrosis at the site of injury and from extension of necrosis into adjacent normal cord (15). T2-weighted images may show increased signal intensity within the spinal cord adjacent to the cyst that could represent gliosis, edema, or myelomalacia (13).

Following decompression, MR imaging shows collapse of an adequately treated syrinx and lack of a flow-void (3). Magnetic resonance imaging can also show the location of a shunt catheter to determine whether it is within the syrinx. The alterations of myelomalacia, often present adjacent to the syrinx, usually remain unchanged following corrective shunting.

REFERENCES

1. Aubin ML, Vignaud J, Jardin C, et al. Computed tomography in 75 clinical cases of syringomyelia. *AJNR* 1981;2:199–204.
2. Ballantine HT Jr, Ojemann RG, Drew JH. Syringohydromyelia. *Progr Neurol Surg* 1971;4:227–45.
3. Barkovich AJ, Sherman JL, Citrin CM, et al. MR of postoperative syringomyelia. *AJNR* 1987;8:319–27.
4. Bradway JK, Kavanagh BF, Houser OW. Post-traumatic spinal-cord cyst: a case report. *J Bone Joint Surg Am* 1986;68A:932–3.
5. Bronskill MJ, McVeigh ER, Kucharczyk W, et al. Syrinx-like artifacts on MR images of the spinal cord. *Radiology* 1988;166:485–8.
6. Castillo M, Quencer RM, Green BA, et al. Syringomyelia as a consequence of compressive extramedullary lesions: postoperative clinical and radiological manifestations. *AJR* 1988;150:391–6.
7. Enzmann DR. Syringomyelia. In: Enzmann DR, DeLaPaz RL, Rubin JB, eds. *Magnetic resonance of the spine.* St. Louis: CV Mosby Co; 1990:540–67.
8. Gardner WJ. Hydrodynamic mechanism of syringomyelia: its relationship to myelocele. *J Neurol Neurosurg Psychy* 1965;28:247–59.
9. Goy AMC, Pinto RS, Raghavendra BN, et al. Intramedullary spinal cord tumors: MR imaging, with emphasis on associated cysts. *Radiology* 1986;161:381–6.
10. Lee BCP, Zimmerman RD, Manning JJ, et al. MR imaging of syringomyelia and hydromyelia. *AJNR* 1985;6:221–8.
11. Levy LM, DiChiro G, Brooks RA, et al. Spinal cord artifacts from truncation errors during MR imaging. *Radiology* 1988;166:479–83.
12. Samuelsson L, Bergstrom K, Thuomas K-A, et al. MR imaging of syringohydromyelia and Chiari malformations in myelomeningocele patients with scoliosis. *AJNR* 1987;8:539–46.
13. Sherman JL, Barkovich AJ, Citrin CM. The MR appearance of syringomyelia: new observations. *AJR* 1987;148:381–91.
14. Sherman JL, Citrin CM, Gangarosa RE, et al. The MR appearance of CSF pulsations in the spinal canal. *AJNR* 1986;7:879–84.
15. Stevens JM, Olner JS, Kendall BE. Post-traumatic cystic and non-cystic myelopathy. *Neuroradiology* 1985;27:48–56.

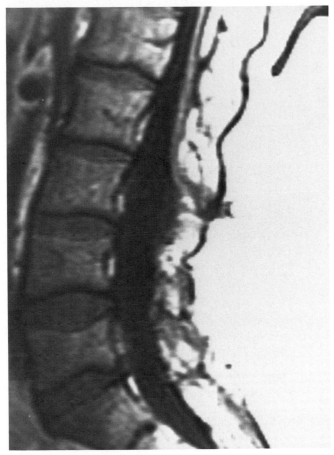

FIG. 37-1A. This 58-year-old man presented with a new onset of leg weakness. Sagittal T1-weighted SE MR image (700/15) of the lumbar spine.

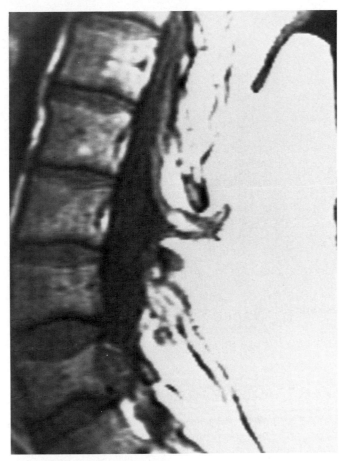

FIG. 37-1B. Sagittal T1-weighted image obtained 5 mm to the left of Fig. 37-1A.

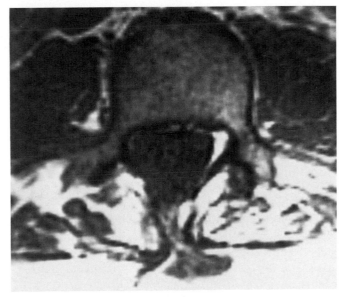

FIG. 37-1C. Axial T1-weighted SE MR image (700/15) at the L3 level.

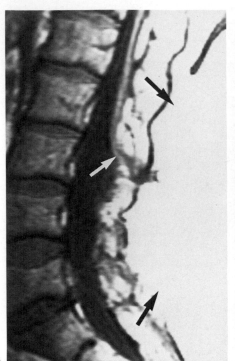
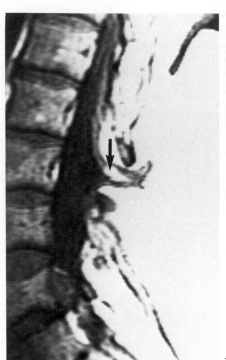
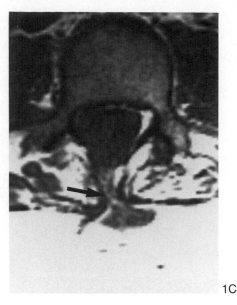

1A   1B   1C

FIG. 37-1A. Lipomyelomeningocele. The spinal cord (*white arrow*) and thecal sac protrude posteriorly into a large subcutaneous lipomatous mass (*black arrows*) of high signal intensity. A disc herniation is present at L5-S1.

FIG. 37-1B. On this image a lipoma (*arrow*) is seen attached to the cord within the protruding thecal sac (meningocele) and extends into the subcutaneous lipomatous mass.

FIG. 37-1C. The thecal sac and neural elements (*arrow*) extend through a dorsal spinal defect into the lipomatous mass.

LIPOMYELOMENINGOCELE

In this case the MR images show the spinal cord and thecal sac protruding posteriorly through an osseous defect into a huge subcutaneous lipomatous mass (Fig. 37-1). This is a lipomyelomeningocele, one of several forms of spinal dysraphism.

Spinal dysraphism indicates a failure of complete fusion of tissues in the dorsal median plane of the developing embryo that leads to anomalies of the skin, bones, dura, spinal cord and nerves. Spinal dysraphism is a complex clinical state that is associated with a broad spectrum of abnormalities that vary in severity and may occur alone or in combination. Some dysraphic conditions such as myeloceles, myelomeningoceles, and many meningoceles are overt (i.e., clearly visible and easily diagnosed on physical examination). Other forms of dysraphism such as lipomyelomeningocele, diastematomyelia, tethered cord and associated intraspinal masses such as lipomas and cysts, are occult (i.e., not visible on physical examination but suspected because of cutaneous and/or neurologic, or-

thopedic, or urologic abnormalities) (2). The cutaneous anomalies in patients with occult dysraphism usually develop in the lower back and include a patch of hair, nevus, lipoma, or dermal sinus (4). Occasionally, occult spinal dysraphism may go undiagnosed until adult life (8). In the overall classification of these disorders we prefer, as do others, the term *spinal dysraphism* to *spina bifida*. Spina bifida (bifid spine) is considered a skeletal dysraphism in which there is a fusion defect of the posterior vertebral elements or, rarely, the vertebral body (Fig. 37-2). The defect varies from a narrow slit of the lamina, detected only by radiography, to splaying or absence of the laminae at several levels. Mild, narrow posterior spina bifida, particularly at L5-S1, is commonly found in asymptomatic patients and is called *spina bifida occulta*. It occurs in approximately 20 percent of the general population and by itself is of no clinical significance (1).

Meningocele is a form of dysraphism in which there is herniation of skin-covered arachnoid and dura

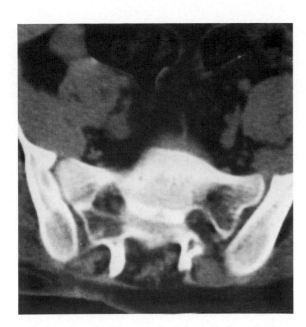

FIG. 37-2. Spina bifida. Axial CT through the proximal sacrum. The laminae are widely splayed, forming a large dorsal bony defect.

through a spina bifida, most often in the lumbosacral region (3). Neural tissue is not present within the protruding sac (4). Vertebral arch defects and widening of the spinal canal are localized and relatively mild. There is no association with syringohydromyelia or Chiari malformation (4).

A myelocele is a severe form of dysraphism in which a plaque of neural tissue representing malformed spinal cord lies exposed and flush with the skin surface (4). Ventral and dorsal nerve roots arising from the neural plaque traverse the subarachnoid space. A myelomeningocele is a myelocele that has been elevated above the skin surface by a protruding arachnoid space (meningocele) (3,4). The term *myelomeningocele* is often used to include both myeloceles and myelomeningoceles (i.e., myeloceles without or with a sac) and is similarly used here. Myelomeningoceles usually develop in the lumbosacral region. These disorders are more devastating than simple meningoceles. Patients with myelomeningocele almost invariably have tethered cord and Chiari II malformation (4). They frequently have hydrocephalus (80 percent) (7) and less often have associated diastematomyelia and/or syringohydromyelia (60 percent) (11). Scoliosis, which may be congenital or acquired, has been reported to occur in 90 percent of patients with myelomeningocele (6). Dysraphic changes in the spine are more extensive in patients with myelomeningocele than those that occur with simple meningocele.

Lipomyelomeningocele is a skin-covered myelomeningocele associated with a subcutaneous lipomatous-connective tissue mass (lipoma). The lipoma attaches to the dorsal surface of the neural plaque and tethers the cord (5). Lipomyelomeningocele accounts for 20–50 percent of cases in patients with occult spinal dysraphism (7,11). Skeletal manifestations of dysraphism are evident. The lipoma may extend into the spinal canal through the dorsal defect (5). Lipomyelomeningoceles are not likely to be associated with a neuromusculoskeletal syndrome at birth (3). Chiari malformation, hydrocephalus, syringohydromyelia, and diastematomyelia are not usually associated with lipomyelomeningocele (4). In both myelomeningocele and lipomyelomeningocele, the dorsal (sensory) nerve roots arise from the placode laterally and the ventral (motor) nerve roots arise more medially (11). The nerve roots continue into the subarachnoid space before exiting their respective neural foramina.

A myelomeningocystocele is a meningocele with a markedly dilated central canal and a lipomyelomeningocystocele is a lipomyelomeningocele with a dilated central canal (10). The spinal cord is positioned more anteriorly and the posterior aspect of the cord is thin and accompanies the meningeal hernia (10).

In patients with spinal dysraphism, the imaging modality utilized varies with the disorder, clinical condition of the patient, the institution, imaging modalities available, and experience of the imaging physician. Most meningoceles are easily diagnosed at birth and, in healthy infants, may be repaired during the first week of life (3). Since they do not as a rule have a tethered cord or Chiari malformation, and surgery is relatively uncomplicated, imaging other than conventional radiography is not usually performed, even though the thecal sac is readily accessible (2,3). However, on occasion a fluctuant mass in the low back may not be a fluid-filled meningocele but rather a lipoma, cystic tumor, or other cystic lesion (3) (Fig. 37-3). When the diagnosis of meningocele is uncertain, imaging with ultrasonography or MR can aid in establishing a diagnosis. Myelomeningocele is easily diagnosed clinically at birth. Most patients are not imaged preoperatively since surgery is performed on viable children as soon as possible (within 30–36 hours after birth) (3), and it is known that patients with myelomeningocele almost invariably have a tethered cord and Chiari II malformation. The goal of surgery is to free the neural plaque, place it into the spinal canal, and reconstruct the dura (2,7). Lipomyelomeningoceles and other forms of occult dysraphism should be imaged when suspected clinically.

Magnetic resonance has revolutionized the imaging evaluation of patients with dysraphism and, in most clinical settings, has virtually replaced CTM and myelography. Magnetic resonance imaging can be used to determine the morphology of the underlying disorder as well as the presence of associated tumor masses, syringohydromyelia, and Chiari malformation. The

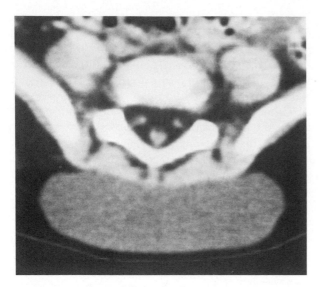

FIG. 37-3. Lymphangioma. This 6-month-old child presented with a palpable mass in the low back that had gradually increased in size since birth. Lower lumbar level CTM reveals a large mass of fluid density in the subcutaneous tissues. The mass did not fill with intrathecal contrast. The laminae are intact, precluding a dysraphic condition (Fig. courtesy of Spencer Borden IV, MD., Philadelphia, Pennsylvania).

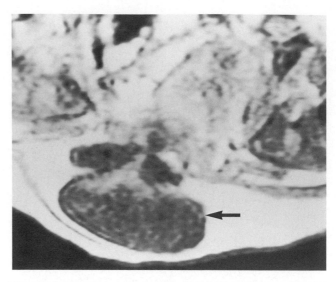

FIG. 37-4. Myelomeningocele. Axial T1-weighted SE MR image (700/20) shows posterior protrusion of the thecal sac (*arrow*) and neural elements through a dorsal bony defect in this 1-month-old infant. Scoliosis is present.

choice of appropriate pulse sequences and planes of imaging are dependent upon the clinical condition and the information desired. In most dysraphic conditions, T1-weighted images are frequently sufficient. The choice of planes of imaging is also dependent upon the clinical condition and information desired. Sagittal images are useful for determining the position of the spinal cord (tethered or not) or the presence of a Chiari malformation. They are usually sufficient to diagnose the presence and location of a lipomatous mass, although axial images allow for better evaluation of the extent of the mass and its relationship to the spinal cord. Syringohydromyelia can often be diagnosed in the sagittal plane but sometimes partial volume averaging, even with thin slices, may not detect a small syrinx, so that the axial views are important as they not only define the extent of the syrinx related to the cord width, but at times establish the diagnosis. Coronal and axial views are useful for diagnosing diastematomyelia.

With MR imaging, a meningocele is seen as a fluid-filled sac extending from the subarachnoid space. A meningocele does not contain nerve roots. On T1-weighted images the sac has decreased signal and on T2-weighted images has increased signal intensity.

A myelomeningocele is seen as a fluid-filled sac containing cerebrospinal fluid; however, the spinal cord enters the sac and ends as a placode on the surface (Fig. 37-4). On the sagittal view, the normal configuration of the conus is replaced by a wider, flatter configuration of the neural plaque (9). The cord can be fol-

lowed through the dorsal defect to where the plaque attaches to the skin surface (Fig. 37-5). The nerve roots originating from the neural plaque traverse the dilated subarachnoid space in a dorsal-ventral direction. On T1-weighted images, nerve roots are slightly lower in signal intensity than spinal cord, possibly because of

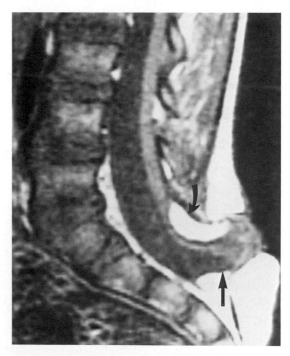

FIG. 37-5. Myelomeningocele. Sagittal T1-weighted SE MR image (600/20) shows the spinal cord and thecal sac (*straight arrow*) protruding through a dorsal bony defect into the subcutaneous tissues. A lipoma (*curved arrow*) is seen adjacent to the low-lying spinal cord.

some partial volume averaging with cerebrospinal fluid (9). On axial views, the tip of the conus and the filum terminale are usually not visualized as separate structures from the cauda equina. The nerve roots are better seen with T2-weighted images which produce a myelographic effect; however, this pulse sequence does not usually add important diagnostic information. Chiari malformation is invariably present and syringohydromyelia is present in 60 percent of cases (11). Following surgical closure of the lesion, the neural plaque may end freely in the dilated subarachnoid space surrounded by cerebrospinal fluid (9). The location of the cord immediately following surgical correction is almost always at the same rostral-caudal location as it was preoperatively (11), although it is slightly more ventral in position (9).

A lipomyelomeningocele appears as a myelomeningocele with the spinal cord extending through the dorsal defect and ending in a subcutaneous lipomatous mass (Fig. 37-6). The fat tissue of the lipomatous mass is easily identified on T1-weighted images as a mass with high signal intensity. However, it may be difficult to determine its exact borders when adjacent to normal subcutaneous fat because of similar signal intensity. Occasionally, a fibrous capsule of low signal intensity on T1-weighted images may be observed separating the lipoma from adjacent subcutaneous tissue (9). Following surgical release, the placode and adjacent fatty tissue lie free in the distal thecal sac. Small adhesions that might be enough to retether the cord might not be visible with MR imaging (9).

Magnetic resonance imaging can be used to differentiate myelomeningocele from myelomeningocystocele and lipomyelomeningocystocele. In patients with myelomeningocystocele and lipomyelomeningocystocele, two fluid-filled compartments can be identified. In one reported case, the outer, more rostral component (cystocele) had a slightly higher signal intensity compared with the inner, more caudal meningocele sac because of greater protein content (10).

In patients with myelomeningocele, MR imaging may be helpful for the evaluation of postsurgical complications. Retethering of the cord may develop as the placode becomes adherent to the dura, dural graft, or subcutaneous tissue adjacent to the surgical site (11). Following myelomeningocele repair, retethering of the cord is found in 3 percent of cases and almost all cases of retethering occur at the site of surgical closure (6). Retethering of the cord may be difficult to assess as the spinal cord usually remains at its preoperative level (6,11). The observation of cerebrospinal fluid between the placode and the posterior aspect of the thecal sac suggests that the cord is not tethered. Additionally, cord tethering is associated with decreased cord motion as evaluated by phase imaging techniques (11). Retethering can be suggested if neural tissue is attached to the repair site by a scar or there is an inclusion mass or thickened filum restricting movement. The incidence of infection is related to the amount of time before repair of the defect. Infection of the ventricles occurs in about 7 percent of cases following early closure (less than 48 hours after birth) and in approximately 37 percent of those repaired after 48 hours (6). Inclusion dermoids are found in 16 percent of patients operated upon for release of a tethered neural placode (6). They form from residual epithelial tissue trapped in the surgical scar or not completely removed from the placode.

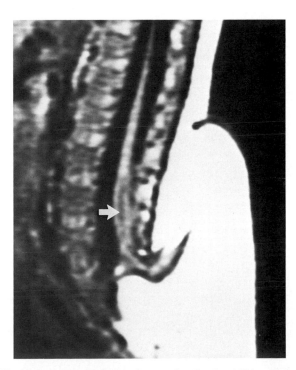

FIG. 37-6. Lipomyelomeningocele. Sagittal T1-weighted SE MR image (600/25) of the lumbosacral spine in a 4-month-old infant. The spinal cord and thecal sac extend through a dorsal bony defect into a large lipomatous mass. There is a syrinx (arrow) noted within the distal cord.

REFERENCES

1. Boone D, Parsons D, Lachmann SM, et al. Spina bifida occulta: lesion or anomaly? *Clin Radiol* 1985;36:159–61.
2. Fitz CR. Midline anomalies of the brain and spine. *Radiol Clin North Am* 1982;20:95–104.
3. French BN. Midline fusion defects and defects of formation. In: Youmans JR, ed. *Neurological surgery.* vol 3. Philadelphia: WB Saunders; 1982:1236–380.
4. Naidich TP, McLone DG, Harwood-Nash DC. Spinal dysraphism. In: Newton TH, Potts DG, eds. *Computed tomography of the spine and spinal cord.* San Anselmo: Clavadel Press; 1983: 299–353.
5. Naidich TP, McLone DG, Mutluer S. A new understanding of dorsal dysraphism with lipoma (lipomyeloschisis): radiologic evaluation and surgical correction. *AJR* 1983;140:1065–78.

6. Nelson MD, Bracchi M, Naidich TP, et al. The natural history of repaired myelomeningocele. *RadioGraphics* 1988;8:695–706.

7. Schut L, Bruce DC, Sutton LN. The management of the child with a lipomyelomeningocele. *Clin Neurosurg* 1983;30:464–76.

8. Sostrin RD, Thompson JR, Rouhe SA, et al. Occult spinal dysraphism in the geriatric patient. *Radiology* 1977;125:165–9.

9. Traill MR, Runge VM, Wolpert SM: Dysraphism: MRI strategies. *MRI Decisions* 1988;July/August:2–9.

10. Vade A, Kennard D. Lipomeningomyelocystocele. *AJNR* 1987;8:375–7.

11. Zimmerman RA, Bilaniuk LT, Bury EA. Magnetic resonance of the pediatric spine. *Mag Res Quart* 1989;5:169–204.

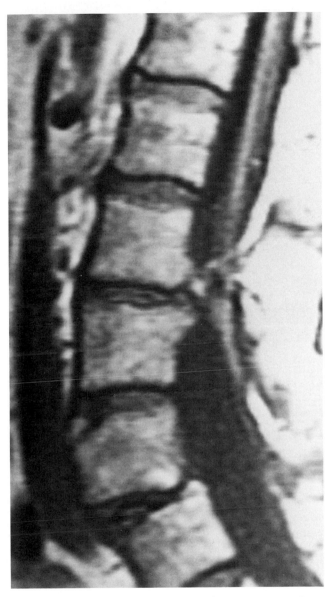

FIG. 38-1A. A 65-year-old woman was evaluated for a possible mass lesion within the spinal canal that was suspected when a CT study performed elsewhere had reportedly showed an enlarged thecal sac. The patient has a history of carcinoma of the breast. Sagittal T1-weighted SE MR image (700/15) obtained in the midline.

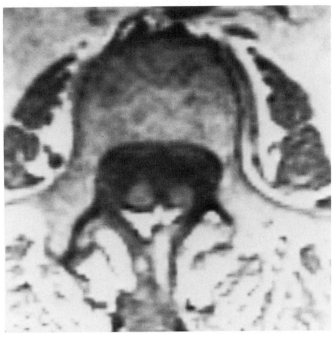

FIG. 38-1B. Axial T1-weighted SE MR image (700/15) obtained at L2.

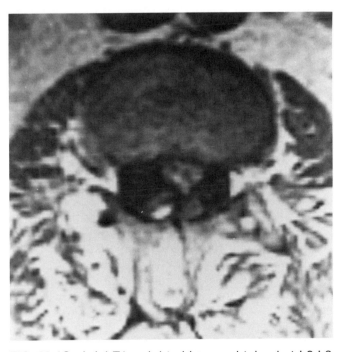

FIG. 38-1C. Axial T1-weighted image obtained at L2-L3.

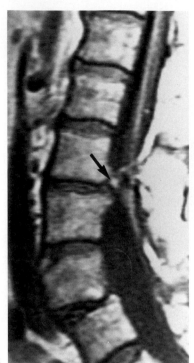
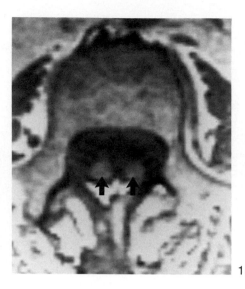
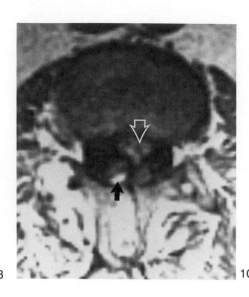

FIG. 38-1A. Diastematomyelia. A large bony spur (*arrow*) is seen at L2-L3. The osseous septum has increased signal intensity on the T1-weighted image because of the presence of fatty marrow. The spinal cord is tethered. There is Grade I spondylolisthesis at L4-L5 incidentally noted.

FIG. 38-1B. At L2 there are two hemicords (*arrows*) in this patient with diastematomyelia.

FIG. 38-1C. The osseous septum (*white arrow*) is seen in the midline. A small lipoma (*black arrow*) of the right hemicord is noted.

DIASTEMATOMYELIA

The sagittal T1-weighted MR image shows a large bony spur of high signal intensity at the L2-L3 level (Fig. 38-1A). An axial image at L2 reveals two round hemicords of intermediate signal intensity (Fig. 38-1B). At L2-L3 the axial image shows the central osseous septum (Fig. 38-1C). A small lipoma is also identified and its presence confirmed on a sagittal image obtained to the right of the midline (Fig. 38-2A). Proton density- and T2-weighted images in the midline further characterize the appearance of the bony septum (Figs. 38-2B, 2C). These findings are characteristic of diastematomyelia.

Diastematomyelia is a form of occult spinal dysraphism in which the spinal cord, conus medullaris, and/or filum terminale are partially or completely divided sagittally into two nearly equal hemicords (8). Each hemicord contains a central canal and an ipsilateral dorsal and ventral horn. The two hemicords usually rejoin caudally into a single cord (6). In 50–80 percent of cases of diastematomyelia, the two hemicords lie within a common subarachnoid space enclosed within a single arachnoid and dura (8,10,11). This form of diastematomyelia has no fibrous septum or osseous cartilaginous spur separating the two hemicords (8). In the other 20–50 percent of cases, the two hemicords each lie within their own separate subarachnoid space covered by their own separate arachnoid and dura (8,10,11). This form of diastematomyelia nearly always has a fibrous septum or osseous cartilaginous spur separating the two dural tubes, each of which contains a hemicord (8). The fibrous septum or bony spur may tether the spinal cord.

Clinically, the signs and symptoms of diastematomyelia may be similar to those of other forms of spinal dysraphism and frequently include a cutaneous abnormality of the back such as a patch of hair, skin dimple, or nevus; abnormal gait; leg weakness; abnormal lower extremity reflexes; scoliosis; and urinary and fecal incontinence (6,11). In one large series, diastematomyelia was found in 28 percent of children examined by CTM because of dysraphism (10). Diastematomyelia occurs in 5 percent of patients with congenital scoliosis

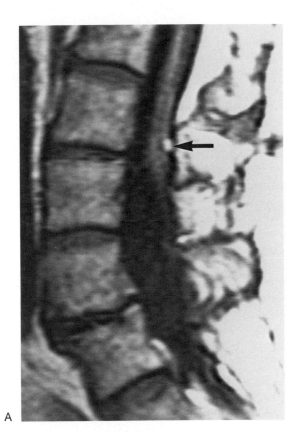

A

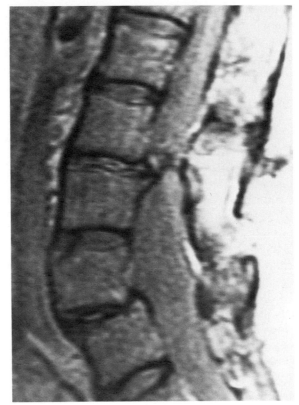

B

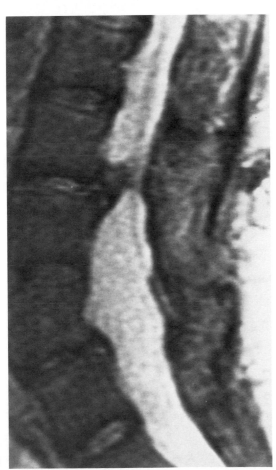

C

FIG. 38-2. Diastematomyelia. Same patient as Fig. 38-1. **A**: Sagittal T1-weighted SE MR image (700/15) obtained 5 mm to the right of the midline shows a small lipoma (*arrow*). Midsagittal proton density-weighted (2000/35) (**B**) and T2-weighted (2,000/70) (**C**) SE MR images further characterize the osseous septum. Note that the septum follows signal characteristics of fatty marrow on all pulse sequences.

and should be excluded in this clinical setting (4). Diastematomyelia is usually discovered in children and is rare in adults (2). It is frequently located in the lumbar region and is rare in the cervical spine.

Once diastematomyelia is suspected clinically, conventional radiographs of the entire spine in AP and lateral projections frequently show spinal abnormalities, the most common being anomalies of the laminae and pedicles occurring in approximately 90 percent of cases (6). Spina bifida, vertical fusion of the laminae, and focal widening of the interpedicular distance are good predictors of the site of cord splitting (6). A calcified spur, although visible in only 30 percent of cases (11), is diagnostic of this disorder and also locates the site of cord splitting (6). Computed tomography can also show the osseous spur as well as other bony abnormalities.

Imaging of patients with diastematomyelia should include identification of the site and extent of cord splitting, demonstration of the presence or absence of a fibrous or osseous cartilaginous spur, and evaluation of associated abnormalities. Conventional myelography followed by CTM can show various features of diastematomyelia (Fig. 38-3) and other frequently associated disorders (1,8,11,14). However, with the advent of MR imaging, these patients can be examined by a noninvasive method that can be used in conjunction with conventional radiography or CT (12,13,15).

Magnetic resonance imaging of many dysraphic conditions is best performed by T1-weighted sagittal images, but because of the parallel orientation of the two

hemicords, axial scans may be necessary to make the diagnosis of diastematomyelia (3,12,13). The two hemicords can be well seen on axial T1-weighted images and appear as intermediate signal intensity structures within the lower-signal cerebrospinal fluid. Coronal T1-weighted images can also be useful, especially when significant scoliosis is present (12). Should severe kyphosis or lordosis be present, however, only small sections of the hemicords can be seen on each successive coronal image, limiting the effectiveness of this imaging plane. In some cases, diastematomyelia may be initially misdiagnosed as a focal area of syringohydromyelia on sagittal T1-weighted images (3). Axial images may be useful for making this differentiation. Diastematomyelia is seen as two adjacent, round intermediate signal hemicords, while syringohydromyelia appears as a central cavity of low signal intensity within a single elliptical cord (3). In some cases of diastematomyelia, cavitation may be found within a hemicord (15). Rarely, double diastematomyelia is present (7).

The identification of a septum may be difficult on T1-weighted images if the septum is fibrous or if an osseous septum lacks fatty marrow (3,12,15). In these cases, the septum has low signal intensity which may be indistinguishable from cerebrospinal fluid on T1-weighted images. T2-weighted axial images may be used to differentiate the septum, which remains of low signal intensity from cerebrospinal fluid which has bright signal with this pulse sequence (3). A bony septum that in part contains fatty marrow may be identified on the T1-weighted images because of the bright signal intensity of fat (5,15). In these cases, sagittal T1-weighted images are useful in localizing the site of spur formation. Regrowth of a previously resected bony spur has been described (9).

Diastematomyelia is associated with other anomalies, some that are well visualized with MR imaging and others that are better seen with conventional radiography or CT. Dural ectasia, tethered cord, caudal lipoma, myelomeningocele, and syringohydromyelia may be found in association with diastematomyelia and are well seen with MR imaging (3,5,15). Osseous abnormalities such as butterfly vertebrae, hemivertebrae, and other anomalies of the laminae and pedicles may be identified with MR imaging, but are generally better seen with conventional radiography or CT.

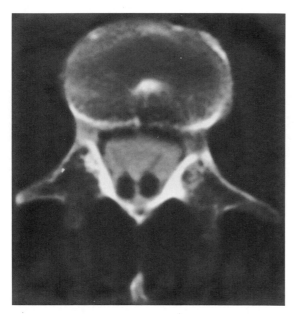

FIG. 38-3. Diastematomyelia; CTM of the lumbar spine shows two hemicords.

REFERENCES

1. Arredondo F, Haughton VM, Hemmy DC, et al. The computed tomographic appearance of the spinal cord in diastematomyelia. *Radiology* 1980;136:685–8.
2. Beyerl BD, Ojemann RG, Davis KR, et al. Cervical diastematomyelia presenting in adulthood. *J Neurosurg* 1985;62:449–53.

3. Davis PC, Hoffman JC Jr, Ball TI, et al. Spinal abnormalities in pediatric patients: MR imaging findings compared with clinical, myelographic, and surgical findings. *Radiology* 1988;166: 679–85.

4. Giordano GB, Cerisoli M. Diastematomyelia and scoliosis: usefulness of CT examination. *Spine* 1983;8:111–2.

5. Han JS, Benson JE, Kaufman B, et al. Demonstration of diastematomyelia and associated abnormalities with MR imaging. *AJNR* 1985;6:215–9.

6. Hilal SK, Marton D, Pollack E. Diastematomyelia in children. *Radiology* 1974;112:609–21.

7. McClelland RR, Marsh DG. Double diastematomyelia. *Radiology* 1977;123:378.

8. Naidich TP, Harwood-Nash DC. Diastematomyelia: hemicord and meningeal sheaths; single and double arachnoid and dural tubes. *AJNR* 1983;4:633–6.

9. Pang D, Parrish RG. Regrowth of diastematomyelic bone spur after extradural resection: case report. *J Neurosurg* 1983;59: 887–90.

10. Pettersson H, Harwood-Nash DCF. *CT and myelography of the spine and cord: techniques, anatomy and pathology in children.* Berlin: Spinger-Verlag; 1982.

11. Scotti G, Musgrave MA, Harwood-Nash DC, et al. Diastematomyelia in children: Metrizamide and CT metrizamide myelography. *AJR* 1980;135:1225–32.

12. Traill MR, Runge VM, Wolpert SM. Dysraphism: MRI strategies. *MRI Decisions*. 1988;2:2–9.

13. Walker HS, Dietrich RB, Flannigan BD, et al. Magnetic resonance imaging of the pediatric spine. *RadioGraphics* 1987;7: 1129–52.

14. Weinstein MA, Rothner AD, Duchesneau P, et al. Computed tomography in diastematomyelia. *Radiology* 1975;118:609–11.

15. Zimmerman RA, Bilaniuk LT, Bury EA. Magnetic resonance of the pediatric spine. *Mag Res Quart* 1989;5:169–204.

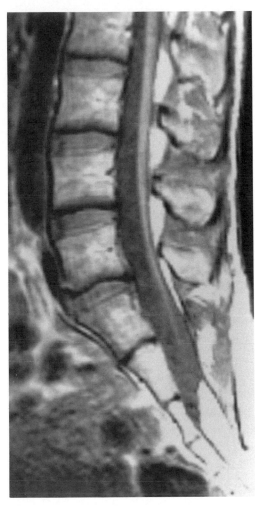

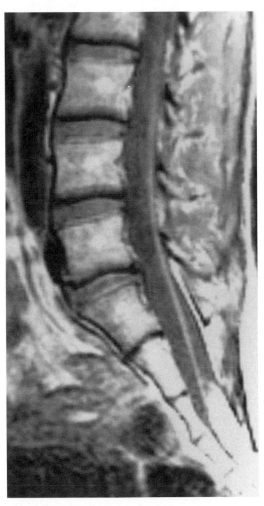

FIG. 39-1A. This 23-year-old man was examined because of bowel and bladder incontinence. Sagittal T1-weighted SE MR image (800/20) in the midline.

FIG. 39-1B. Sagittal T1-weighted image obtained 4 mm to the right of Fig 39-1A.

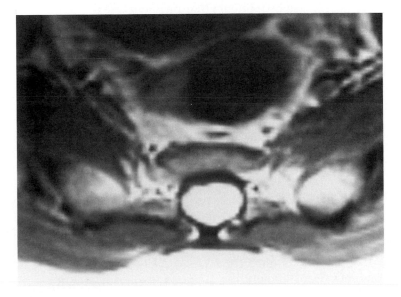

FIG. 39-1C. Axial T1-weighted SE MR image (800/20) at the S3-S4 level.

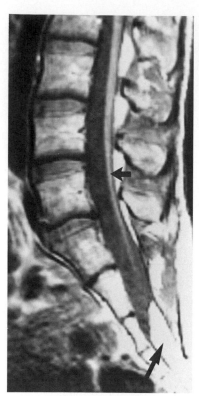

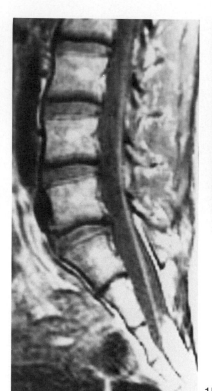

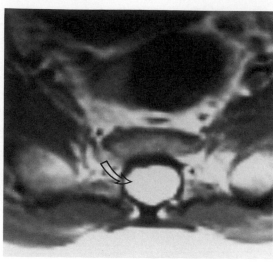

FIG. 39-1A. Tethered cord with lipoma. The spinal cord (*short arrow*) is low lying. There is an intradural lipoma at S3-S4 (*long arrow*) that has very bright signal on the T1-weighted image.

FIG. 39-1B. The conus can be visualized to the S3 level and is tethered by the lipoma. Mild disc bulging is incidentally noted at L5-S1.

FIG. 39-1C. At the S3-S4 level the intradural lipoma (*arrow*) fills the spinal canal and has bright signal intensity on the T1-weighted image because of the short T1 relaxation time of fat.

TETHERED CORD WITH LIPOMA

This patient has a tethered cord that is well seen on sagittal T1-weighted images (Figs. 39-1A, 1B). The cord is tethered by a lipoma that displays bright signal intensity on T1-weighted sagittal and axial (Fig. 39-1C) images. On T2-weighted images, the lipoma appears less bright than on T1-weighted images (Fig. 39-2).

During gestation, the vertebral column develops at a more rapid rate than the spinal cord. Consequently, the conus medullaris "ascends" from the level of the coccyx to approximately the lower border of L2 at birth (2). Two months after birth the conus is at its adult level which is most often opposite L1 or L2 but may be anywhere from T12 to the L2-L3 intervertebral disc (2) (Fig. 39-3). Some authors have suggested that the diagnosis of tethered cord is established if the spinal cord lies below the level of the L2-L3 intervertebral disc after the age of 5 years (4). Others, studying a large series of children with MR imaging, have found that the conus attains the adult level during the first few months of life and that a conus level at L2-L3 or above should be considered normal at any age (13). In patients with tethered cord, the spinal cord is usually fixed (tethered) by one or more abnormalities such as a short, thickened filum terminale; an intradural lipoma; lipomatous infiltration; or fibrous adhesions (9). The cord may also be tethered by the septum in diastematomyelia, by the neural plaque of myelomeningocele, or by adhesions that form at the site of a myelomeningocele repair (5,9). The tethering anomalies cause compression or longitudinal traction on the spinal cord (6,10), and traction may lead to cord ischemia, a possible cause of symptoms (4).

The tethered cord syndrome usually presents during childhood, but milder cases may go undetected until the adult years (1,6,9). Clinically there may be unexplained spastic gait, lower-extremity weakness, scoliosis, foot deformity, or neurogenic bladder or bowel dysfunction (4). Cutaneous manifestations of spinal dysraphism are frequent (4,9).

Conventional radiographs reveal varying degrees of

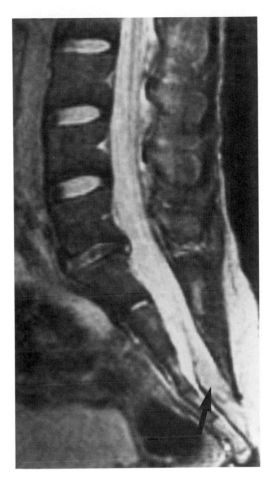

FIG. 39-2. Sagittal T2-weighted SE MR image (2000/70) in same patient as in Fig. 39-1. Signal intensity of the lipoma (*arrow*) is less bright on the T2-weighted image than on the T1-weighted images.

spina bifida, usually mild, involving at least one level in all cases (5,9). A widened spinal canal and posterior scalloping may be present (6) but are not frequent. Magnetic resonance imaging is an excellent method of evaluating patients with tethered spinal cord syndrome. This modality provides a noninvasive, multiplanar method of demonstrating the location of the tip of the conus, causes of the tethering, and osseous dysraphic abnormalities. Sagittal and axial T1-weighted images provide anatomic detail needed to determine the site of the conus. The axial study helps differentiate the conus from adjacent nerve roots of the cauda equina that may be inseparable on the sagittal images. Coronal T1-weighted images are useful when scoliosis is present, and in differentiating a low conus from a thickened filum (13).

Frequently, the cause of tethering is a spinal lipoma, a term which includes intramedullary lipoma, lipoma of the filum terminale, and lipomyelomeningocele. Other causes of tethered spinal cord syndrome include tight filum terminale, diastematomyelia, and myelomenin-

gocele. Intramedullary lipoma appears as a mass of high signal intensity on T1-weighted images (Fig. 39-4). A fatty filum terminale (Fig. 39-5) is found in 1 percent of adults and 6 percent of children studied for occult spinal dysraphism (8). This may be found with or without associated tethered cord. A fatty filum terminale with a normal position of the conus is most likely an asymptomatic finding, although it may be symptomatic. An irregularly thickened fatty filum terminale, however, is likely to be symptomatic, especially when associated with a low conus (8). The presence of a short, thickened filum terminale and a low-lying conus is described as the tight filum terminale syndrome (11). The thickness of the filum terminale is best measured on axial images at the L5-S1 level since at the midlumbar levels the filum may appear normal in width due to stretching. In one study of patients with tethered spinal cord syndrome, the filum was greater than 2 mm in 94 percent of patients (11). Some of these

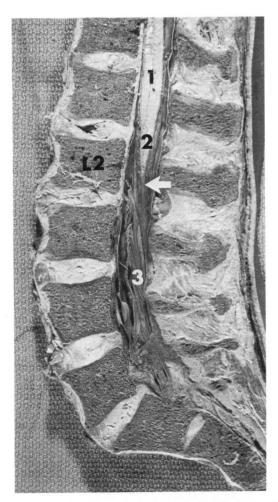

FIG. 39-3. Sagittal section of a gross adult specimen showing the normal level of the conus medullaris. *1,* spinal cord; *2,* conus medullaris; *3,* cauda equina; *arrow,* filum terminale.

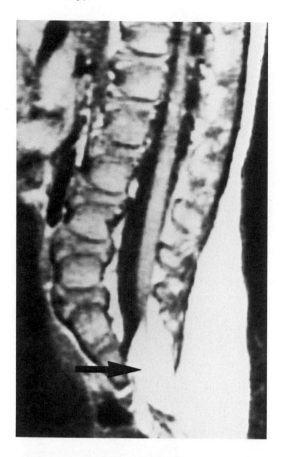

FIG. 39-4. Tethered cord with lipoma. Sagittal T1-weighted SE MR image (400/25) in a 1-year-old girl. A lipoma (*arrow*) is well seen and tethers the cord to the S1 level.

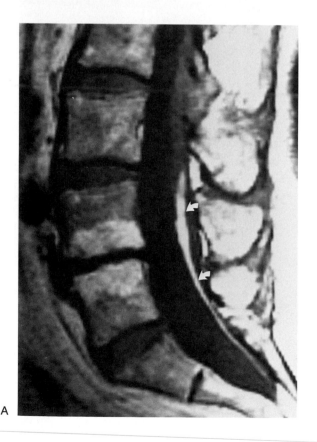

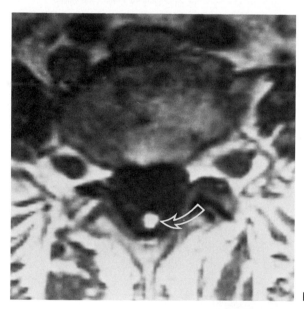

FIG. 39-5. Fatty infiltration of the filum terminale in a 68-year-old woman. **A**: Sagittal T1-weighted SE MR image (700/15) shows bright signal intensity of the filum caused by fatty infiltration (*arrows*). Incidentally noted are degenerative changes of the inferior vertebral body endplate of L4 and the superior endplate of L5 with increased signal intensity caused by fatty replacement. **B**: Axial T1-weighted SE MR image (700/15) again reveals fatty filum terminale (*arrow*).

patients had associated lipoma. Patients with tethered spinal cord syndrome have a normal position of the conus in 16 percent of cases (11). In this circumstance, the diagnosis of tethered cord is made by demonstrating an abnormal filum or a tethering lesion. In one study (12) of pediatric patients evaluated for closed spinal dysraphism, tethered cord was found in 13 percent. Of these patients, 86 percent had a low conus and 64 percent had a thickened filum.

MR imaging may also show sites of syringohydromyelia or myelomalacia within the conus or in the cord adjacent to a tethering lesion (11) (Fig. 39-6). These are best seen on axial T1-weighted images and appear as low signal intensity within the cord, typically measuring 10–40 mm in length and 1–5 mm in diameter (11).

Magnetic resonance imaging may be used to evaluate pediatric patients with scoliosis. In one study (7), 53 percent of children with scoliosis had MR demonstra-

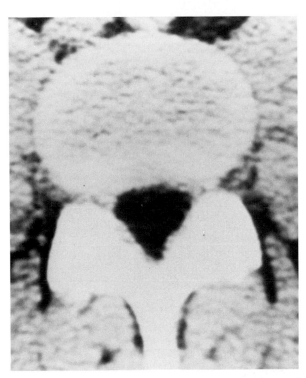

FIG. 39-7. Intradural lipoma. Axial CT of the lumbar spine shows an intradural lipoma of negative CT attenuation value that fills the spinal canal. This patient had an associated tethered cord.

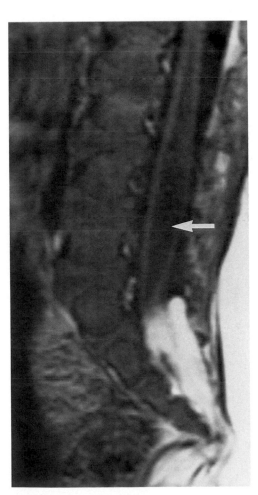

FIG. 39-6. Syrinx within tethered spinal cord. Sagittal T1-weighted SE MR image (400/16) shows the spinal cord tethered to L5-S1 by a lipoma of high signal intensity. A syrinx (arrow) is seen as low signal intensity within the enlarged, low-lying spinal cord.

tion of neuropathologic abnormalities associated with their scoliosis. Of the various neuropathic conditions found, tethered cord was the most common, occurring in 25 percent of children with scoliosis (7). Children with prior meningomyelocele repair can be evaluated with MR imaging. Typically, the conus and/or the neural placode is seen below the L2 level. The diagnosis of tethering is made when neural tissue is attached by scar to the repair site, or is restricted by a tethering mass or thickened filum terminale (3). It may be difficult to confirm the presence of tethering when the neural placode is flat, dorsally positioned, and indistinct from the adjacent thecal sac (3).

Although MR imaging is the study of choice for the evaluation of the tethered cord syndrome, both conventional myelography and CTM can show the presence of cord tethering, thickened filum terminale, intradural mass (4,6), and other causes of cord tethering such as diastematomyelia, myelomeningocele, and lipomyelomeningocele. The position of the conus and the thickness of the filum terminale can be determined by CTM. A low-lying thin cord can be differentiated from a thickened filum terminale if nerve roots are seen arising from the cord. With CTM or CT, intradural lipoma and lipomatous infiltration of the filum or conus can be specifically diagnosed by the negative attenuation coefficient of fat tissue (Fig. 39-7).

REFERENCES

1. Balagura S. Late neurological dysfunction in adult lumbosacral lipoma with tethered cord. *Neurosurgery* 1984;15:724–6.
2. Barson AJ. The vertebral level of termination of the spinal cord during normal and abnormal development. *J Anat* 1970;106:489–97.
3. Davis PC, Hoffman JC Jr, Ball TI, et al. Spinal abnormalities in pediatric patients: MR imaging findings compared with clinical, myelographic, and surgical findings. *Radiology* 1988;166:679–85.
4. Fitz CR, Harwood-Nash DC. The tethered conus. *AJR* 1975;125:515–23.
5. Heinz ER, Rosenbaum AE, Scarff TB, et al. Tethered spinal cord following meningomyelocele repair. *Radiology* 1979;131:153–60.
6. Kaplan JO, Quencer RM. The occult tethered conus syndrome in the adult. *Radiology* 1980;137:387–91.
7. Nokes SR, Murtagh FR, Jones JD III, et al. Childhood scoliosis: MR imaging. *Radiology* 1987;164:791–97.
8. Okumura R, Minami S, Asato R, et al. Fatty filum terminale: assessment with MR imaging. *J Comput Assist Tomogr* 1990;14:571–3.
9. Pang D, Wilberger JE Jr. Tethered cord syndrome in adults. *J Neurosurg* 1982;57:32–47.
10. Sarwar M, Virapongse C, Bhimani S. Primary tethered cord syndrome: a new hypothesis of its origin. *AJNR* 1984;5:235–42.
11. Raghavan N, Barkovich AJ, Edwards M, et al. MR imaging in the tethered spinal cord syndrome. *AJNR* 1989;10:27–36, *AJR* 1989;152:843–52.
12. Scatliff JH, Kendall BE, Kingsley DPE, et al. Closed spinal dysraphism: analysis of clinical, radiological, and surgical findings in 104 consecutive patients. *AJNR* 1989;10:269–77, *AJR* 1989;152:1049–57.
13. Wilson DA, Prince JR. MR imaging determination of the location of the normal conus medullaris throughout childhood. *AJNR* 1989;10:259–62, *AJR* 1989;152:1029–32.

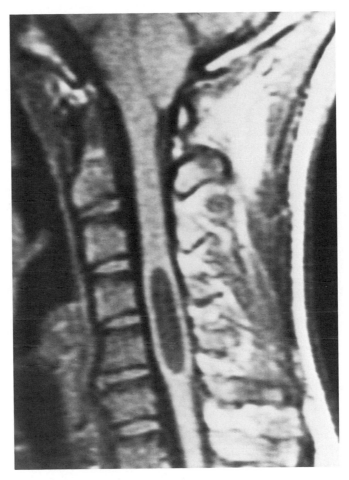

FIG. 40-1. This 18-year-old man had a syrinx seen on this sagittal T1-weighted SE MR image (600/25). What additional diagnosis can be made?

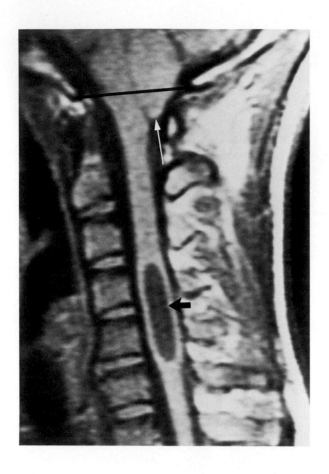

FIG. 40-1. Chiari I malformation. The cerebellar tonsil (*white arrow*) extends below the level of the foramen magnum (*long black arrows*). The syrinx (*short black arrow*) is causing widening of the spinal cord at C4 and C5 and appears as low signal intensity on this T1-weighted image.

CHIARI MALFORMATION

In addition to having syringohydromyelia, this patient has a Chiari I malformation with the cerebellar tonsils seen below the level of the foramen magnum (Fig. 40-1).

The Chiari malformation is a constellation of congenital anomalies including protrusion of the hindbrain into the cervical canal. The cerebellar tonsils and sometimes the inferior vermis protrude through the foramen magnum in the Chiari I malformation (7) (Fig. 40-2). The tonsils lie dorsal and lateral to the cervical cord and usually extend to the level of C1 or C2 while the medulla and fourth ventricle are in their normal position (6). Syringohydromyelia occurs frequently with Chiari I malformation, whereas hydrocephalus is less common. Severe spinal abnormalities and myelomeningocele are not associated with Chiari I malformation (7).

Chiari II malformation is more extensive and severe than Chiari I malformation and almost invariably presents in children with a myelomeningocele. Magnetic resonance imaging is ideally suited to show the many features of Chiari II (5,8). There are varying degrees of downward protrusion of the medulla, pons, fourth ventricle, and cerebellar vermis through the foramen magnum into the cervical canal (6). The medulla may

displace the cervical cord inferiorly or it may lie posterior to the cord. When pronounced, protrusion of the medulla causes a "kink" at the cervicomedullary junction (7), a finding noted in 79 percent of cases (4) (Fig. 40-3). Herniation of small cerebellar hemispheres and tonsils is variable. The relatively large cerebellar vermis may lie dorsal to the medulla. Compression of the cervical cord or protruding structures may develop.

The upper cervical canal is widened in Chiari II patients. At birth, obliteration of the subarachnoid space and scalloping of the odontoid process occurs because of pressure from herniated structures, and can be seen with MR imaging (3). During childhood growth, the spinal canal continues to enlarge, and along with dorsal displacement of neural tissue, leads to marked widening of the anterior space (3). When Chiari II patients are divided into an asymptomatic group and those with brainstem or long-tract symptoms, the level of hindbrain descent is critical. In one study (3), 67 percent of the symptomatic patients had a cervicomedullary kink at C4 or lower, whereas none of the asymptomatic group had the fourth ventricle, medulla, or kink below C3-C4. Associated hydromyelia or diastematomyelia can also be evaluated by MR imaging in patients with Chiari II. In addition to hindbrain abnormalities, pa-

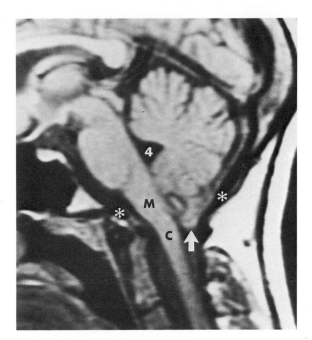

FIG. 40-2. Chiari I malformation. T1-weighted SE MR image shows cerebellar tonsil (*arrow*) caudad to level of foramen magnum (*asterisks*). A syrinx can be seen at the C3 and C4 levels. *C,* spinal cord; *M,* medulla; *4,* fourth ventricle.

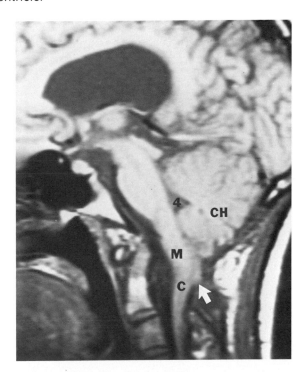

FIG. 40-3. Chiari II malformation. This 23-year-old woman had a history of myelomeningocele repair at birth. She now presented with severe headaches and weakness of the upper extremities. Sagittal T1-weighted SE MR image (600/20) includes upper cervical spine. The medulla (*M*) lies below the foramen magnum and is kinked (*arrow*) on the spinal cord (*C*). The cerebellar hemisphere (*CH*) and fourth ventricle (*4*) are more caudad than normal and there is enlargement of the lateral ventricles. There has been partial resection of the occipital bone.

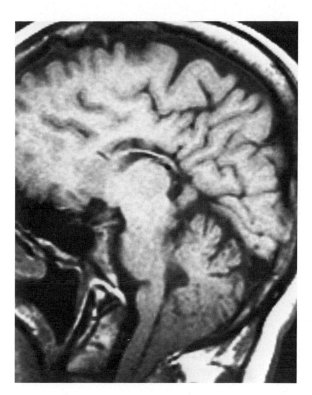

FIG. 40-4. Chiari II malformation. Sagittal T1-weighted SE MR image (600/15) shows downward displacement of the cerebellar tonsils to the level of C2-C3. The medulla is low in position and there is dysgenesis of the corpus callosum.

tients with Chiari II malformation have anomalies of the supratentorial brain that are well seen with cranial MR imaging (Fig. 40-4).

Magnetic resonance imaging is the preferred method of investigation of Chiari malformation. The position of the foramen magnum is determined by a line drawn from the inferior tip of the clivus (basion) to the inferior border of the posterior lip of the foramen magnum (opisthion) (see Fig. 40-1). The basion and the opisthion are seen as low-signal cortical bone. The basion is readily identified on T1-weighted images because of the high signal of the marrow of the clivus and fat tissue around the basion. It is more difficult to identify the opisthion. On T1-weighted sagittal MR images, the tonsils are well seen approximately 5 mm lateral to the midline (5).

The frequency of low-lying cerebellar tonsils varies as different criteria are used for diagnosis. In one study (5), sagittal T1-weighted images were used to determine the location of the cerebellar tonsils in relation to surrounding structures in normal individuals. The tonsils were located high above the foramen magnum in 14 percent of cases; just on or close to the upper border of the posterior lip of the foramen magnum in 78 percent of cases; and close to the line of the foramen magnum in 8 percent of cases. No cases were observed with the tonsils below the line of the foramen magnum in this series. However, others (2) have observed the tonsils anywhere from 8 mm above to 5 mm below the foramen magnum in normal patients. These investigators found that tonsilar ectopia of 2 mm or less is unlikely to be of clinical significance in the absence of syringohydromyelia. Still others (1) have concluded that 3 mm or less tonsillar displacement below the foramen magnum is within normal limits and greater than 5 mm displacement is considered abnormal.

REFERENCES

1. Aboulezz AO, Sartor K, Geyer CA, et al. Position of cerebellar tonsils in the normal population and in patients with Chiari malformation: a quantitative approach with MR imaging. *J Comput Assist Tomogr* 1985;9:1033–6.
2. Barkovich AJ, Wippold FJ, Sherman JL, et al. Significance of cerebellar tonsillar position on MR. *AJNR* 1986;7:795–9.
3. Curnes JT, Oakes WJ, Boyko OB. MR imaging of hindbrain deformity in Chiari II patients with and without symptoms of brainstem compression. *AJNR* 1989;10:293–302.
4. El Gammal T, Mark EK, Brooks BS. MR imaging of Chiari II malformation. *AJR* 1988;150:163–70.
5. Ishikawa M, Kikuchi H, Fujisawa I, et al. Tonsillar herniation on magnetic resonance imaging. *Neurosurgery* 1988;22:77–81.
6. Naidich TP, McLone DG, Fulling KH. The Chiari II malformation: part IV: the hindbrain deformity. *Neuroradiology* 1983;25:179–97.
7. Northfield DWC. *The surgery of the central nervous system.* London: Blackwell Scientific Publications; 1973.
8. Wolpert SM, Anderson M, Scott RM, et al. Chiari II malformation: MR imaging evaluation. *AJNR* 1987;8:783–92, *AJR* 1987;149:1033–42.

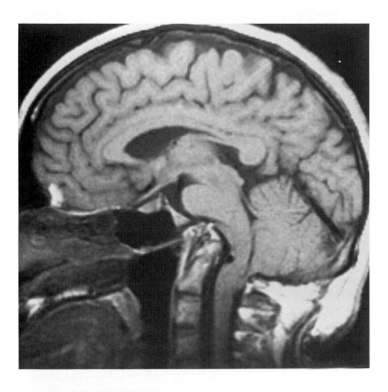

FIG. 41-1A. Sagittal T1-weighted SE MR image (600/15) of the brain and upper cervical spine in a 28-year-old man with a known underlying disorder.

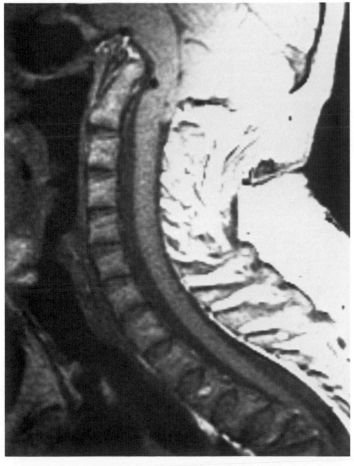

FIG. 41-1B. Sagittal T1-weighted SE MR image (700/15) of the cervical and upper thoracic spine.

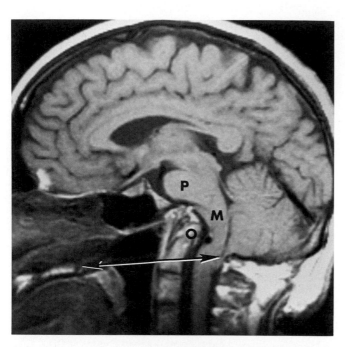

FIG. 41-1A. Osteogenesis imperfecta with basilar invagination. The tip of the odontoid process (*O*) is 15 mm above the approximate location of McGregor's line (*arrows*). The pons (*P*) and medulla (*M*) are draped over the odontoid and the medulla is compressed. There is deformity of the 4th ventricle.

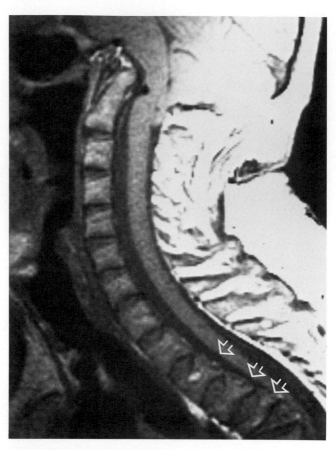

FIG. 41-1B. Basilar invagination with compression of the medulla is again seen. The cerebellar tonsils lie below the level of the foramen magnum. In addition, there are multiple compression fractures of the upper thoracic spine (*arrows*) in this patient with osteogenesis imperfecta.

OSTEOGENESIS IMPERFECTA WITH BASILAR INVAGINATION

This patient has basilar invagination that has occurred secondary to osteogenesis imperfecta (Fig. 41-1). Basilar invagination (basilar impression) is a rare disorder. It is a deformity of bony structures at the base of the skull in the region of the foramen magnum in which the margins of the foramen magnum are turned upward, reducing the volume of the posterior cranial fossa (4,7). The odontoid process and cervical spine then assume a more craniad location. The odontoid process may protrude into the foramen magnum and encroach upon or compromise the brainstem (6), and even the vertebral arteries.

Basilar invagination may occur in association with congenital anomalies of the spine or with disorders that lead to bone softening. Basilar invagination associated with congenital disorders is the more common type, often accompanied by other anomalies such as Klippel-Feil syndrome, hypoplasia of the atlas, atlantoaxial fu-

sion, occipitalization of the atlas, odontoid abnormalities, or block vertebra. Familial basilar invagination has been reported (2). Paget's disease is the most frequent cause of basilar invagination associated with disorders of bone softening at the base of the skull (3). In one series (10), basilar invagination occurred in 30 percent of cases of Paget's disease. Other bone softening disorders include osteoporosis, osteomalacia, rickets, cretinism, osteogenesis imperfecta, and renal osteopathy.

Basilar invagination is difficult to evaluate radiographically. Several methods have been used to measure basilar invagination, each with its advantages and limitations. They include: McGregor's line; McRae's line; Chamberlain's line; Bull's angle; and digastric line. Only McGregor's and McRae's lines will be discussed here.

McGregor's line is drawn from the upper surface of

228

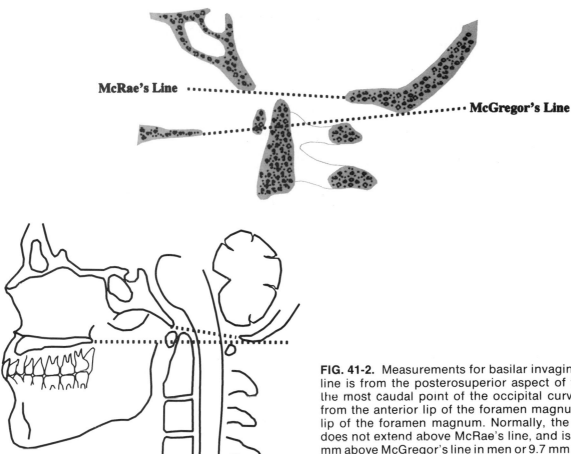

FIG. 41-2. Measurements for basilar invagination. McGregor's line is from the posterosuperior aspect of the hard palate to the most caudal point of the occipital curve. McRae's line is from the anterior lip of the foramen magnum to the posterior lip of the foramen magnum. Normally, the odontoid process does not extend above McRae's line, and is not more than 8.0 mm above McGregor's line in men or 9.7 mm above McGregor's line in women (see text).

the posterior edge of the hard palate to the most caudal point of the occipital curve in the true lateral projection (Fig. 41-2). McGregor found that the mean value for the position of the odontoid process was 1.3 mm below the line (SD 2.62 mm), and a measurement of the odontoid 4.5 mm or greater above the line was considered to be abnormal (6). Hinck et al. (4) studied a normal population and found that the mean value for the position of the odontoid was 0.33 mm above the line (SD 3.81 mm) for men, and 3.67 mm above the line (SD 2.62 mm) for women. They determined measurements of the odontoid 8.0 mm above the line in men, or 9.7 mm above the line in women to be abnormal. The measurements obtained were significantly different from those of McGregor because of technical factors and racial differences in the population studied (4).

McRae's line (foramen magnum line) is drawn from the anterior lip of the foramen magnum (basion) to the posterior lip of the foramen magnum (opisthion) on the lateral view (see Fig. 41-2). Basilar invagination is present "if the line of the occipital squama is convexed upward or if it lies above the line of the foramen magnum or if the occipital condyles lie on or above the line of the foramen magnum." (8) Basilar invagination

should not be confused with platybasia or cranial settling. *Platybasia* is the anthropologists' term referring to the degree of obtuseness of the basal angle of the skull. *Cranial settling* is the term describing upward movement of the odontoid process on C1 caused by destruction and collapse of the occipito-atlantal and atlanto-axial articulations and lateral masses of C1 as may be seen in rheumatoid arthritis.

Basilar invagination can usually be determined by utilizing craniometric lines and angles on the conventional radiograph of the skull. In cases where this is difficult to assess, conventional tomography may be helpful. However, because basilar invagination may be associated with neurologic symptoms, MR imaging is very useful in evaluating these patients. With MR imaging, the craniocervical region and posterior fossa can be seen in multiple planes without the artifacts that occur with CT evaluation of this area. Magnetic resonance imaging can show compression of the medulla, pons, cerebellum, and spinal cord in addition to bony alterations (2) (Fig. 41-3A). T1-weighted images are usually sufficient to evaluate the presence and degree of basilar invagination as well as any compromise on neural structures. Computed tomography is useful in

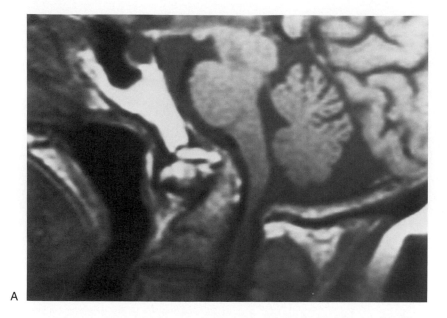

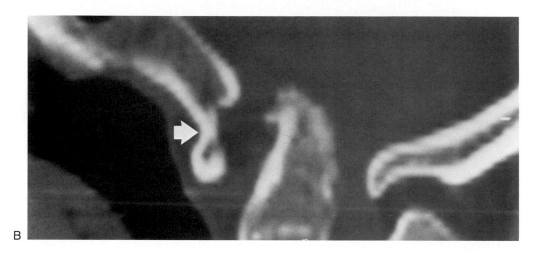

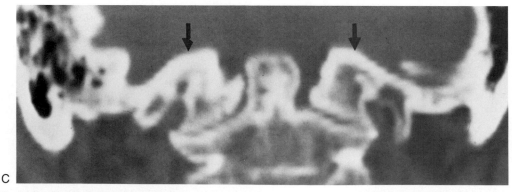

FIG. 41-3. Basilar invagination in a patient with occipitalization of C1. **A**: Sagittal T1-weighted SE MR image (600/20) shows basilar invagination with the odontoid seen above the foramen magnum. The odontoid is compressing the medulla and the spinal cord. Developmental abnormality of the clivus and the anterior arch of C1 is noted. The posterior arch of C1 is not seen. **B**: Sagittal reconstruction of axial CT images shows basilar invagination, fusion of the clivus with the anterior arch of C1 (*arrow*), atlanto-axial subluxation, and narrowing of the spinal canal. **C**: Coronal reconstruction of axial CT images shows fusion of the occiput with the lateral masses of C1 (*arrows*).

evaluating the congenital osseous causes of basilar invagination (Figs. 41-3B, 3C).

Osteogenesis imperfecta is a rare, non-sex-linked, autosomal dominant, hereditary, congenital disorder, probably resulting from defects in the molecular structure of collagen (9). It is classically characterized by fragile bones, blue sclerae, and otosclerosis (5). However, these findings may occur alone or in combination and, in fact, may not be clinically evident (5,9). As with many congenital disorders, there is a congenita form which is clinically more devastating, and a tarda form which is clinically more benign, with patients living into adult life and having mild osseous changes. Osteogenesis imperfecta may be associated with basilar invagination (11) because of the soft nature of the skull base.

Vertebral collapse is frequent in patients with osteogenesis imperfecta because of softness and fragility of the bones. Biconcave vertebrae are also frequent and occur because of the effect of an elastic nucleus pulposus on the soft vertebrae (1). Microfractures may occur near the endplates and interfere with normal growth, causing deformity. Scoliosis may develop because of the laxity of spinal ligaments, and possibly vertebral compression (1).

In patients with osteogenesis imperfecta, vertebral collapse and osteopenia can be readily identified with conventional radiography; however, MR is helpful in evaluation of any patient with signs and symptoms of spinal cord compression secondary to vertebral fractures and kyphosis.

REFERENCES

1. Benson DR, Donaldson DH, Millar EA. The spine in osteogenesis imperfecta. *J Bone Joint Surg (Am)* 1978;60A:925–9.
2. Bewermeyer H, Dreesbach HA, Hunermann B, et al. MR imaging of familial basilar impression. *J Comput Assist Tomogr* 1984; 8:953–6.
3. Dolan KD. Cervicobasilar relationships. *Radiol Clin N Am* 1977; 15:155–66.
4. Hinck VC, Hopkins CE, Savara BS. Diagnostic criteria of basilar impression. *Radiology* 1961;76:572–85.
5. Levin EJ. Osteogenesis imperfecta in the adult. *AJR* 1964;91: 973–8.
6. McGregor M. The significance of certain measurements of the skull in the diagnosis of basilar impression. *Br J Radiol* 1948; 21:171–81.
7. McRae DL. The significance of abnormalities of the cervical spine. *AJR* 1960;84:3–25.
8. McRae DL, Barnum AS. Occipitalization of the atlas. *AJR* 1953; 70:23–46.
9. Paterson CR, McAllion S, Miller R. Osteogenesis imperfecta with dominant inheritance and normal sclerae. *J Bone Joint Surg (Br)* 1983;65B:35–9.
10. Poppel MH, Jacobson HG, Duff BF, et al. Basilar impression and platybasia in Paget's disease. *Radiology* 1953;61:639–44.
11. Pozo JL, Crockard HA, Ransford AO. Basilar impression in osteogenesis imperfecta: a report of three cases in one family. *J Bone Joint Surg (Br)* 1984;66B:233–8.

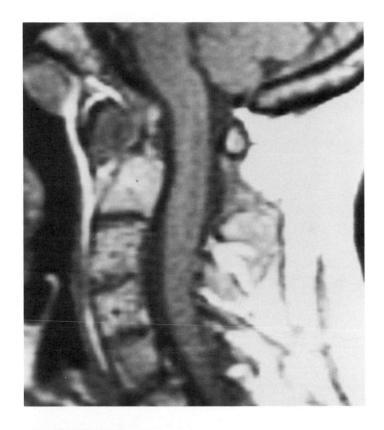

FIG. 42-1A. This 46-year-old woman has suboccipital neck pain that is most severe when the neck is in flexion. Sagittal T1-weighted SE MR image (500/11) of the cervical spine with the neck in neutral position.

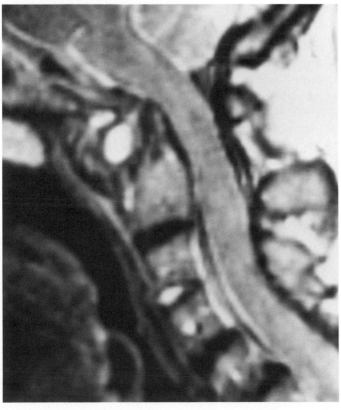

FIG. 42-1B. Sagittal T2-weighted SE MR image (2500/80) with the neck in flexion.

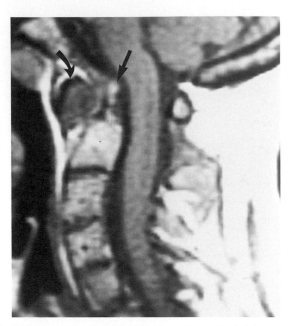

FIG. 42-1A. Rheumatoid arthritis. The odontoid process is severely eroded (*straight arrow*). There is a round mass of intermediate signal intensity pannus surrounding the anterior arch of C1 (*curved arrow*). Anterior C1-C2 subluxation is present and there is compression of the anterior subarachnoid space.

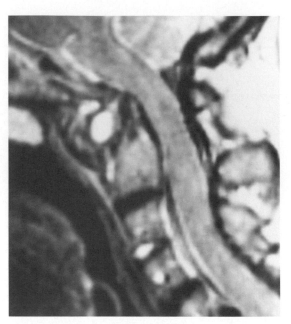

FIG. 42-1B. The predental mass shows heterogeneous signal intensity on the T2-weighted image. The pannus has intermediate signal, whereas other areas of high signal intensity reflect increased water content, compatible with synovial fluid and/or pannus. Narrowing of the spinal canal is again noted and there is slight impression on the spinal cord with the neck in flexion.

RHEUMATOID ARTHRITIS

The MR examination shows an anterior subluxation of C1 in relation to the odontoid process of C2, erosion of the odontoid, and pannus surrounding the anterior arch of C1 (Fig. 42-1). This patient has rheumatoid arthritis.

Normally, the strong transverse ligament helps prevent posterior displacement of the odontoid process. This ligament arches posterior to the odontoid process and attaches to tubercles on the medial aspect of the lateral masses of C1 (Figs. 42-2, 42-3). Anterior subluxation occurs as a result of laxity or rupture of the transverse ligament caused by the rheumatoid process. At the C1-C2 level, anterior subluxation is the most frequent type of subluxation, and occurs in 35 percent of patients with rheumatoid arthritis. The incidence and degree of severity of atlanto-axial subluxation may parallel several factors including the severity and duration of rheumatoid arthritis, seropositivity, steroid treatment, and the presence of rheumatoid nodules (7). Atlanto-axial subluxation is diagnosed when the distance between the anterior arch of C1 and the odontoid process exceeds 3 mm in an adult or 5 mm in a child (8) (Fig. 42-4). This evaluation can be made with conventional radiography, conventional tomography, CT, or MR imaging. Some patients with rheumatoid arthritis

develop lateral, posterior, or superior subluxation at C1-C2. Atlanto-axial subluxation may also occur in psoriatic arthritis, juvenile rheumatoid arthritis, and less commonly in ankylosing spondylitis, Down's syndrome, and Marfan's syndrome. Subluxation at C1-C2 may also occur following trauma.

Many patients with rheumatoid arthritis are neurologically asymptomatic despite abnormalities of the craniocervical junction. Nevertheless, spinal cord compression with myelopathy may occur and is usually secondary to anterior C1-C2 subluxation exceeding 9 mm or secondary to cranial settling (superior subluxation) (12). The degree of C1-C2 subluxation can be correlated with spinal cord pathology. In one study (5), 39 percent of patients with C1-C2 subluxation greater than 9 mm had spinal cord compression. Subluxation measuring between 6 mm and 9 mm caused spinal cord compression in 6 percent and obliteration of the subarachnoid space in 28 percent, whereas 5 mm or 6 mm subluxation was not associated with compression of the cord or subarachnoid space. Atlanto-axial subluxation may be accentuated with the neck in the flexion position. In one series, atlanto-axial subluxation was fixed in only about one-third of the cases (4). Most MR examinations are performed in the neutral position so

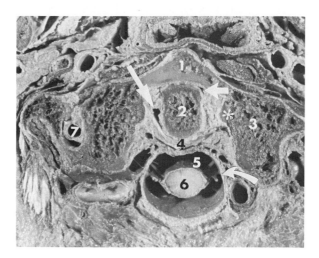

FIG. 42-2. Normal anatomic specimen, transaxial section. The anterior arch of C1 (*1*) is in close approximation to the odontoid process of C2 (*2*). The lateral masses of C1 (*3*) have tubercles along their medial wall (*asterisk*), that act as attachments for the transverse ligament (*4*). Two synovial membrane-lined joints are located about the odontoid process and are partially visualized on this section. The larger joint lies posterolaterally between the odontoid and the transverse ligament (*long straight arrow*). The smaller anterior joint is found between the anterior arch of C1 and the odontoid (*short straight arrow*). This section displays other pertinent anatomy such as the dura (*curved arrow*), subarachnoid space (*5*), spinal cord (*6*), and vertebral artery (*7*) within the foramen transversarium.

that mild instability may not be elicited; however, these alterations may be seen when the MR examination is performed in flexion (Fig. 42-5).

Normally, the odontoid process displays increased

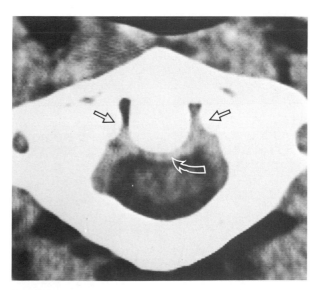

FIG. 42-3. Normal transverse ligament. Computed tomography shows the transverse ligament (*curved arrow*) arching posterior to the odontoid process and attaching to tubercles on the medial aspect of the lateral masses of C1 (*straight arrows*).

signal intensity on T1-weighted images characteristic of fat marrow (1) and the apical portion of the dens usually has heterogeneous signal (5). Partial volume effect can render the tip of the odontoid process as intermediate signal intensity. Occasionally, in the parasagittal plane, normal individuals can have an apparent enlargement of the odontoid process which is caused by normal ligamentous tissues, synovial joint, and dura (10). In patients with rheumatoid arthritis, the signal intensity of the odontoid process on T1-weighted images correlates with the density of the odontoid seen with conventional tomography in 67 percent of patients studied (3). As the dens becomes more sclerotic, the signal intensity decreases on T1-weighted images. Osteopenia of the dens on tomography correlates with increased signal on T1-weighted MR images (3).

An important anatomic consideration is the presence of two synovial-lined joints about the odontoid process. The smaller joint lies between the anterior arch of C1 and the odontoid while the larger posterolateral joint is located between the odontoid and the transverse ligament (see Fig. 42-2). Erosion of the odontoid process is a frequent finding in rheumatoid arthritis and occurs as a result of synovial inflammation (pannus) arising in these peridental joint spaces. Some authors believe that erosions of the odontoid are equally well seen with MR imaging and CT (1–3), both being superior to conventional radiography (1). In one study, sixty patients with cervical rheumatoid arthritis and atlanto-axial subluxation of at least 5 mm, or cranial settling as determined by McRae's line, were evaluated with MR imaging (5). The most common abnormalities identified with MR imaging were erosion of the odontoid process (88 percent), which occurs most often on the dorsal aspect, and the presence of pannus (87 percent) (5) (see Fig. 42-1), which forms around the odontoid process in the pre- and postdental joint spaces. Pannus is frequently present in patients with mobile atlanto-axial subluxation (7). It is seen as intermediate signal and is often discrete (5). In one study (4), 66 percent of patients with atlanto-axial subluxation from rheumatoid arthritis had pannus greater than 3 mm. Extensive pannus formation may cause compression of the upper spinal cord and medulla oblongata (7) (Fig. 42-6). The pannus not only represents rheumatoid inflammatory tissue, but also fibrous granulation tissue produced by chronic mechanical irritation caused by the instability (11). Sometimes, almost the entire odontoid process is replaced by fluid or a mass of pannus (1). Rarely, a pathologic fracture of the odontoid process may occur.

Magnetic resonance imaging is the best method for evaluating the spinal cord in patients with atlanto-axial and subaxial subluxations. It can show the presence, location, and degree of compression of the spinal cord

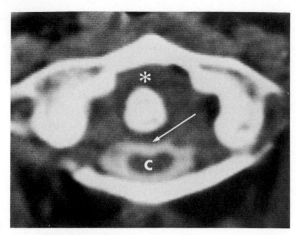

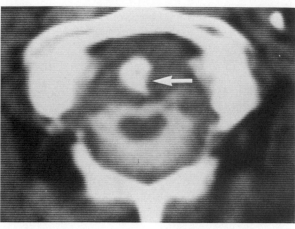

FIG. 42-4. Rheumatoid arthritis with atlantoaxial subluxation. Axial CTM at C1-C2 in a 47-year-old man with a three week history of numbness and weakness of the extremities. **A**: There is widening of the space between the anterior arch of C1 and the odontoid process of C2 (*asterisk*). This distance measures 9 mm (normal distance is less than 3 mm in adults). The anterior C1-C2 subluxation is causing compression and displacement of the anterior subarachnoid space (*arrow*) and spinal cord (*C*). **B**: Erosion of the odontoid process is present (*arrow*). The anterior subluxation of C1-C2 can once again be seen causing spinal cord compression.

as well as the presence of edema or myelomalacia within the cord. Compression of the medulla and upper cervical cord is caused by atlanto-axial subluxation as well as pannus formation (7). Spinal cord or brainstem abnormalities are seen in all patients with neurologic symptoms (1). About 19 percent of patients with rheumatoid arthritis develop cervical myelopathy (4). Myelopathy is less common in the mid- and lower cervical spine but may be caused by marked subluxation or abundant granulation tissue in the posterior portion of the spinal canal encroaching on the spinal cord.

Compression of the upper cervical spinal cord is identified on T1-weighted images when there is indentation of the cord by the odontoid process or by pannus. In patients with pannus, spinal cord diameter decreases with flexion and remains unchanged in extension compared with the neutral position (4). In one functional MR study (4), most patients with my-

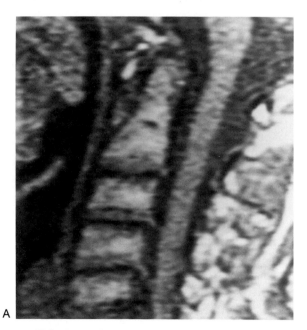

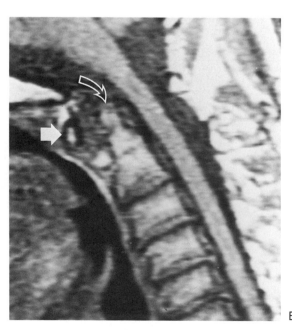

FIG. 42-5. Rheumatoid arthritis with atlantoaxial subluxation. **A**: T1-weighted SE MR image (600/20) with the neck in extension. The atlanto-axial interval and the odontoid appear normal. There is no evidence of spinal cord compression. **B**: T1-weighted SE MR image (600/20) with the neck in the flexion position. The space between the anterior arch of C1 (*straight arrow*) and the odontoid process (*curved arrow*) is widened and there is slight narrowing of the anterior subarachnoid space without compression of the spinal cord. Flexion can accentuate atlanto-axial subluxation.

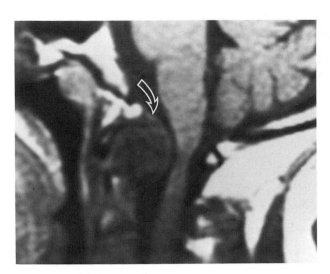

FIG. 42-6. Rheumatoid arthritis with extensive pannus and spinal cord compression. Sagittal T1-weighted MR image (600/10) of the upper cervical spine in a 45-year-old woman. There is a large mass of intermediate signal intensity surrounding the odontoid process. This mass is caused by extensive predental, retrodental, and supradental pannus (*arrow*) that is causing spinal cord compression. Anterior C1-C2 subluxation is present.

elopathy had a spinal cord diameter of less than 6 mm, as seen only in the flexion position. These investigators concluded that it is important to obtain MR images in the sagittal plane during flexion and extension in patients with atlanto-axial instability from rheumatoid arthritis. None of the thirty-four patients in this study had an increase in symptoms during flexion (4). Others (5), however, believe that a functional MR examination is unnecessary and poses an undue risk to the patient. Surgical treatment of patients with rheumatoid arthritis depends upon demonstrating cord compression. Fol-

lowing surgery, compression of the medulla and/or spinal cord may remain, but pannus decreases in size due to atlanto-axial immobility, and eventually disappears (7).

Cranial settling is probably the most serious complication of rheumatoid arthritis. It occurs when pannus from the inflamed synovial joints leads to erosion and collapse of the lateral masses of C1 and, to a lesser extent, erosion of the occipital condyles and superior articular facets of C2 (3). These pathologic changes permit the skull to settle at a lower level on the cervical spine, causing the odontoid process to be above the level of the foramen magnum. This can be determined by using McRae's or McGregor's lines. The body of C2 may be seen within the ring of C1 and is another important diagnostic feature of cranial settling (Figs. 42-7, 42-8). Magnetic resonance imaging or CT is indicated if confirmation of cranial settling is required or if there are signs of cord compression.

Cranial settling occurs in 5–8 percent of patients with rheumatoid arthritis (6). Neurologic symptoms such as paresthesias, paresis, or micturition disturbances occur in 30 percent of patients with rheumatoid arthritis and cranial settling (9). There is a statistical correlation between the severity of superior subluxation and the presence of neurologic symptoms (9). In addition, patients with cranial settling are more likely to have neurologic symptoms when there is narrowing of the sagittal diameter of the canal at C1 to less than 13 mm (9). Cranial settling typically occurs in patients with long-standing rheumatoid arthritis. Follow-up examination of these patients reveals progression of the superior subluxation in 80 percent of cases (9). Odontoid compression of the medulla and spinal cord has led to death in some patients with cranial settling, and vertebral artery occlusion has been implicated as a cause of death in others (6).

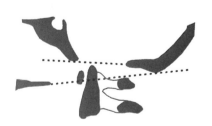
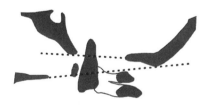

Normal   *Cranial Settling*

FIG. 42-7. Comparison of the position of the odontoid process of C2 relative to the foramen magnum, and the anterior arch of C1 relative to the odontoid, in normal individuals and in patients with rheumatoid arthritis and cranial settling. *Dotted lines* show position of McRae's line and McGregor's line. Normally the odontoid lies below the foramen magnum, and the anterior arch of C1 articulates with the upper portion of the odontoid. In patients with rheumatoid arthritis and cranial settling, erosion and collapse of the lateral masses of C1 permit the skull to settle at a lower level on the cervical spine. The odontoid may lie above the foramen magnum, and the anterior arch of C1 articulates with the lower portion of the odontoid or the body of C2. When the odontoid is severely eroded, its position relative to the foramen magnum may not be observable, and the clue to the diagnosis of cranial settling may be the position of the anterior arch of C1 relative to the odontoid.

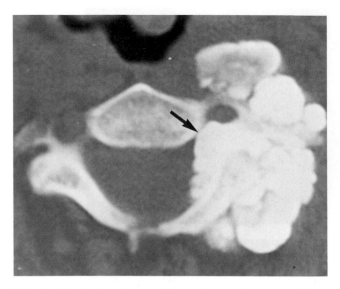

FIG. 43-1A. Scleroderma. There is massive amorphous calcification causing encroachment upon the spinal canal and neural canal (*arrow*).

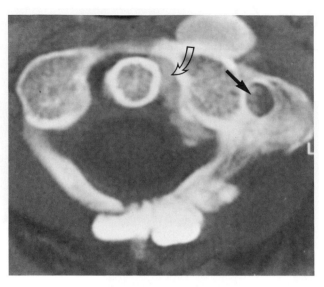

FIG. 43-1B. Extensive calcification is causing narrowing of the foramen transversarium (*straight arrow*) and the space between C1 and the odontoid process (*curved arrow*).

SCLERODERMA WITH MASSIVE CALCIFICATION

Massive intraspinal and paraspinal calcifications are present with extension into the neural foramen, foramen transversarium and the C1-C2 articulation (Fig. 43-1). Additional CT sections showed that this process extended from C1 to C3. These findings are due to dystrophic accumulation of hydroxyapatite crystals. The diagnosis of scleroderma was established in this patient approximately 1 year after the initial CT examination, as the clinical features of this disorder became apparent. This patient developed sclerodactyly and telangiectasia. Small focal calcifications in the subcutaneous tissues of the fingers were discovered radiographically.

The calcifications found in patients with scleroderma consist of hydroxyapatite crystals. These calcifications may develop within subcutaneous tissues, tendon sheaths, bursae, and joints; and may appear punctate, amorphous, or linear (4). Frequent sites of calcification include the hands, elbows, forearms, shoulders, and hips. Calcifications within the spine are rare.

In the case presented there are massive intraspinal and paraspinal calcifications. Although rare, similar CT demonstrations of massive calcific deposits at the craniovertebral junction have been reported in one patient with calcium pyrophosphate deposition disease (1) and in another with systemic lupus erythematosus (5). In those cases, spinal cord compression and osseous erosion were seen with CT; MR imaging reveals a large area of signal void at the site of massive calcification (5). Other patients with the clinical diagnosis

of scleroderma have had CT demonstration of large, lobulated calcific masses centered at the apophyseal joints in the mid- and lower cervical spine (5). Osteolysis around the joints and osseous erosions were seen with CT in these cases. Extensive heterotopic new bone formation may occur in the cervical spine in patients with fibrodysplasia ossificans progressiva (myositis ossificans progressiva) (3) and in patients who have sustained previous head injury (2).

Patients with massive paraspinal and intraspinal calcification in the cervical spine may have radiculopathy, focal pain, or stiffness. Computed tomography is useful in delineating the calcific masses earlier than conventional radiography and is helpful in treatment planning in those cases in which surgical intervention is contemplated (3).

REFERENCES

1. El-Khoury GY, Tozzi JE, Clark CR, et al. Massive calcium pyrophosphate crystal deposition at the craniovertebral junction. *AJR* 1985;145:777–8.
2. Groswasser Z, Reider-Groswasser I. Heterotopic new bone formation in the cervical spine following head injury: case report. *J Neurosurg* 1986;64:513–5.
3. Reinig JW, Hill SC, Fang M, et al. Fibrodysplasia ossificans progressiva: CT appearance. *Radiology* 1986;159:153–7.
4. Resnick D, Niwayama G. *Diagnosis of bone and joint disorders: with emphasis on articular abnormalities.* vol 2. Philadelphia: WB Saunders; 1981.
5. Schweitzer ME, Cervilla V, Manaster BJ, et al. Cervical paraspinal calcification in collagen vascular diseases. *AJR* 1991;157:523–5.

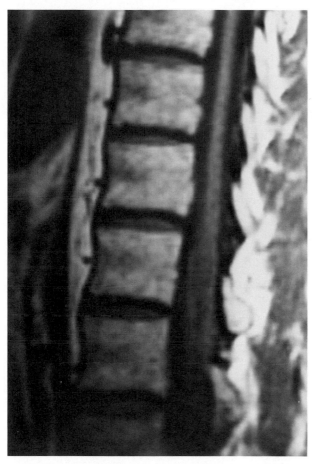

FIG. 44-1A. This 26-year-old man had an abnormal chest radiograph. Sagittal T1-weighted SE MR image (800/20) of the thoracolumbar spine.

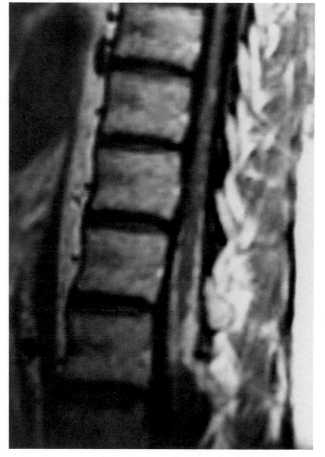

FIG. 44-1B. Sagittal T1-weighted SE MR image (800/20) after the intravenous injection of gadopentetate dimeglumine.

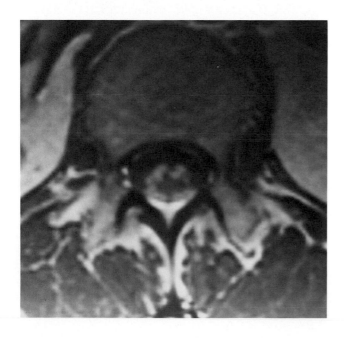

FIG. 44-1C. Axial T1-weighted SE MR image at the level of the conus after injection of gadopentetate dimeglumine.

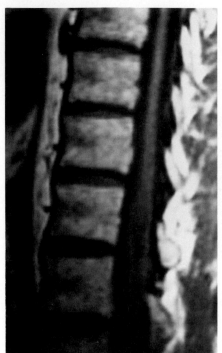

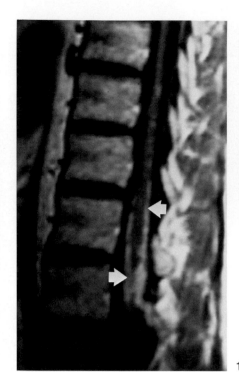

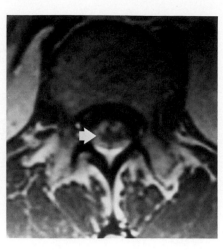

1A

1B

1C

FIG. 44-1A. Sarcoidosis. The precontrast T1-weighted image shows normal signal intensity of the spinal cord.

FIG. 44-1B. There is patchy, linear enhancement along the surface of the spinal cord and conus (*arrows*) after the injection of gadopentetate dimeglumine.

FIG. 44-1C. The axial image shows leptomeningeal enhancement (*arrow*) after the injection of the paramagnetic agent.

SARCOIDOSIS

The precontrast T1-weighted MR image is unremarkable (Fig. 44-1A). Patchy, linear enhancement of the leptomeninges is seen after the intravenous injection of gadopentetate dimeglumine (Figs. 44-1B, 44-1C). This is an abnormal but nonspecific finding. However, in light of the history of interstitial lung disease, the diagnosis of neurosarcoidosis should be considered. This patient was known to have sarcoidosis, and MR imaging of the brain showed extensive meningeal enhancement (Fig. 44-2).

Sarcoidosis is a systemic granulomatous disease of unknown etiology that is characterized by the widespread presence of noncaseating granulomas. It often affects young adults and occurs more frequently in women and the black population. Chest radiography may reveal bilateral hilar and paratracheal lymphadenopathy and interstitial lung disease. Skin or eye lesions may be present.

Approximately 5 percent of patients with sarcoidosis have neurologic involvement, with almost half of these having a neurologic presentation (8). Cranial neuropa-

thy, especially a peripheral facial nerve palsy, is the most frequent neurologic manifestation. Others include aseptic meningitis, hydrocephalus, parenchymatous disease of the central nervous system, peripheral neuropathy, and myopathy (8). Magnetic resonance imaging of the brain may show hydrocephalus secondary to basal arachnoiditis and periventricular and multifocal white matter lesions indistinguishable from multiple sclerosis (5). Enhanced CT or MR imaging of the brain may show diffuse meningeal involvement (7). Less often, sarcoidosis may involve the spinal cord or spinal leptomeninges. This involvement may present as an intramedullary mass, arachnoiditis, or as intradural extramedullary or extradural lesions (3,6). In a review of the literature (6), 48 histologically confirmed cases of spinal cord or leptomeningeal sarcoidosis were evaluated with 35 percent predominantly intramedullary, 35 percent extramedullary, and 23 percent combined intramedullary and extramedullary. Only 2 percent were extradural with a small remaining number of cases unspecified in the literature.

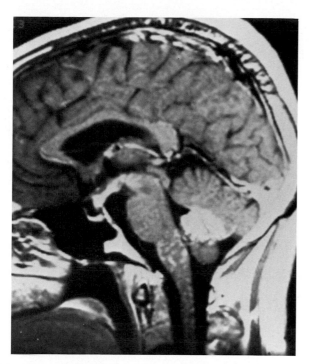

FIG. 44-2. Sarcoidosis. Same patient as in Fig. 44-1. Sagittal T1 weighted SE MR image of the brain after the injection of gadopentetate dimeglumine reveals extensive leptomeningeal enhancement surrounding the inferior vermis, medulla, and upper cervical spinal cord.

section evaluation of biopsy specimens of spinal cord sarcoidosis may be mistaken for an astrocytoma (3). Resection of spinal cord sarcoidosis is associated with increased morbidity and mortality when compared to steroid-treated patients (4).

Some investigators have used gadopentetate dimeglumine in the evaluation of spinal cord sarcoidosis (6,7). Enhancement in these cases may be patchy, multifocal, and broad-based along the surface of the spinal cord (6). In addition, more subtle linear enhancement may be seen along the surface of the spinal cord, corresponding to leptomeningeal involvement. These enhancement features may be useful in suggesting the diagnosis of sarcoidosis and in differentiating it from astrocytoma and ependymoma. Leptomeningeal involvement is unusual for astrocytoma and patchy infiltrative cord involvement is not typical of ependymoma (6). Peripheral multifocal enhancement is unusual for both. The patchy peripheral enhancement pattern of the cord is nonspecific and may be seen in other disorders such as multiple sclerosis and mycobacterial or fungal myelitis (6). In some cases of spinal sarcoidosis, the diagnosis is suggested only on the contrast-enhanced images (7).

After steroid therapy, patients may improve clinically, and follow-up MR imaging may reveal a spinal cord of normal size and signal intensity (2).

With myelography and CTM, spinal sarcoidosis may be seen as an intramedullary mass (2,4). Nodularity may be detected in the subarachnoid space (2). On a rare occasion, spinal involvement in sarcoidosis may be limited to infiltration of a nerve root with noncaseating granulomata that appear on CT as a fusiform soft tissue mass within the neural foramen (1). With MR imaging, the T1-weighted images may show only fusiform widening of the spinal cord (3), although patchy areas of decreased signal intensity may be seen within the cord (6). On T2-weighted images, diffuse increase in signal intensity of the cord over multiple vertebral levels may be seen (3). The appearance of spinal cord sarcoidosis with myelography, CTM, and unenhanced MR imaging may simulate more common spinal cord masses such as astrocytoma or ependymoma. This has additional significance since on occasion the frozen-

REFERENCES

1. Baron B, Goldberg AL, Rothfus WE, et al. CT features of sarcoid infiltration of a lumbosacral nerve root. *J Comput Assist Tomogr* 1989;13:364–5.
2. Cooper SD, Brady MB, Williams JP, et al. Neurosarcoidosis: evaluation using computed tomography and magnetic resonance imaging. *CT* 1988;12:96–9.
3. Kelly RB, Mahoney PD, Cawley KM. MR demonstration of spinal cord sarcoidosis: report of a case. *AJNR* 1988;9:197–9.
4. Martin CA, Murali R, Trasi SS. Spinal cord sarcoidosis: case report. *J Neurosurg* 1984;61:981–2.
5. Miller DH, Kendall BE, Barter S, et al. Magnetic resonance imaging in central nervous system sarcoidosis. *Neurology* 1988;38:378–83.
6. Nesbit GM, Miller GM, Baker HL Jr, et al. Spinal cord sarcoidosis: a new finding at MR imaging with Gd-DTPA enhancement. *Radiology* 1989;173:839–43.
7. Seltzer S, Mark AS, Atlas SW. CNS sarcoidosis: evaluation with contrast-enhanced MR imaging. *AJNR* 1991;12:1227–33, *AJR* 1992;158:391–7.
8. Stern BJ, Krumholz A, Johns C, et al. Sarcoidosis and its neurological manisfestations. *Arch Neurol* 1985;42:909–17.

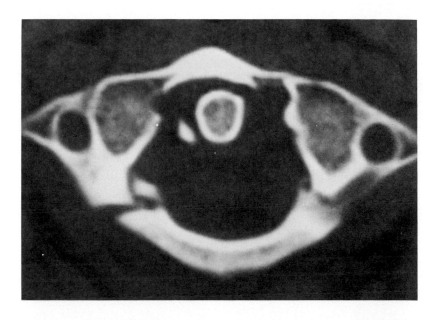

FIG. 45-1A. Axial CT at the level of C1 in a 20-year-old patient who sustained trauma to the cervical spine from a motor vehicle accident.

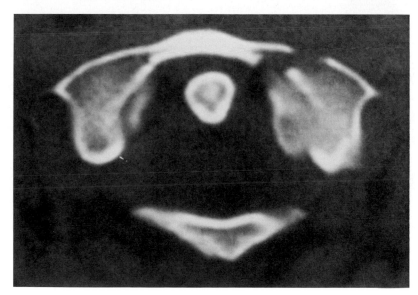

FIG. 45-1B. Axial CT 4 mm cephalad to Fig. 45-1A.

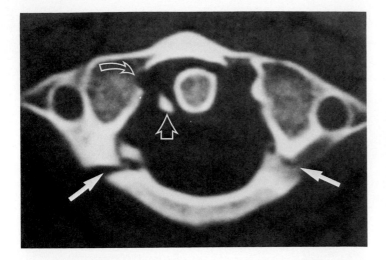

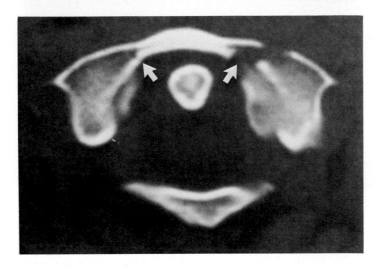

FIG. 45-1A. Jefferson fracture. There are bilateral fractures of the posterior arch of C1 (*closed arrows*) with a displaced fragment noted on the right. There is also a fracture of the medial tubercle of the lateral mass of C1 on the right (*curved arrow*) with displacement of a fragment into the canal (*straight open arrow*). The medial tubercle is the site of attachment of the transverse ligament. Widening of the space between the odontoid and the lateral masses of C1 can be appreciated.

FIG. 45-1B. There are bilateral fractures of the anterior arch of C1 (*arrows*). The fracture on the right is subtle and nondisplaced.

JEFFERSON FRACTURE

There are bilateral fractures of the posterior and anterior arches of C1 (Fig. 45-1). A fracture of the medial tubercle of the lateral mass of C1 can also be seen. Coronal reconstruction of the axial images shows lateral offset of the lateral masses of C1 in relation to the superior articular surfaces of C2 (Fig. 45-2). This is a Jefferson fracture.

The Jefferson fracture is an injury that occurs from a direct blow to the vertex of the skull with the head held erect, resulting in compressive forces between the

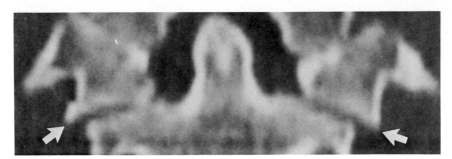

FIG. 45-2. Jefferson fracture. Same patient as Fig. 45-1. Coronal reconstruction of the axial images shows lateral offset of the lateral masses of C1 (*arrows*) in relation to the superior articular surfaces of C2.

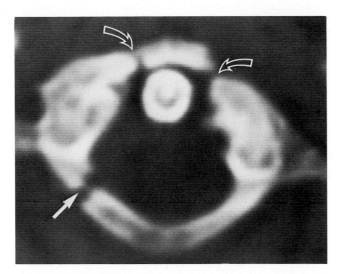

FIG. 45-3. Fractures of the atlas. Axial CT through C1 shows bilateral fractures of the anterior arch (*curved arrows*) and fracture of the right posterior arch (*straight arrow*).

occiput and the articular surfaces of C2 (4,5). Because of the oblique plane of the articular surfaces, the transmitted force is directed laterally, leading to lateral spread of the lateral masses of C1 (5). This may in turn lead to tension fracture of the anterior and posterior arches of C1. The classic Jefferson fracture includes bilateral lateral offset of C1 and bilateral fractures of the posterior and anterior arches of C1. However, depending upon the degree of force and the position of the

head at the time of injury, fractures may be unilateral or may be limited to the posterior or anterior arch (5). Lateral offset is usually bilateral but may be unilateral (4). Although some patients with Jefferson fracture die immediately at the time of injury, those patients presenting for clinical and radiographic evaluation of a Jefferson fracture usually do not have neurologic loss or compromise of the spinal cord.

Fractures of the atlas comprise 5 percent of all cervical fractures and dislocations (4). In a review of a large series of atlas fractures (7), 15 percent were diagnosed as an unstable Jefferson variant fracture, 83 percent were considered a stable Jefferson variant fracture, and only 2 percent were the classic Jefferson fracture. The unstable Jefferson variant fracture is an injury that most likely occurs by the same mechanism as the classic Jefferson fracture but has less than four fractures in the atlas and is more often associated with neurologic injury. The bilateral anterior arch fracture is the pattern that is associated with the most severe spinal cord injury. The unstable Jefferson variant fracture may have associated tear of the transverse ligament and C1-C2 subluxation. Isolated single and bilateral posterior arch Jefferson variant fractures are stable injuries not associated with neurologic deficit (7). Fracture of the lateral mass of C1 is usually associated with additional fractures of the atlas. Less common fractures of the atlas include fracture of the transverse process and isolated fracture of the lateral mass.

Conventional radiography can show lateral offset of the lateral masses of C1 in relation to the superior artic-

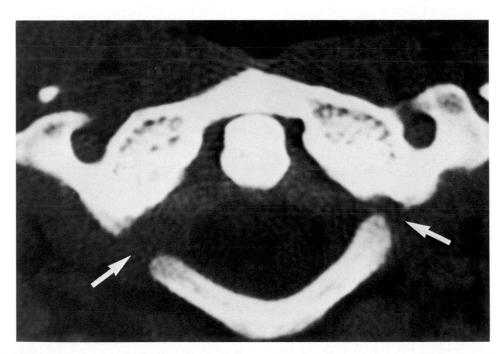

FIG. 45-4. Posterior clefts of atlas. Axial CT through C1 reveals bilateral posterior clefts (*arrows*). The smooth, rounded margins of the posterior arch help differentiate these congenital clefts from fractures, which typically have a more irregular, jagged appearance.

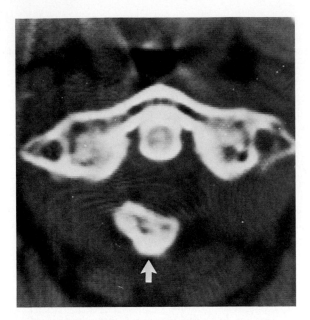

FIG. 45-5. Partial aplasia of the posterior arch of C1. This patient had sustained trauma to the neck. Abnormal radiographs of the cervical spine led to this CT examination. There is partial aplasia of the posterior arch of C1 with a persistent posterior tubercle (*arrow*).

ular surfaces of C2 as visualized with the open-mouth view. Fractures of the atlas may be identified with radiography. However, the fractures of the C1 ring usually occur near the junction of the arches and the lateral masses and are frequently not appreciated (4). Conventional tomography may also fail to reveal the fractures or may be inconclusive (8). Computed tomography is ideally suited for evaluating fractures of the atlas since the fractures through the ring of the atlas occur perpendicular to the plane of the CT scan and can thus be readily identified (Fig. 45-3). The presence of a bone fragment within the spinal canal, one of the few indications for surgery in this injury, can be best seen with CT (6). Lateral displacement of the lateral masses of C1 may be visualized on the transaxial scans as well as with coronal reformation. When the lateral offset exceeds 7 mm, there is probably an associated tear of

the transverse ligament (2). In the present case, fracture of the medial tubercle of the lateral mass of C1 is noted. This is the site of attachment of the transverse ligament.

The differential diagnosis of a Jefferson fracture includes congenital clefts, aplasia of the arch of the atlas, and pseudospread of the atlas. Congenital clefts are rare (Fig. 45-4). Posterior clefts occur more frequently than anterior clefts and are most often in the midline (3). Should lateral offset occur, it is limited to 1–2 mm (3). Aplasia of the posterior arch of C1 may be partial or complete. Partial posterior aplasia may have a persistent posterior tubercle (Fig. 45-5) (1). Clefts and aplasia can be differentiated from fracture by their smooth cortical margins (1). Pseudospread of the atlas occurs in children aged 3 months to 4 years, most frequently in the second year (9). Pseudospread results from more rapid growth of C1 in relation to C2, leading to apparent lateral offset of C1 as visualized on AP open-mouth radiographs (9). In comparison, the Jefferson fracture is rare in children.

REFERENCES

1. Dorne HL, Just N, Lander PH. CT recognition of anomalies of the posterior arch of the atlas vertebra: differentiation from fracture. *AJNR* 1986;7:176–7.
2. Fielding JW, Cochran GVB, Lawsing JF, et al. Tears of the transverse ligament of the atlas: a clinical and biomechanical study. *J Bone Joint Surg (Am)* 1974;56A:1683–90.
3. Gehweiler JA Jr, Daffner RH, Roberts L Jr. Malformations of the atlas vertebra simulating the Jefferson fracture. *AJNR* 1983; 4:187–90; *AJR* 1983;140:1083–6.
4. Gehweiler JA Jr, Duff DE, Martinez S, et al. Fractures of the atlas vertebra. *Skeletal Radiol* 1976;1:97–102.
5. Jefferson G. Fracture of the atlas vertebra: report of four cases, and a review of those previously recorded. *Brit J Surg* 1920;7: 407–22.
6. Kershner MS, Goodman GA, Perlmutter GS. Computed tomography in the diagnosis of an atlas fracture. *AJR* 1977;128:688–9.
7. Lee C, Woodring JH. Unstable Jefferson variant atlas fractures: an unrecognized cervical injury. *AJNR* 1991;12:1105–10, *AJR* 1992;158:113–8.
8. Steppe R, Bellemans M, Boven F, et al. The value of computed tomography scanning in elusive fractures of the cervical spine. *Skeletal Radiol* 1981;6:175–8.
9. Suss RA, Zimmerman RD, Leeds NE. Pseudospread of the atlas: False sign of Jefferson fracture in young children. *AJNR* 1983;4: 183–6; *AJR* 1983;140:1079–82.

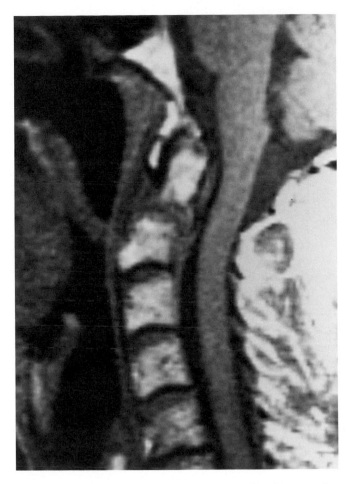

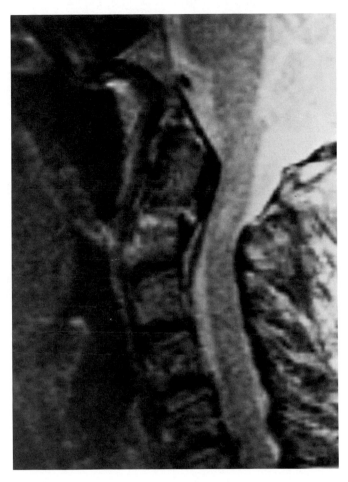

FIG. 46-1A. This 75-year-old woman sustained trauma to her neck. Sagittal T1-weighted SE MR image (700/15) of the cervical spine.

FIG. 46-1B. Sagittal T2-weighted SE MR image (2400/70).

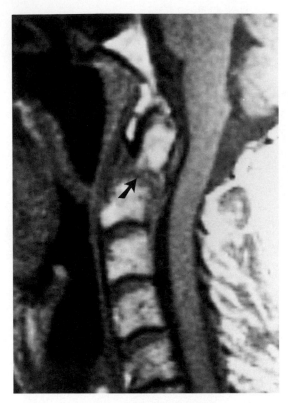

FIG. 46-1A. Fracture of the odontoid process of C2. There is a horizontal fracture through the base of the odontoid process of C2 (*arrow*). Intermediate signal intensity is seen at the fracture site as well as anterior and posterior to C2 and the odontoid.

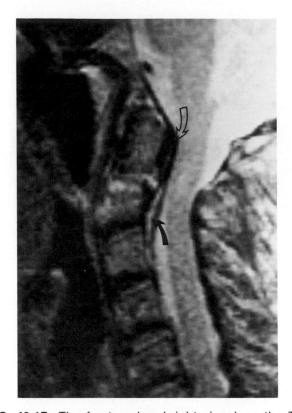

FIG. 46-1B. The fracture has bright signal on the T2-weighted image caused by edema. Increased signal of the C2 vertebral body is also noted. Posteriorly there are areas of high-signal edema (*solid arrow*), and low-signal acute hematoma with deoxyhemoglobin (*open arrow*), causing compression of the anterior subarachnoid space. A small area of bright signal within the spinal cord may be caused by cord edema.

FRACTURE OF C2

In this case, sagittal T1- and T2-weighted MR images show a fracture of the odontoid process as well as soft tissue edema and hematoma (Fig. 46-1). Bright signal intensity at the fracture site is seen on T2-weighted images and is caused by edema. Magnetic resonance imaging can also show displacement of the fracture fragments, disruption of the ligaments, and spinal cord compression (Fig. 46-2).

The odontoid process is the most frequently fractured segment of the C2 vertebra, and these fractures account for 13 percent of cervical spine fractures (7). These fractures may go undetected with conventional radiographic studies, and further evaluation with CT or MR imaging may be needed. Computed tomography may also fail to show an odontoid fracture, especially when the fracture is horizontal and nondisplaced (2). In this setting the plane of scanning is parallel to the fracture line, and the nondisplaced fracture may not be visualized on the axial scan. In some cases, sagittal

and coronal reconstruction views may be the best or only way to identify these fractures with CT (Fig. 46-3). Thin section axial scans (1.5 mm or 2.0 mm) are needed to obtain best quality reconstruction. Axial CT and sagittal reconstruction views can help evaluate displacement of a fracture and the degree of spinal canal and spinal cord compromise (Fig. 46-4). Patient cooperation is particularly important when studying odontoid fractures since patient movement significantly detracts from the reformatted image (Fig. 46-5).

Odontoid fractures are classified into three types (1). Type I fractures are uncommon, stable avulsion fractures located at the tip of the odontoid process. Type II fractures occur at the junction of the odontoid process and the body of C2. This is the most common type of odontoid fracture. It is unstable and has a high incidence of nonunion when treated conservatively (1). Nonunion may develop whether the fracture is displaced or nondisplaced. Fractures that are initially

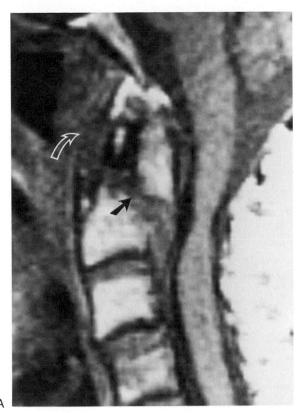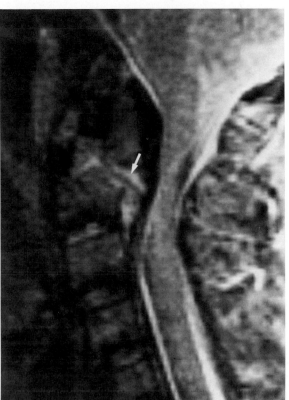

A   B

FIG. 46-2. Fracture of the odontoid process with posterior displacement. **A**: Sagittal T1-weighted SE MR image (700/15) of the cervical spine shows a fracture through the base of the odontoid process (*black arrow*) with posterior displacement of the odontoid. Compression of the spinal cord can be seen. Note disruption of the anterior longitudinal ligament (*white arrow*) and prevertebral edema. **B**: Sagittal T2-weighted SE MR image (2609/70) shows bright signal of edema at the fracture site (*arrow*) as well as anterior and posterior to C2. Spinal cord compression is again noted.

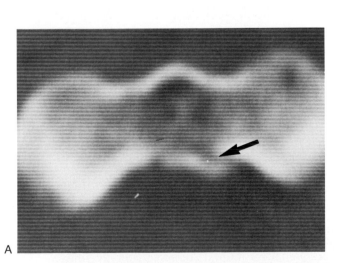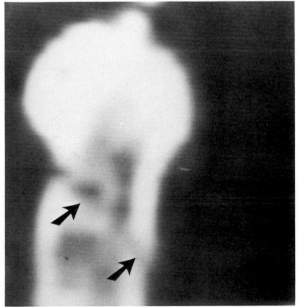

A   B

FIG. 46-3. Fracture at the base of the odontoid process. **A**: Axial CT at the base of the odontoid process suggests a subtle fracture (*arrow*). This injury could not be further delineated by additional axial scans. **B**: Sagittal reconstruction of the axial images. In this case, the use of sagittal reconstruction permitted better visualization of the fracture and its orientation. The fracture is not displaced and has an oblique course (*arrows*).

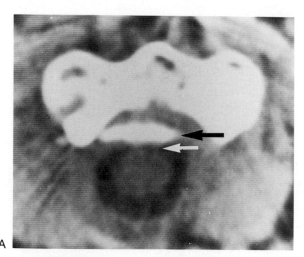
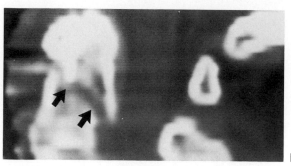

FIG. 46-4. Odontoid fracture. **A**: Axial CT shows a fracture at the base of the odontoid process. The posteriorly displaced fracture fragment (*black arrow*) abuts the anterior subarachnoid space (*white arrow*) without compressing or displacing the spinal cord. **B**: Sagittal reconstruction of the axial images. The oblique course of the fracture is apparent (*arrows*), with the fracture involving both the odontoid and the body of C2 (type III odontoid fracture).

nondisplaced frequently become displaced if fusion is not performed (1). The type III fracture extends into the body of C2. This fracture leads to nonunion in 40 percent of cases when the displacement is more than 5 mm and in 22 percent of cases when angular deformity is greater than 10 degrees (3). Fracture of the odontoid may be associated with the Jefferson-type fracture of C1 or atlanto-axial subluxation and should be sought when these injuries are present (10) (see Fig. 46-5).

The second most common fracture of C2 is the so-called hangman's fracture, with bilateral fractures of the pedicles of C2 occurring anterior to the inferior articular processes (Fig. 46-6). This injury results from acute hyperextension of the skull upon the cervical spine and accounts for 7 percent of cases of fracture and/or dislocation of the cervical spine (5). The bilateral fracture through the pedicles may or may not be associated with anterior displacement of the C2 vertebral body on C3 (traumatic spondylolisthesis of the axis). Anterior slippage of C2 occurs as a result of disruption of the anterior longitudinal ligament. In addition, there may be an avulsion fracture of the anterior inferior aspect of the C2 vertebral body or the anterior superior margin of C3 (4). Much less often there may be atypical fractures of the neural arch of C2 with frac-

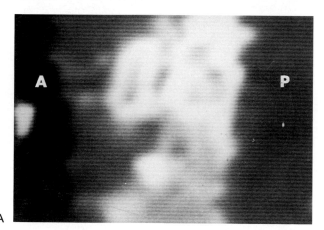
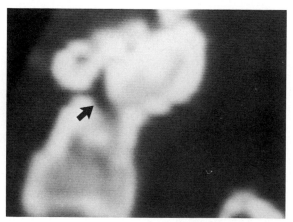

FIG. 46-5. Fracture of the odontoid process. **A**: Unsatisfactory sagittal reconstruction because of an inability of the patient to cooperate. A Jefferson fracture of C1 was diagnosed with axial CT in this uncooperative trauma victim. Considerable patient motion detracted from the image quality and prevented adequate reconstruction of the axial images. Although no fracture of the odontoid process could be seen, a repeat examination was recommended. *A*, anterior; *P*, posterior. **B**: A repeat examination was obtained when the patient was able to cooperate. An oblique angulated fracture of the odontoid could now be seen (*arrow*). This case demonstrates the need for patient cooperation in obtaining diagnostic reconstruction views.

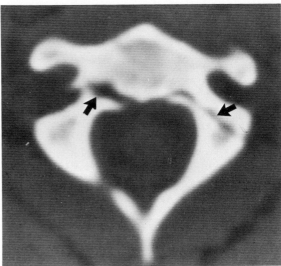

FIG. 46-6. Hangman's fracture. Bilateral fracture of the pedicles of C2 (*arrows*) shown on CT. This type of injury may be associated with traumatic spondylolisthesis of the axis.

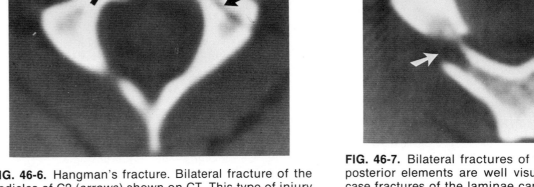

FIG. 46-7. Bilateral fractures of the laminae of C2. The posterior elements are well visualized with CT. In this case fractures of the laminae can be seen (*arrows*).

ture of both laminae of C2 (Fig. 46-7) or fracture of one pedicle and the opposite lamina. These atypical neural arch fractures as well as the typical bilateral pedicular fractures are considered unstable but are usually not associated with significant neurologic defi-

cit. They usually heal well with conservative management (4–8). Bilateral symmetric fractures of the arch of C2 are usually readily apparent on the lateral radiograph of the cervical spine. However, fractures may be more difficult to detect when they occur asymmetri-

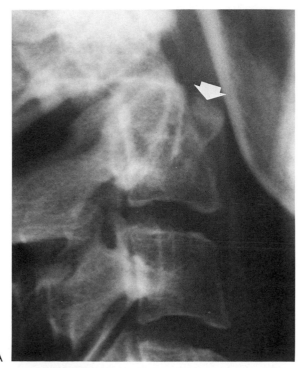

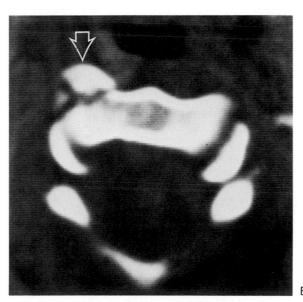

A   B

FIG. 46-8. Fracture of C2. **A**: Lateral radiograph of the upper cervical spine. A suspicious bone density is seen anterior to the C2 vertebral body (*arrow*). There is no soft-tissue swelling. **B**: Axial CT scan at the level of the C2 vertebral body just caudad to the odontoid process. A fracture on the right side of C2 is clearly seen (*arrow*). The anteriorly displaced fracture fragment accounts for the presence of the bone density anterior to C2 as seen on the conventional lateral radiograph.

cally at different sites of the vertebral arch (and are thus obscured by superimposition of solid bone from the opposite side) (9). Questionable abnormalities seen on conventional radiographs can be clarified with the use of CT (Fig. 46-8).

REFERENCES

1. Anderson LD, D'Alonzo RT. Fractures of the odontoid process of the axis. *J Bone Joint Surg (Am)* 1974;56A:1663–74.
2. Brant-Zawadzki M, Miller EM, Federle MP. CT in the evaluation of spine trauma. *AJR* 1981;136:369–75.
3. Clark CR, White AA III. Fractures of the dens: a multicenter study. *J Bone Joint Surg (Am)* 1985;67A:1340–8.
4. Elliott JM, Rogers LF, Wissinger JP, et al. The hangman's fracture: fractures of the neural arch of the axis. *Radiology* 1972; 104:303–7.
5. Gehweiler JA, Clark WM, Schaaf RE, et al. Cervical spine trauma: the common combined conditions. *Radiology* 1979;130: 77–86.
6. Gehweiler JA, Osborne RL, Becker RF. *The radiology of vertebral trauma*. Philadelphia: WB Saunders; 1980.
7. Martinez S, Morgan CL, Gehweiler JA, et al. Unusual fractures and dislocations of the axis vertebra. *Skeletal Radiol* 1979;3: 206–12.
8. Miller MD, Gehweiler JA, Martinez S, et al. Significant new observations on cervical spine trauma. *AJR* 1978;130:659–63.
9. Rogers LF. *Radiology of skeletal trauma*. New York: Churchill Livingstone; 1982.
10. Sherk HH. Fractures of the atlas and odontoid process. *Orthop Clin North Am* 1978;9:973–84.

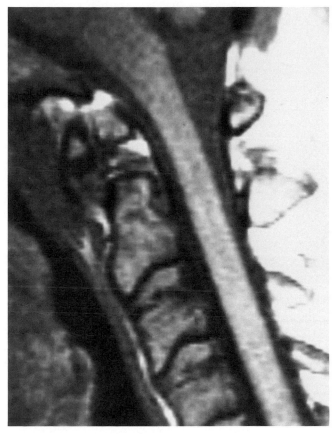

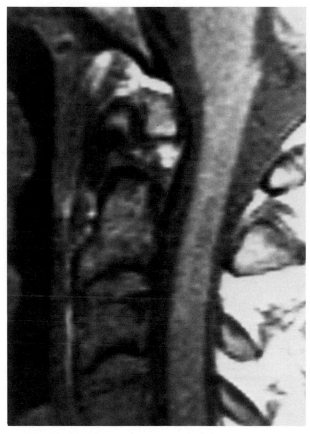

FIG. 47-1A. This 26-year-old man had no history of trauma. Sagittal T1-weighted SE MR image (700/15) of the cervical spine obtained with the neck in flexion.

FIG. 47-1B. Sagittal T1-weighted image with the neck in extension.

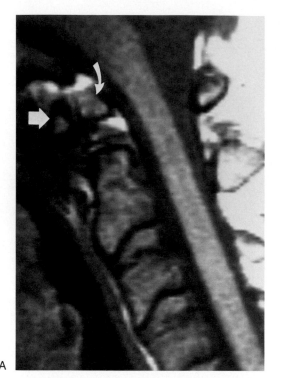 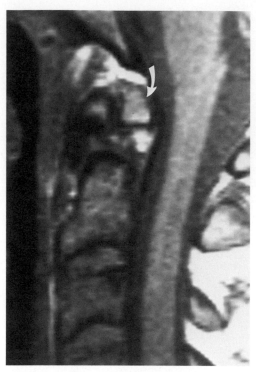

FIG. 47-1A. Os odontoideum. An os odontoideum (*curved arrow*) is seen as an ossicle separate from a hypoplastic odontoid process. Bright signal of fat is seen above and below the os. The anterior arch of C1 is noted (*straight arrow*).

FIG. 47-1B. In extension, the os odontoideum (*arrow*) is displaced posteriorly in relation to the hypoplastic odontoid process. Slight compression of the anterior subarachnoid space can be seen.

OS ODONTOIDEUM

There is an os odontoideum (Fig. 47-1A) that shows motion, with slight impression on the anterior subarachnoid space, when the neck is placed in extension (Fig. 47-1B). As os odontoideum is a small, round or oval, corticated ossicle that is separated from and craniad to a hypoplastic odontoid process. The ossicle may be in a normal position adjacent to the tip of the odontoid process or it may be more cephalad near the basion and either separate or fused to the basion (1). Associated osseous abnormalities of C1 include hypoplasia of the posterior arch and hypertrophy of the anterior arch (5).

Most authors feel that os odontoideum is a congenital anomaly (3,5); however, some believe that it occurs secondary to childhood trauma (1,2). It is usually seen in normal individuals but may also be found in patients with trisomy 21 (Down's syndrome) or Klippel-Feil syndrome (1). Other congenital anomalies of the occipitocervical region may be associated with os odon-

toideum. Cases have been reported following trauma in patients with a previously normal-appearing odontoid process (1,2). Os odontoideum has also been seen after acute ligamentous disruption followed by atlanto-axial instability. Os odontoideum is frequently associated with atlanto-axial instability. Such instability depends on the level of the cleft in the odontoid process (5). If the transverse ligament is in juxtaposition to the os odontoideum, the odontoid process is not able to form a stable relationship with the atlas, thus leading to atlanto-axial instability (5). Although patients with os odontoideum are frequently symptomatic, the symptoms are not attributed to the os odontoideum itself, but rather to the atlanto-axial instability (3). The severity of symptoms is in turn related to the size of the spinal canal (4).

Conventional radiographs with flexion and extension can display the degree of motion of the ossicle, extent of compromise of the spinal canal, and whether the

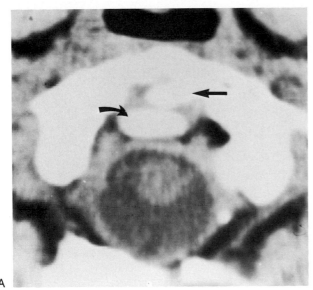
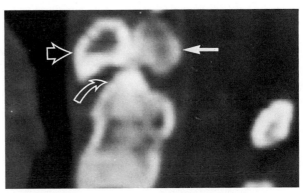

A

B

FIG. 47-2. Os odontoideum. **A**: Axial CT image through the plane of the superior portion of the odontoid process of C2 (*straight arrow*) and the inferior aspect of an os odontoideum (*curved arrow*). **B**: Sagittal reconstruction of axial CT images at C1 and C2 levels. An os odontoideum (*closed arrow*) is seen cephalad to a hypoplastic odontoid process (*curved arrow*). There is hypertrophy of the anterior arch of C1 (*straight open arrow*). In this case the anterior superior aspect of the odontoid lies anterior to the inferior portion of the os odontoideum. This sagittal reconstruction view is helpful in understanding the axial scan shown in (A).

transverse ligament is intact. The osseous anatomy is shown well on CT, including the presence of a corticated ossicle and associated abnormalities of C1 (Fig. 47-2A). Sagittal reconstruction of the axial images is useful in clarifying the axial images (Fig. 47-2B). Magnetic resonance imaging is helpful in determining the degree of compromise of the spinal cord. This can be accomplished with SE T1-weighted images in the sagittal projection and, if necessary, with flexion and extension MR study.

REFERENCES

1. Fielding JW, Hensinger RN, Hawkins RJ. Os odontoideum: *J Bone Joint Surg (Am)* 1980;62A:376–83.
2. Freiberger RH, Wilson PD, Nicholas JA. Acquired absence of the odontoid process. *J Bone Joint Surg (Am)* 1965;47A:1231–6.
3. McRae DL. The significance of abnormalities of the cervical spine. *AJR* 1960;84:3–25.
4. Minderhoud JM, Braakman R, Penning L. Os odontoideum: clinical, radiological and therapeutic aspects. *J Neurol Sci* 1969;8:521–44.
5. Wollin DG. The os odontoideum. *J Bone Joint Surg (Am)* 1963;45A:1459–71,1484.

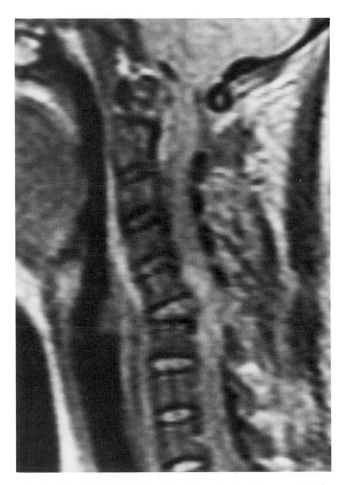

FIG. 48-1A. This 29-year-old man sustained trauma to the cervical spine. Sagittal proton density-weighted SE MR image (2200/40).

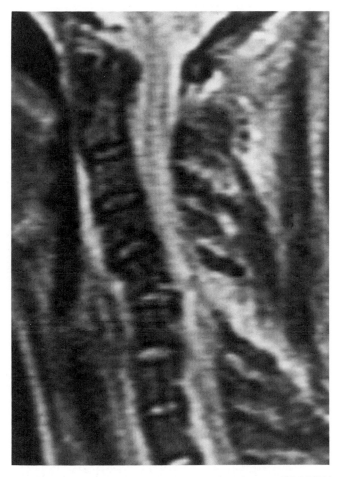

FIG. 48-1B. Sagittal T2-weighted SE MR image (2200/80) of the cervical spine.

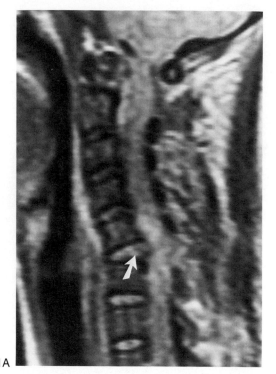 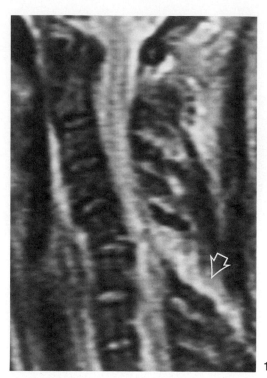

1A 1B

FIG. 48-1A. Cervical flexion injury with dislocation and posterior ligamentous injury. There is widening of the C5-C6 intervertebral disc space (*arrow*) and vertebral body displacement. A previous radiograph had shown dislocation at C5-C6 that was partially reduced at the time of the MR examination. Bright signal of edema is seen within the spinal cord.

FIG. 48-1B. Bright signal intensity can be seen extending through the posterior ligamentous complex (*arrow*), and there is widening of the interspinous distance indicating ligamentous disruption. This is a flexion injury.

CERVICAL FLEXION INJURY WITH DISLOCATION AND DISRUPTION OF THE POSTERIOR LIGAMENTOUS COMPLEX

This patient had a flexion injury with dislocation at C5-C6. At the time of the MR examination, the dislocation was partially reduced; however, widening of the disc space with some angulation and malalignment can be seen (Fig. 48-1A). On the T2-weighted image there is bright signal intensity within the substance of the interspinous ligaments (Fig. 48-1B). Injury to the ligaments such as contusion, hemorrhage, or rupture leads to abnormal signal intensity of the ligaments. The assessment of the extent of ligamentous injury may be helpful in evaluation of spinal instability (3,4). Identification of ligamentous injury, which is best seen with MR imaging, may also assist in our understanding of the mechanism of injury in spinal trauma.

In one study (4), victims of spinal trauma were examined with a low-field-strength magnet within 3 weeks of trauma, and 43 percent had MR demonstration of injury to the posterior ligamentous complex. In this study, increased signal intensity was seen within the interspinous and intertransverse ligaments on T1- and T2-weighted images but was optimally seen on STIR images. Each case that had abnormal signal within the posterior ligamentous complex had associated vertebral column or intraspinal abnormalities, although some patients had intraspinal pathology in the absence of ligamentous signal alterations (4).

Magnetic resonance imaging is also able to show an acute posttraumatic disc herniation, a surgically correctable cause of spinal cord compression that may occur in association with severe flexion or extension injury. In one study (4), disc protrusion was present in 30 percent of patients with recent cervical trauma. Surgical intervention for traumatic disc herniation may prevent a neurologic deficit if undertaken before spinal cord compromise, or may reverse an already existing deficit (9).

Conventional CT without contrast is often used in evaluation of cervical trauma and is helpful in showing

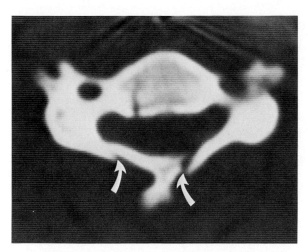

FIG. 48-2. Unstable fracture of C4. Axial CT shows fractures of both laminae of C4 (*arrows*) with some displacement causing spinal canal narrowing. A fracture of the vertebral body is also noted.

the location and configuration of cervical fractures, displacement of fracture fragments, and degree of spinal stenosis (Fig. 48-2). Computed tomography is particularly important in the evaluation of C6, C7, and T1 since these levels may be difficult to evaluate adequately by conventional radiography (10). It is also the best method available for evaluating the posterior elements.

The vertebral arch is the most frequent site of fracture in cervical spine injury. Fractures of the vertebral arch are found in 50 percent of patients with cervical spine fracture and/or dislocation (5). From C3 to C7, the pillar fracture is the most frequent type of vertebral

arch fracture (5). The pillar is a rhomboid structure formed by the fusion of the superior and inferior articular process of each vertebra (e.g., the superior and inferior articular processes of C5 fuse to form the pillars of C5). Fractures through the pillars can be detected by CT even in cases that appear normal with conventional radiography (1,10,11) (Fig. 48-3). However, some cervical pillar fractures may be difficult to detect with axial CT, especially when the fracture is in the horizontal plane (7). These fractures may superficially resemble a normal or distracted facet joint (13). Computed tomographic demonstration of a distracted uncovertebral joint or facet joint without other identified abnormalities suggests the need for further evaluation (e.g., reconstruction views, conventional tomography) (13). Uncovertebral joint subluxation indicates a rotation injury of the vertebral body and is usually accompanied by additional fracture or dislocation at that level. Facet joint subluxation or widening suggests the possibility of associated pillar fracture or locked facet (7,13) (Fig. 48-4).

It is very important to study the conventional radiograph in conjunction with the CT study. Occasionally a unilateral locked facet is better seen with conventional radiography than with CT (10). The CT evaluation of vertebral body subluxation or compression depends on reconstruction views. Patient cooperation and detailed attention to technique are necessary for satisfactory reconstruction. A sagittal reconstruction view is shown in Figure 48-5, which shows an apparent subluxation of C2-C3. This patient had no history of trauma or arthritis and no actual cervical subluxation. This pseudosubluxation was created when a pillow was

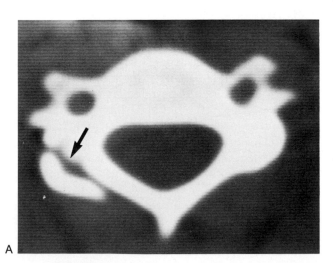

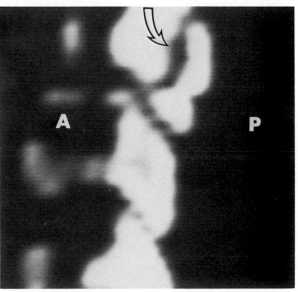

FIG. 48-3. Pillar fracture. **A**: A fracture through the C3 pillar is present on the right (*arrow*). **B**: Parasagittal reconstruction of axial images through the plane of the right articular processes. The fracture can be seen extending vertically through the C3 pillar (*arrow*). *A*, anterior; *P*, posterior.

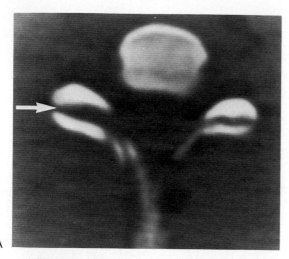 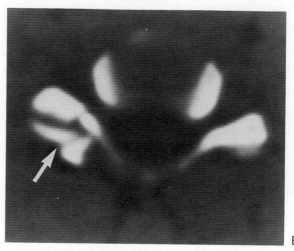

FIG. 48-4. Widening of facet joint and pillar fracture. **A**: There is considerable widening of the right facet joint (*arrow*). Compare with the normal left side. A fracture of the right lamina is present; however, this was better visualized on an adjacent scan. **B**: A comminuted pillar fracture of C6 (*arrow*) is present in this patient who also had widening of the facet joint as shown in (A). The CT demonstration of a pillar fracture may be misinterpreted as a widened facet joint in some cases.

placed behind the patient's head and neck in the middle of the examination in an effort to relieve patient discomfort. With the patient's position altered during the examination, the sagittal reconstruction showed an apparent subluxation. Commonly, the degree of vertebral body subluxation and compression can be better determined by conventional radiography or MR imaging in the sagittal plane.

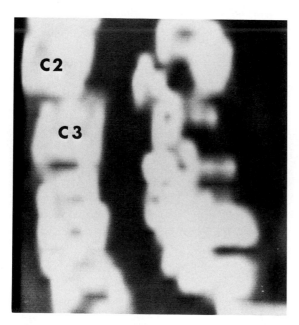

FIG. 48-5. Pseudosubluxation. Sagittal reconstruction of axial images suggests a C2-C3 subluxation. However, no subluxation is present. The apparent subluxation on this reconstruction study occurred because the patient's position was altered during the examination by the placement of a pillow beneath the head and neck.

Cervical nerve root avulsion is another injury to the cervical spine that can be seen with myelography, CTM, and MR imaging. A cervical nerve root avulsion appears on CTM examination as an expanded outpouching of contrast extending ventrolaterally from the thecal sac into the neural foramen (6,8) (Fig. 48-6). This collection of contrast, which represents a meningocele, is sometimes separated from the thecal sac by a thin dural plane measuring 1–2 mm in width (8). At the time of injury the avulsed nerve root retracts and is usually not seen within the meningocele during CTM study. Cervical nerve root avulsion may lead to brachial plexopathy or palsy. The C7, C8, and T1 nerve roots are most commonly involved when the injury occurs while the arm is in abduction (8). Traction is greatest on the C5 and C6 nerve roots when the arm is in adduction (8). Myelography can be used to show cervical nerve root avulsion; however, CTM offers the additional benefit of showing the presence of bone fracture fragments and hematoma, which could be correctable causes of symptoms. Computed tomographic myelography is also useful in diagnosing a dural tear with or without associated nerve root avulsion. The dural laceration leads to contrast escaping outside the subarachnoid space, a finding that is more readily seen with CTM than with conventional myelography in some cases (6).

With cervical nerve root avulsion, the surrounding nerve root sleeve is disrupted and may be enlarged. It contains cerebrospinal fluid that does not pulsate to the same degree as the cerebrospinal fluid surrounding the spinal cord, and is therefore not subjected to the same degree of signal loss caused by pulsatile motion on MR examination (2). Thus, axial T2-weighted MR

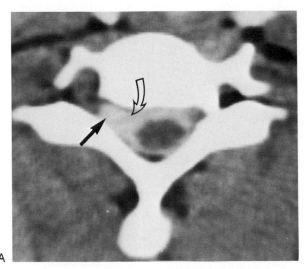 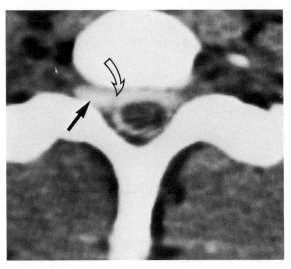

A   B

FIG. 48-6. Cervical nerve root avulsion. **A**: Axial CTM at C6-C7 of a patient who sustained a traumatic brachial palsy. There is an outpouching of contrast (*straight arrow*) within the neural foramen. This collection of contrast represents a meningocele, which occurs from avulsion of the C7 nerve root. The meningocele is separated from the contrast-filled subarachnoid space by a thin dural plane (*curved arrow*). Slight displacement of the spinal cord is noted. **B**: Axial CTM at C7-T1. Avulsion of the C8 nerve root is diagnosed as contrast extends ventrolaterally into the neural foramen at the C7-T1 level (*straight arrow*). Again, a thin dural plane (*curved arrow*) separates the meningocele from the subarachnoid space.

images obtained without flow compensation show relatively higher signal intensity of fluid within the meningoceles than is seen within pulsatile cerebrospinal fluid surrounding the spinal cord. Traumatic lumbar meningoceles are uncommon. However, like the more common cervical meningoceles, they can be evaluated with myelography, CTM, and MR imaging (12). Avulsion of a nerve root can be determined with these various imaging modalities by showing the absence of a nerve root within a meningocele. However, in one case described, the continuity of the nerve roots could only be assessed by axial T1-weighted MR images (12).

REFERENCES

1. Coin CG, Pennink M, Ahmad WD, et al. Diving-type injury of the cervical spine: contribution of computed tomography to management. *J Comput Assist Tomogr* 1979;3:362–72.
2. Enzmann DR, Rubin JB, DeLaPaz R, et al. Cerebrospinal fluid pulsation: benefits and pitfalls in MR imaging. *Radiology* 1986; 161:773–8.
3. Goldberg AL, Rothfus WE, Deeb ZL, et al. The impact of magnetic resonance in the diagnostic evaluation of acute cervicothoracic spinal trauma. *Skeletal Radiol* 1988;17:89–95.
4. Kerslake RW, Jaspan T, Worthington BS. Magnetic resonance imaging of spinal trauma. *Brit J Radiol* 1991;64:386–402.
5. Miller MD, Gehweiler JA, Martinez S, et al. Significant new observations on cervical spine trauma. *AJR* 1978;130:659–63.
6. Morris RE, Hasso AN, Thompson JR, et al. Traumatic dural tears: CT diagnosis using metrizamide. *Radiology* 1984;152: 443–6.
7. Pech P, Kilgore DP, Pojunas KW, et al. Cervical spinal fractures: CT detection. *Radiology* 1985;157:117–20.
8. Petras AF, Sobel DF, Mani JR, et al. CT myelography in cervical nerve root avulsion. *J Comput Assist Tomogr* 1985;9:275–9.
9. Post MJD, Green BA. The use of computed tomography in spinal trauma. *Radiol Clin North Am* 1983;21:327–75.
10. Post MJD, Green BA, Quencer RM, et al. The value of computed tomography in spinal trauma. *Spine* 1982;7:417–31.
11. Steppe R, Bellemans M, Boven F, et al. The value of computed tomography scanning in elusive fractures of the cervical spine. *Skeletal Radiol* 1981;6:175–8.
12. Verstraete KLA, Martens F, Smeets P, et al. Traumatic lumbosacral nerve root meningoceles: the value of myelography, CT and MRI in the assessment of nerve root continuity. *Neuroradiology* 1989;31:425–9.
13. Yetkin Z, Osborn AG, Giles DS, et al. Uncovertebral and facet joint dislocations in cervical articular pillar fractures: CT evaluation. *AJNR* 1985;6:633–7.

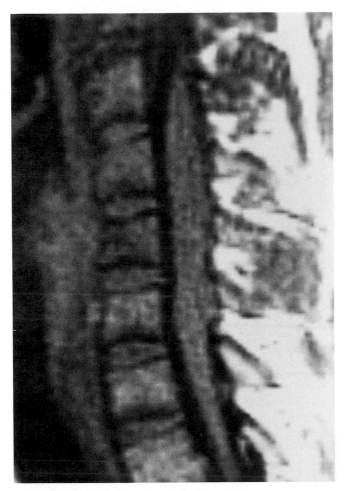

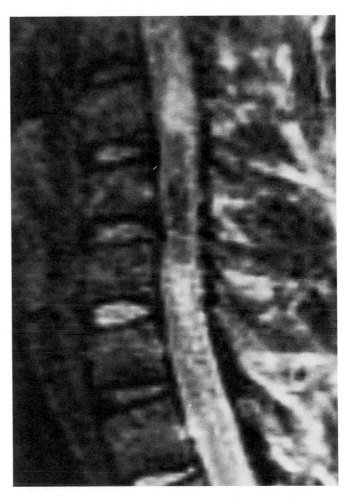

FIG. 49-1A. Sagittal T1-weighted SE MR image (700/15) of the cervical spine obtained with a 1.5-T magnet. This 24-year-old man had sustained trauma to the cervical spine.

FIG. 49-1B. Sagittal T2-weighted SE MR image (2143/70).

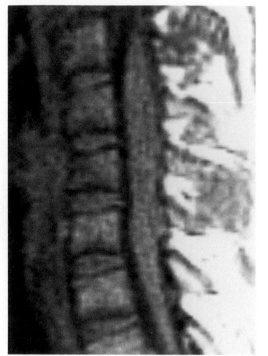 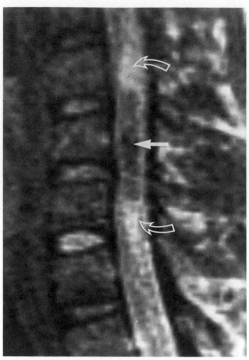

FIG. 49-1A. The spinal cord is widened and remains of normal signal intensity. There is corresponding narrowing of the subarachnoid space.

FIG. 49-1B. On the T2-weighted image there is a large area of very low signal intensity within the spinal cord caused by the presence of deoxyhemoglobin in an acute spinal cord hematoma (*straight arrow*). The bright signal intensity above and below the hematoma is caused by edema (*curved arrows*).

HEMATOMA AND EDEMA OF THE SPINAL CORD

In this case there is an acute spinal cord hematoma that is isointense relative to the spinal cord on T1-weighted MR images (Fig. 49-1A) and hypointense to the cord on T2-weighted images (Fig. 49-1B) because of the presence of deoxyhemoglobin within the hematoma. Edema of the cord is present both superior and inferior to the hemorrhage and is seen as areas of increased signal intensity on T2-weighted images. The hematoma has very low signal intensity on the axial GRE images (Fig. 49-2).

Magnetic resonance imaging is a useful method of evaluating patients with spinal cord injury. It can show both extrinsic compression on the cord (such as occurs secondary to fracture fragments or disc herniation) and intrinsic abnormalities of the cord (such as hemorrhage or edema).

The MR appearance of hematoma in the brain has been well described (2). The appearance of intracranial hematoma depends on the age of the hematoma and on the field strength of the magnet (3). Hematoma is classified as acute (<1 week old), subacute (>1 week and <1 month old), and chronic (>1 month old). Using a low-field-strength magnet (<0.5-T), acute hematomas are isointense with the surrounding brain, whereas subacute and chronic hematomas have increased signal intensity on all pulse sequences.

The appearance of intracranial hematomas differs when they are studied with a 1.5-T, high-field-strength magnet. In the acute phase, the hematoma will remain isointense on T1-weighted images, but will have marked central hypointensity on T2-weighted images because of the presence of deoxyhemoglobin within intact red blood cells. This hypointensity on T2 is thought to be caused by local heterogeneity in magnetic susceptibility, which results in a preferential T2 proton relaxation enhancement (2,3). Subacute hematomas initially have peripheral hyperintensity on T1- and hypointensity on T2-weighted images due to the presence of intracellular methemoglobin. Later, hyperintensity can be seen on both T1- and T2-weighted images because of the presence of free methemoglobin which occurs after red blood cell lysis (2). Macrophages digest the red blood cells in the periphery of the hematoma and produce hemosiderin, which is seen as a pe-

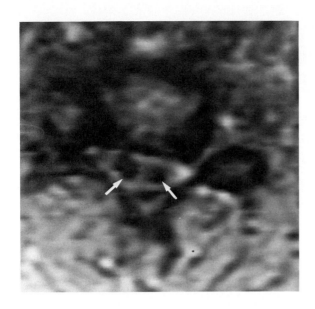

FIG. 49-2. Spinal cord hematoma. Same patient as Fig. 49-1. Axial GRE image (GRASS, 24/13 with 8-degree flip angle) obtained through the area of spinal cord hematoma shown in Fig. 49-1B. Note very low signal intensity within the spinal cord caused by the presence of deoxyhemoglobin (*arrows*). Gradient-echo images are particularly sensitive to magnetic susceptibility effects and are therefore sensitive to the presence of deoxyhemoglobin (and hemosiderin, not shown).

ripheral rim of markedly decreased signal intensity on T2-weighted images. In the chronic stage, the central portion of the hematoma also shows increased signal intensity on both T1- and T2-weighted images because of the presence of free methemoglobin. The peripheral rim of hemosiderin remains. Eventually the hematoma may appear as a slit of hemosiderin, with low signal intensity that is most obvious on T2-weighted images. The hypointensity patterns of deoxyhemoglobin and hemosiderin are proportional to the square of the magnitude of the mean magnetic field (2,3). This explains why central decreased signal intensity of deoxyhemoglobin in the acute stage, and the peripheral rim of decreased signal intensity of hemosiderin in the subacute and chronic stages, are seen with high-field-strength magnets and not with low-field-strength magnets. Edema can be seen at the periphery of acute and subacute hematomas as increased signal intensity on the T2-weighted images and is visualized with both high- and low-field-strength magnets.

The MR images of an intradural spinal hematoma are shown in Figs. 49-3 and show the evolution of signal intensity changes over a 5-week period similar to those described for intracranial hematomas. This patient was a pregnant woman who had an acute onset of severe sacral and coccygeal pain caused by an epedymoma that bled. In addition to the intradural hematoma, a subarachnoid hemorrhage was seen on the initial images (Figs. 49-3A to 3C). Follow-up examinations were obtained at 6 days (Figs. 49-3D, 3E) and 5 weeks (Figs. 49-3F, 3G). Four months later (Figs. 49-3H, 3I), the hematoma had resolved and the ependymoma enhanced after the injection of gadopentetate dimeglumine.

Magnetic resonance imaging of acute spinal cord injury has been studied with animal experimentation using a high-field-strength magnet (4). Images were obtained within 3–5 hours after experimentally induced spinal cord injury. Markedly low signal intensity was seen on the T2-weighted images, and is caused by deoxyhemoglobin. Surrounding edema and possible necrosis were seen as areas of increased signal intensity on the T2-weighted images. This experimentation suggests that MR imaging can be used to differentiate presumably irreversible damage caused by hemorrhage from potentially reversible damage due to edema (4).

In a clinical study using a high-field-strength magnet (1.5-T), MR signal characteristics of spinal cord injury were compared to the patient's initial neurologic examination (7). The Frankel classification (1) was used to identify the spectrum of spinal cord injury (Table 49-1). When MR imaging showed an intramedullary hematoma with deoxyhemoglobin causing decreased signal intensity on the T2-weighted images, 93 percent of the patients had complete motor and sensory loss distal to the lesion (Frankel A), while one patient (7 percent) had only preserved crude sensation distal to the level of injury (Frankel B) (7). This MR pattern of decreased signal intensity on the T2-weighted images was associated with the most severe neurologic deficit. A second type of signal pattern was seen as high signal intensity on the T2-weighted images, and was thought to represent petechial hemorrhages and intraparenchymal edema. When this pattern extended for more than one spinal segment, 82 percent were Frankel A or B injuries. When the petechial hemorrhages and edema extended for less than one spinal segment, only 21 percent were within the Frankel A or B category. Patients with cervical spine injury and a normal spinal cord signal pattern had Frankel E injuries in 75 percent of cases and Frankel D injuries in 18 percent. In this study the MR appearance could be correlated with the patient's

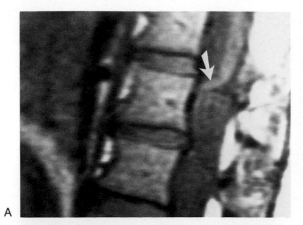

A

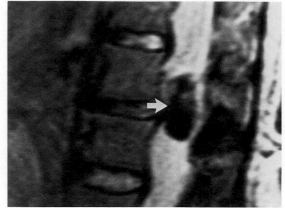

B

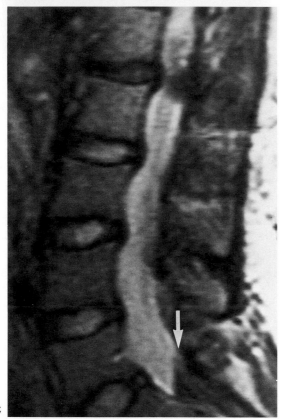

C

FIG. 49-3. Intradural hematoma and subarachnoid hemorrhage due to an ependymoma that bled. An emergency MR examination was performed with a 1.5T magnet for this 30-year-old woman who was in her 28th week of pregnancy and presented with severe sacral and coccygeal pain radiating into both legs (Figs. A-C). Follow-up examinations were obtained 6 days (Figs. D, E), 5 weeks (Figs. F, G), and 4 months (Figs. H, I) after the initial examination. **A**: Sagittal T1-weighted SE MR image (800/20) of the upper lumbar spine shows displacement of the conus (*arrow*). Just inferior to the conus there is minimal alteration in signal intensity. **B**: Sagittal T2-weighted SE MR image (2000/70) shows an intradural hematoma (*arrow*) adjacent to the conus, with very low signal intensity due to deoxyhemoglobin. **C**: Sagittal T2-weighted image obtained 6 mm to the right of Fig. (B) shows a fluid-fluid level (*arrow*) due to subarachnoid hemorrhage. The cerebrospinal fluid has bright signal and the deoxyhemoglobin has low signal on the T2-weighted image. The patient's supine position accounts for the plane of the fluid level.

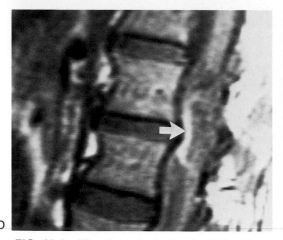

D

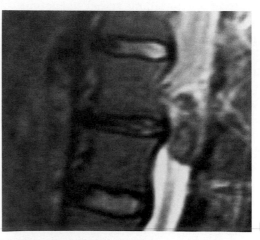

E

FIG. 49-3. (*Continued*). **D**: Sagittal T1-weighted SE MR image (700/15) shows bright signal intensity at the periphery of the hematoma (*arrow*) due to intracellular methemoglobin. **E**: Sagittal T2-weighted SE MR image (2000/70) shows hypointense hematoma.

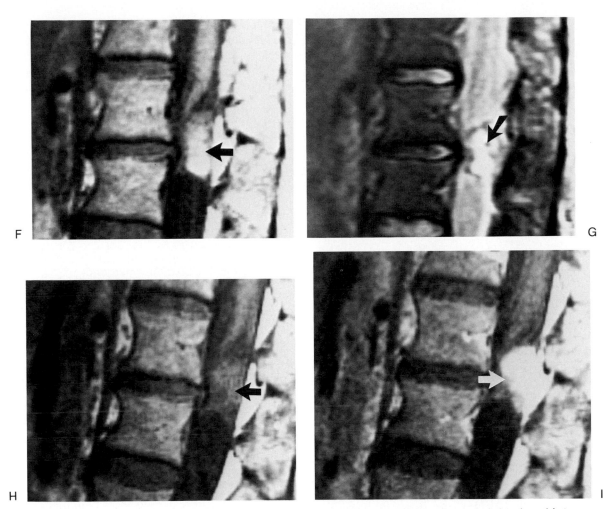

FIG. 49-3. (*Continued*). **F**: Sagittal T1-weighted SE MR image (700/15) shows bright signal intensity of the hematoma (*arrow*). **G**: Sagittal T2-weighted SE MR image (2000/70) shows bright signal intensity of the hematoma (*arrow*). The bright signal on both T1- and T2-weighted images is caused by the presence of extracellular (free) methemoglobin. **H**: Sagittal T1-weighted SE MR image (600/15) shows a mass (*arrow*) that is adjacent to the conus and is of intermediate signal intensity. **I**: Sagittal T1-weighted SE MR image (650/20) obtained after the intravenous injection of gadopentetate dimeglumine shows marked enhancement of the mass (*arrow*). This proved to be an ependymoma.

presenting neurologic status, with intramedullary hematomas and extensive areas of contusion and edema being associated with the most severe neurologic deficits, whereas the appearance of small focal contusions and edema or a normal spinal cord were associated with less severe deficit or no neurologic deficit (7).

In other studies (5,6) the MR pattern of spinal cord injury was compared to the neurologic recovery experienced by the patient. In these studies, three patterns of MR signal intensity were described for spinal cord lesions. The first pattern was found in 33 percent of patients with traumatic spinal cord abnormalities seen with MR imaging (5). In this pattern, the acute phase (<3 days) was characterized by a large area of decreased signal intensity relative to the normal spinal cord on T2-weighted images, caused by deoxyhemo-

globin. Axial T2-weighted images may show bilateral areas of hypointensity at the junction of the grey and white matter. Importantly, patients with this pattern failed to have significant neurologic recovery (5,6). T1-weighted images may show focal areas of asymmetric cord enlargement but fail to show abnormal signal intensity in the acute stage. Between days 3 and 7 there

TABLE 49-1. *Frankel classification of spinal cord injury*

Classification	Neurologic status
A	Complete motor and sensory loss
B	Preserved sensation only
C	Preserved motor (nonfunctional)
D	Preserved motor (functional)
E	Complete neurologic recovery

From ref. 1, with permission.

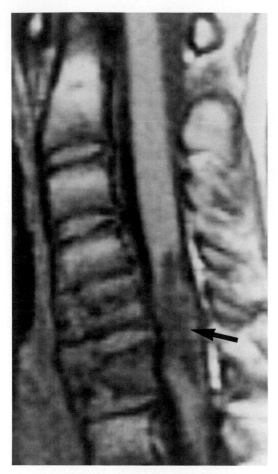

FIG. 49-4. Posttraumatic myelomalacia/syrinx. This 13-year-old boy had sustained fractures of C5 and C6 1 year before this examination. Sagittal T1-weighted SE MR image (700/20) shows low signal intensity within the spinal cord (*arrow*) thought to be caused by myelomalacia or possibly a syrinx. Note compression and low signal intensity of the C5 and C6 vertebral bodies.

edema. This pattern showed rapid resolution on follow-up MR images and often resolved between 1 and 3 weeks after injury (6). Patients with this MR pattern were neurologically normal or experienced significant neurologic recovery from initial neurologic deficits (5,6).

The third pattern was seen in 12 percent of cases with MR-demonstrated post-traumatic spinal cord abnormalities, and is thought to represent a mixed type of injury (5). On T2-weighted images, this pattern showed a small area of decreased signal intensity centrally, with a larger area of surrounding increased signal intensity. This is thought to represent a small central hemorrhage with surrounding edema. These patients have a variable prognosis, with some neurologic recovery possible.

In summary, MR performed with a 1.5-T magnet can be used to differentiate spinal cord hemorrhage from edema and small petechial contusions. The MR signal intensity characteristics can be correlated with the patient's presenting neurologic deficit and with prognosis for neurologic recovery.

MR imaging is also used in the evaluation of chronic spinal cord injury and can show the presence of myelomalacia (Fig. 49-4), syringohydromyelia, and spinal cord atrophy. Both myelomalacia and syringohydromyelia show alterations within the cord, having low signal on T1- and high signal on T2-weighted images. The proton density-weighted images may be useful in differentiating myelomalacia from a small syrinx, since myelomalacia typically has intermediate to high signal and syringohydromyelia has low signal intensity with this pulse sequence.

is increased signal intensity in the peripheral portion of the lesion, and decreased signal intensity centrally on T2-weighted images. The T1-weighted images may also show increased signal intensity on the periphery of these lesions due to the presence of free methemoglobin.

The second MR pattern of spinal cord injury was that of increased signal intensity on T2-weighted images in the acute stage. This pattern was found in approximately 55 percent of patients with MR-demonstrated cord abnormalities and is thought to be the result of edema and small petechial hemorrhages (5). Linear hyperintensity can be seen extending superiorly and inferiorly from the lesion and is thought to represent

REFERENCES

1. Frankel HL, Hancock DO, Hyslop G, et al. The value of postural reduction in initial management of closed injuries of the spine with paraplegia and tetraplegia. *Paraplegia* 1969;7:179–92.
2. Gomori JM, Grossman RI, Goldberg HI, et al. Intracranial hematomas: imaging by high-field MR. *Radiology* 1985;157:87–93.
3. Gomori JM, Grossman RI, Yu-Ip C, et al. NMR relaxation times of blood: dependence on field strength, oxidation state and cell integrity. *J Comput Assist Tomogr* 1987;11:684–90.
4. Hackney DB, Asato R, Joseph PM, et al. Hemorrhage and edema in acute spinal cord compression: demonstration by MR imaging. *Radiology* 1986;161:387–90.
5. Kulkarni MV, Bondurant FJ, Rose SL, et al. 1.5 tesla magnetic resonance imaging of acute spinal trauma. *Radio Graphics* 1988; 8:1059–82.
6. Kulkarni MV, McArdle CB, Kopanicky D, et al. Acute spinal cord injury: MR imaging at 1.5-T. *Radiology* 1987;164:837–43.
7. Schaefer DM, Flanders A, Northrup BE, et al. Magnetic resonance imaging of acute cervical spine trauma: correlation with severity of neurologic injury. *Spine* 1989;14:1090–5.

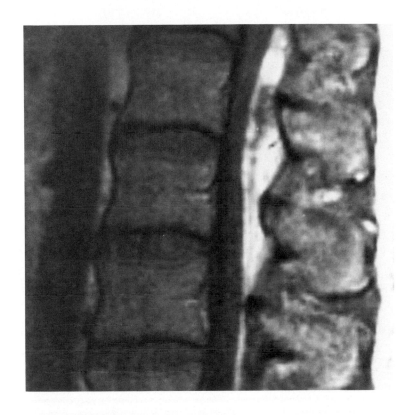

FIG. 50-1A. Magnetic resonance imaging was performed for a 59-year-old man who injured his back while performing construction work and developed low back pain and radiculopathy. Sagittal T1-weighted SE MR image (600/15) from T12 to L3, obtained with 1.5-T superconducting magnet.

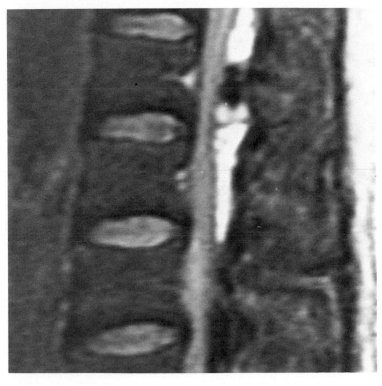

FIG. 50-1B. T2-weighted SE MR image (2000/70) obtained at the same level.

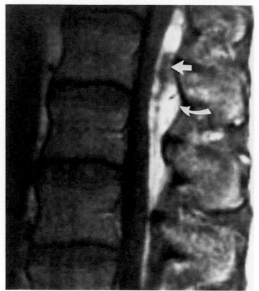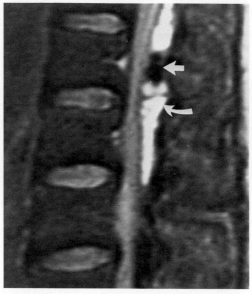

1A   1B

FIG. 50-1A. Epidural hematoma. There is a posterior epidural hematoma from the inferior aspect of T11 to L2. This has bright signal intensity on the T1-weighted images (*curved arrow*) because of the presence of extracellular (free) methemoglobin. Note the biconvex configuration of the hematoma, as well as compression on the thecal sac. Within the central portion of the hematoma is an area of intermediate signal intensity on this T1-weighted image (*straight arrow*).

FIG. 50-1B. On the T2-weighted image the extracellular methemoglobin has bright signal intensity (*curved arrow*). The central portion of the hematoma has markedly low signal intensity on the T2-weighted image because of the presence of deoxyhemoglobin (*straight arrow*). The extracellular methemoglobin represents a subacute stage of the hematoma, whereas the deoxyhemoglobin represents an acute stage.

EPIDURAL HEMATOMA

There is an epidural hematoma that shows high signal intensity on T1- and T2-weighted MR images because of the presence of extracellular (free) methemoglobin (Fig. 50-1). Within the center of the hematoma is an area of low signal intensity on the T2-weighted images, caused by deoxyhemoglobin. Axial T1-weighted images show compression of the thecal sac by the posteriorly located hematoma (Fig. 50-2).

Epidural hematoma may occur after spinal surgery or lumbar puncture, or in association with trauma, infection, neoplasm, coagulopathy, or anticoagulant therapy (2,11,13,14). Occasionally epidural hematoma may occur spontaneously (1,7,12). Clinically an acute epidural hematoma represents an emergency which can lead to severe neurologic complications and possibly death if not treated promptly. Patients present with severe back or neck pain which occurs suddenly and is often radicular. This may progress to weakness and urinary retention and then lead to paraplegia or quadriplegia (11). Although treatment for an acute epidural hematoma usually requires decompressive laminectomy with immediate evacuation of the hematoma, occasionally an epidural hematoma may resolve sponta-

neously (2). Epidural hematoma has been found in approximately 0.2 percent of patients who have had spinal surgery for lumbar disc herniation (4). These patients may have an immediate symptom-free postoperative period lasting approximately 1 day which is followed by persistent, painless paresthesias over the dermatome of the effected nerve root (4).

Magnetic resonance is now considered the imaging modality of choice for diagnosis of epidural hematoma. Long segments of the spinal canal can be studied, which is helpful since epidural hematomas may extend for several vertebral body segments (1,10,12). Magnetic resonance imaging can also be used for follow-up evaluation. In one patient with a posttraumatic epidural hematoma that extended for several cervical levels, nearly complete resolution of the hematoma was seen 4 days after the injury (10).

With MR imaging, blood products can be identified and an epidural location of the hematoma can be determined (Fig. 50-3). Several cases of epidural hematoma have been studied by MR imaging within the first 3 days of the patient's symptoms (1,3,10,12,13). The MR signal characteristics have been variable. On the T1-

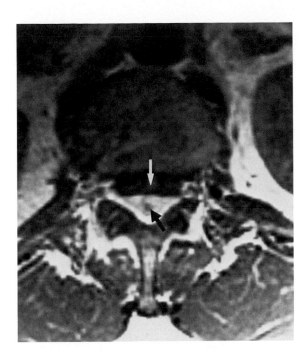

FIG. 50-2. Posterior epidural hematoma. Same patient as in Fig. 50-1. Axial T1-weighted SE MR image (750/15) shows a high signal intensity posterior epidural hematoma (*black arrow*) compressing the thecal sac with its low-signal-intensity cerebrospinal fluid (*white arrow*).

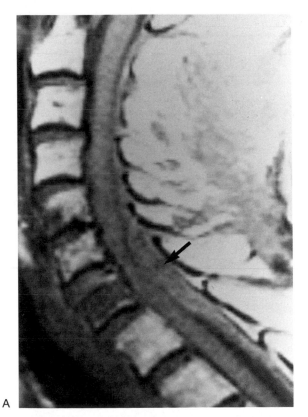

A

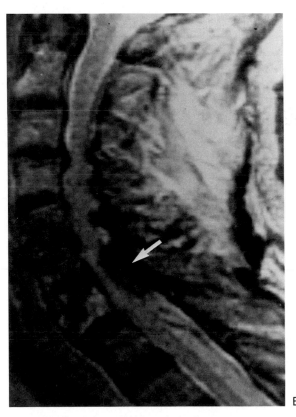

B

FIG. 50-3. Posterior epidural hematoma of the lower cervical and upper thoracic spine. **A**: Sagittal T1-weighted SE MR image (700/15) shows an epidural hematoma (*arrow*) of intermediate signal intensity compressing the spinal cord, most severely from C6 to T1. The C7 vertebral body has low signal intensity. **B**: Sagittal T2-weighted SE MR image (2338/70). There is markedly decreased signal intensity of the epidural hematoma at the level of C7 (*arrow*). This represents deoxyhemoglobin and is indicative of an acute stage of the hematoma. The C7 vertebral body has increased signal intensity suggesting posttraumatic bone marrow edema. Degenerative changes of the cervical spine are incidently noted.

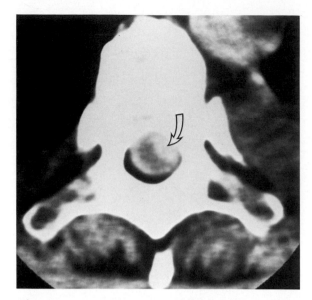

FIG. 50-4. Acute epidural hematoma and subarachnoid hemorrhage. This patient had a history of anticoagulant therapy and experienced bilateral lower extremity weakness. The CT study of the thoracic spine shows a lenticular-shaped high-density epidural hematoma (*arrow*) causing compression of the spinal cord. Hemorrhage is also noted in the subarachnoid space (courtesy Jeffrey Blinder, M.D., Allentown, Pennsylvania).

gins that are usually present (12). Cerebrospinal fluid or dura may be seen separating the hematoma from the spinal cord, especially on axial images (1,12). The axial images may also reveal a unilateral distribution of the hematoma. Compression of the thecal sac and spinal cord is readily assessed by MR imaging. Enhancement of thickened meninges can be seen after the intravenous injection of gadopentetate dimeglumine (3).

Computed tomography can also be used in the diagnostic workup of a patient in whom epidural hematoma is suspected (7–9,11,14). A biconvex high-density epidural mass can be identified (Fig. 50-4). If an intravenous injection of iodinated contrast is given, rim enhancement may be seen (9). In some cases the high-density hematoma may fill the entire canal. However, the CT study has been unrewarding in several cases in which MR imaging clearly showed the hematoma (1,13). In addition, a clinical spinal level cannot be determined in some patients. In the subacute stage, an epidural hematoma may be isodense with the thecal sac with conventional CT. In these cases, a myelogram followed by CTM may establish the diagnosis but represents an invasive, less desirable technique when compared to MR imaging.

weighted images, the acute epidural hematoma may be isointense to the spinal cord or may show increased signal. On the T2-weighted images, the reported epidural hematomas have had increased or heterogeneous signal intensity. Those hematomas that appear inhomogeneous on T2-weighted images may have areas of low signal intensity due to the magnetic susceptibility effect of deoxyhemoglobin when studied with high-field-strength magnets (5). Areas of increased signal suggest high protein or high water content. Acute spinal cord injury was induced and studied in animals using a high-field-strength magnet (6). In this study, images were obtained 3–5 hours after injury. Acute epidural hematomas had high signal intensity on T1-weighted images and were isointense on the T2-weighted images. These findings differed from the signal intensity characteristics of spinal cord hemorrhage which revealed isointensity or slight hypointensity relative to the normal spinal cord on T1-weighted images, and marked decreased signal intensity on T2-weighted images (6). Epidural hematomas that have been present between 1 week and 1 month have shown increased signal intensity on both T1- and T2-weighted images (1,2,13). This corresponds to the findings described in cases of subacute intracerebral hematomas, which have increased signal intensity on T1- and T2-weighted images because of the presence of free methemoglobin (5).

The epidural location of a spinal hematoma may be suggested by the well-defined, tapered, convex mar-

REFERENCES

1. Avrahami E, Tadmor R, Ram Z, et al. MR demonstration of spontaneous acute epidural hematoma of the thoracic spine. *Neuroradiology* 1989;31:89–92.
2. Bernsen PLJA, Haan J, Vielvoye GJ, et al. Spinal epidural hematoma visualized by magnetic resonance imaging. *Neuroradiology* 1988;30:280.
3. Crisi G, Sorgato P, Colombo A, et al. Gadolinium-DTPA-enhanced MR imaging in the diagnosis of spinal epidural haematoma. *Neuroradiology* 1990;32:64–6.
4. DiLauro L, Poli R, Bortoluzzi M, et al. Paresthesias after lumbar disc removal and their relationship to epidural hematoma. *J Neurosurg* 1982;57:135–6.
5. Gomori JM, Grossman RI, Goldberg HI, et al. Intracranial hematomas: imaging by high-field MR. *Radiology* 1985;157:87–93.
6. Hackney DB, Asato R, Joseph PM, et al. Hemorrhage and edema in acute spinal cord compression: demonstration by MR imaging. *Radiology* 1986;161:387–90.
7. Haykal HA, Wang A-M, Zamani AA, et al. Computed tomography of spontaneous acute cervical epidural hematoma. *J Comput Assist Tomogr* 1984;8:229–31.
8. Kaiser MC, Capesius P, Ohanna F, et al. Computed tomography of acute spinal epidural hematoma associated with cervical root avulsion. *J Comput Assist Tomogr* 1984;8:322–3.
9. Laissy J-P, Milon P, Freger P, et al. Cervical epidural hematomas: CT diagnosis in two cases that resolved spontaneously. *AJNR* 1990;11:394–6.
10. Pan G, Kulkarni M, MacDougall DJ, et al. Traumatic epidural hematoma of the cervical spine: diagnosis with magnetic resonance imaging—case report. *J Neurosurg* 1988;68:798–801.
11. Post MJD, Seminer DS, Quencer RM. CT diagnosis of spinal epidural hematoma. *AJNR* 1982;3:190–2.
12. Rothfus WE, Chedid MK, Deeb ZL, et al. MR imaging in the diagnosis of spontaneous spinal epidural hematomas. *J Comput Assist Tomogr* 1987;11:851–4.
13. Tarr RW, Drolshagen LF, Kerner TC, et al. MR imaging of recent spinal trauma. *J Comput Assist Tomogr* 1987;11:412–7.
14. Zilkha A, Irwin GAL, Fagelman D. Computed tomography of spinal epidural hematoma. *AJNR* 1983;4:1073–6.

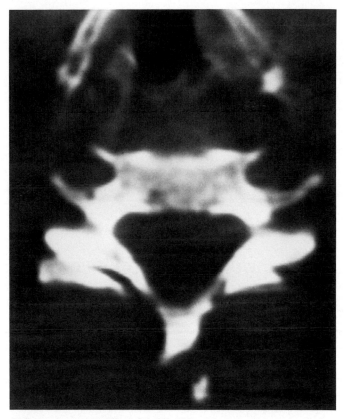

FIG. 51-1. Axial CT at C6-C7. This 44-year-old trauma victim sustained injury to the cervical spine. Conventional radiographs showed anterior subluxation of the C6 vertebral body in relation to C7.

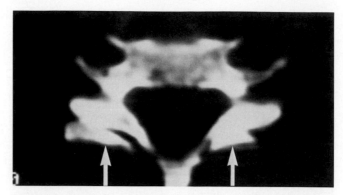

FIG. 51-1. Bilateral locked facets. The superior articular processes of C7 (*arrows*) lie posterior to the inferior articular processes of C6. Note that the superior articular processes have a half-moon shape with a flat posterior margin. Normally, the inferior articular processes of the vertebra above lie posteriorly and have a rounded posterior configuration.

BILATERAL LOCKED FACETS

The superior articular processes of C7 lie posterior to the inferior articular processes of C6 (Fig. 51-1). This is an example of bilateral locked facets. The injury is thought to occur from combined flexion and distraction forces, which cause separation of the spinous processes and disruption of the posterior ligaments (3). The inferior articular processes of the vertebra above become locked in position anterior to the superior articular processes of the vertebra below. Bilateral locking of the facets requires at least 50 percent anterior displacement of one vertebra upon the next lower vertebra (1,4).

Bilateral locked facets have a typical CT appearance. Normally, the inferior articular processes of the vertebra above lie posterior to the superior articular processes of the vertebra below and have rounded posterior margins. When locking of the facets occurs, the half-moon-shaped superior articular processes lie posterior to the inferior articular processes and have flat posterior margins (6) (see Fig. 51-1). Parasagittal or oblique reconstruction through the plane of the articular processes further demonstrates the locked facet (Fig. 51-2). Bilateral locked facets is considered an unstable injury and is frequently associated with spinal cord compromise (1,4).

Unilateral locking of the facets occurs as a result of flexion, distraction, and rotation forces and is associated with less than 50 percent vertebral body displacement (1). One facet joint acts as a fulcrum for the rotational forces. Simultaneous flexion and rotation leads to dislocation of the contralateral facet joint (4). The correct diagnosis of unilateral locked facet is overlooked on the initial radiographic examination in ap-

proximately 50 percent of cases (2). On a true lateral radiograph, the left and right articular processes below the dislocation lie symmetrically parallel to each other, whereas above the dislocation two distinct sets of articular processes are seen at each level (5) (Fig. 51-3). The processes above the level of dislocation appear to

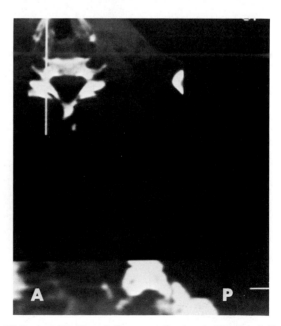

FIG. 51-2. Locked facet. Same patient as in Fig. 51-1. Parasagittal reconstruction of the axial CT images obtained through the plane of the right articular processes. Above: the plane of reconstruction is shown by the *white line.* Below: Reconstruction clearly shows the anteriorly locked position of the inferior articular process of C6 in relation to the superior articular process of C7. *A,* anterior; *P,* posterior.

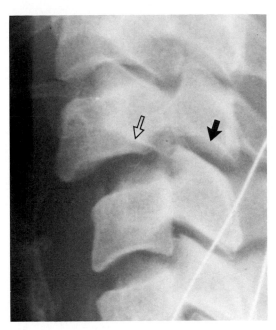

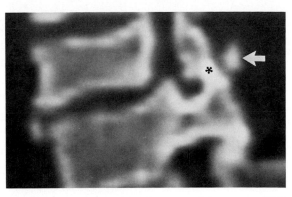

FIG. 51-5. Unilateral locked facet and fracture. Oblique reconstruction of the axial CT images through the plane of the articular processes shows a locked facet. The superior articular process of C6 (*asterisk*) lies posterior to the inferior articular process of C5. An articular process fracture fragment is present posteriorly (*arrow*). Reconstruction views may be useful in evaluating complex pathology that is difficult to assess in the axial plane alone.

FIG. 51-3. Unilateral locked facet. Lateral radiograph of the midcervical spine. There is a unilateral locked facet at C4-C5. One inferior articular process of C4 is dislocated anteriorly (*open arrow*) whereas the other remains in normal position (*closed arrow*) articulating with a superior articular process of C5.

be in an oblique position because of the presence of rotation. Difficult diagnostic problems can be clarified by CT or conventional tomography. Computed tomography shows normal articulation of the articular processes on one side and a reverse relationship of the processes on the opposite side, with the superior artic-

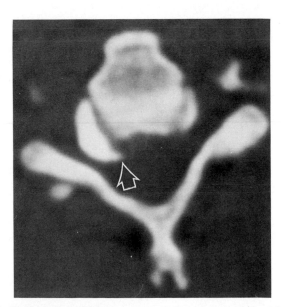

FIG. 51-4. There is distraction of the uncovertebral joint on the right (*arrow*). This patient also had a unilateral locked facet. Computed tomographic demonstration of uncovertebral joint distraction should raise the index of suspicion for a possible locked facet or pillar fracture.

ular process seen posteriorly. Associated distraction of the uncovertebral joint (Fig. 51-4) or fractures of the vertebral body and vertebral arch may be present (6) (Fig. 51-5). The spinous process is rotated toward the abnormal side in one-third of cases (5). Unilateral locked facet is found in 16 percent of patients with trauma to the cervical spinal cord, with approximately 80 percent of these injuries occurring at C4-C5 or C5-C6 (5). It is considered a stable injury (1,2) and is less often associated with neurologic deficit than is the bilateral locked facet injury (3). However, if the diagnosis is not made promptly, reduction becomes difficult and recovery is hindered (2,5).

In addition to showing bilateral or unilateral locked facets, CT can be used to diagnose facet joint subluxation as well as perching of the facets. Facets are described as "perched" when the tip of the inferior articular process above rests on the tip of the superior articular process below. This injury may occur bilaterally or unilaterally. Axial CT reveals a "naked" facet with the superior and inferior articular processes imaged at different levels (6).

REFERENCES

1. Beatson TR. Fractures and dislocations of the cervical spine. *J Bone Joint Surg (Br)* 1963;45B:21–35.
2. Braakman R, Vinken PJ. Old luxations of the lower cervical spine. *J Bone Joint Surg (Br)* 1968;50B:52–60.
3. Gehweiler JA Jr, Osborne RL Jr, Becker RF. *The radiology of vertebral trauma.* Philadelphia: WB Saunders; 1980.
4. Harris JH Jr. Acute injuries of the spine. *Semin Roentgenol* 1978; 13:53–68.
5. Scher AT. Unilateral locked facet in cervical spine injuries. *AJR* 1977;129:45–8.
6. Yetkin Z, Osborn AG, Giles DS, et al. Uncovertebral and facet joint dislocations in cervical articular pillar fractures: CT evaluation. *AJNR* 1985;6:633–7.

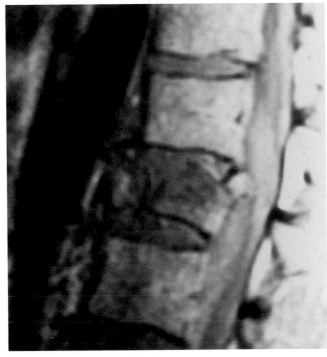

FIG. 52-1A. This 39-year-old man sustained trauma to the thoracic spine. Sagittal T1-weighted SE MR image (600/ 10) of lower thoracic spine.

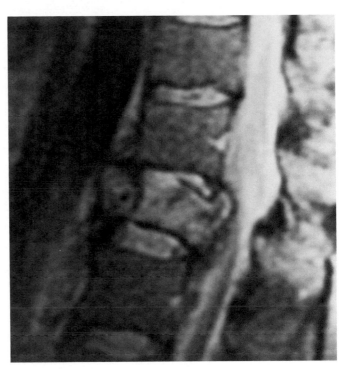

FIG. 52-1B. Sagittal T2-weighted SE MR image (2195/70).

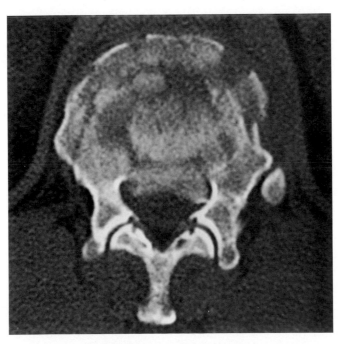

FIG. 52-1C. Axial CT at T12.

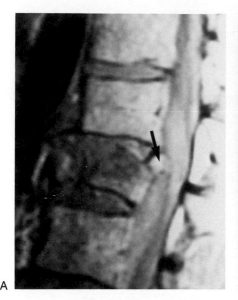
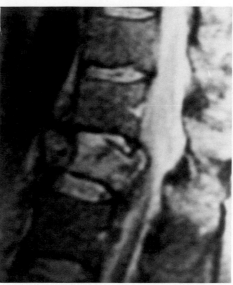
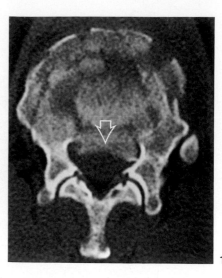

1A

1B

1C

FIG. 52-1A. Burst fracture of T12. There is compression of the T12 vertebral body with posterior displacement of a fracture fragment (*arrow*). The vertebra has low signal intensity in this acute stage. Hematoma is seen posterior to T12.

FIG. 52-1B. The posteriorly displaced fragment is well seen on the T2-weighted image and is compressing the conus.

FIG. 52-1C. Computed tomography shows the comminuted fracture of the T12 vertebral body. The large posteriorly displaced fracture fragment (*arrow*) is well seen. The posterior elements, which are best seen with CT, are intact.

BURST FRACTURE

This is an example of a burst fracture of the T12 vertebral body. Magnetic resonance imaging shows the vertebral body fracture, the fracture fragments displaced posteriorly into the spinal canal, the degree of stenosis, and hematoma in the canal (Figs. 52-1A, 1B). Computed tomography provides excellent bony detail and shows the displaced fracture fragments (Fig. 52-1C). The posterior elements are well seen with CT. This patient had fractures of two noncontiguous vertebrae, a finding that was established by conventional radiography and further clarified by CT and MR imaging (Fig. 52-2).

The spine can be divided into three columns for purposes of evaluation of thoracolumbar fractures (3,5,15). The anterior column consists of the anterior two-thirds of the vertebral body, the anterior annulus, and the anterior longitudinal ligament. The middle column comprises the posterior third of the vertebral body, the posterior annulus, and the posterior longitudinal ligament. The posterior column includes the laminae, the spinous process, the articular processes, the facet joint capsules, the ligamenta flava, and the supraspinous and interspinous ligaments. Determination of the integrity of these three columns is useful in the evaluation of stability.

The simple anterior wedge fracture of the thoracolumbar spine involves the anterior column only, usually with less than 50 percent compression. This is a stable injury without neurologic deficit (15) and has a typical appearance in the axial view, with an arch of irregular bone density displaced circumferentially from the anterior portion of the vertebral body (13) (Fig. 52-3). More than 50 percent compression of the anterior column may indicate additional injury to the posterior elements, with possible progression of spinal deformity and neurologic compromise (5).

The more significant burst fracture is an axial compression injury with fracture of the vertebral endplate of sufficient force to cause the nucleus pulposus to be thrust into the vertebral body, producing comminution of the latter (8). This leads to failure of the anterior and middle columns under compression (3). Typically there is a single sagittally oriented fracture through the inferior endplate of the vertebral body (Fig. 52-4A) with broadening and comminution of the fracture as it is seen more superiorly (13,14) (Fig. 52-4B).

280

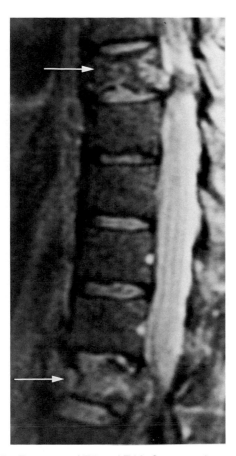

FIG. 52-2. Fracture of T7 and T12. Same patient as in Fig. 52-1. Fractures of two noncontiguous vertebrae are well seen with MR (*arrows*).

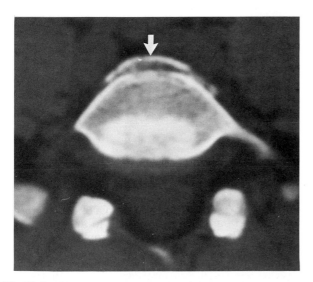

FIG. 52-3. Simple anterior wedge fracture. Computed tomography shows a crescentic arc of bone (*arrow*) that is displaced anteriorly from the vertebral body. No additional fracture is present. This is a characteristic CT appearance of a wedge fracture.

Varying degrees of retropulsion of the posterior fracture fragments may be observed with resultant compromise of the spinal canal (Figs. 52-5, 52-6). Usually the fragment is derived from the superior posterior aspect of the vertebral body. The retropulsed fragment may have intrafragment fracture, anterior rotation, and/or cephalad or caudad displacement (7). The fragment can be evaluated by CT, and the discovery of one or more of these findings may alert the surgeon to the possibility of increased difficulty in obtaining adequate reduction of the fragment (7). The axial CT examination is supplemented by sagittal reconstruction views, which further delineate the fragment and the degree of spinal canal compromise (Fig. 52-7). However, some authors believe that there is no correlation between the amount of preoperative spinal canal narrowing and the degree of neurologic impairment (1,15,17). Coronal reconstruction graphically displays the bursting nature of this injury (Fig. 52-8).

A fracture is unstable if it may lead to progressive spinal deformity or increased neurologic deficit. Although there is some controversy concerning the stability of different fractures, a burst fracture is clearly unstable when there is subluxation, dislocation, or fracture-dislocation of the articular processes (3,5). Some authors believe there is a high probability of progressive spinal deformity or neurologic compromise when the middle column has been disrupted and bone has been displaced into the canal (3,5). Minimally displaced vertical fractures of the laminae, on the other hand, may not necessarily indicate instability (9).

The initial evaluation of patients with suspected thoracolumbar injury begins with AP and lateral radiographs of the spine. The burst fracture is identified by conventional radiography; however, about 20 percent of posterior element fractures are not seen in this manner (11) and are better evaluated by CT (14,15). In patients with significant x-ray or neurologic findings, the preliminary radiographs may be followed by CT examination. CT is more useful than conventional radiography in helping to determine the presence of instability and determining the extent of spinal canal compromise (1,11,16). Computed tomographic evaluation for instability and spinal canal compromise adds important information which, when used in conjunction with the clinical assessment of the patient, helps determine the appropriate therapeutic approach. This includes the possible need for stabilization or decompression.

The use of CT in addition to conventional radiography eliminates the need for conventional tomography in the evaluation of most burst fractures (2,4,11). This is advantageous because conventional tomography almost always requires repositioning of the patient into a lateral decubitus position, which may increase neurologic deficit in a patient with an unstable fracture. The CT examination, on the other hand, is conducted with radiographs are studied for clues to this injury. On the AP radiograph a break may be seen in the continuity of the cortex of the pedicles and/or the spinous processes (4). Also on the AP view, distraction forces lead to separation and elevation of the posterior elements, with posterior elements no longer superimposed over the corresponding vertebral body (4). On the lateral radiograph the horizontal fracture through the posterior structures may be identified. The spinous processes are widely separated if ligamentous injury is present. An optimal lateral view, however, is often difficult to obtain in the injured patient, and CT may be performed to better delineate the abnormalities. The finding of disappearing laminae on the axial images is a clue to the presence of a horizontal fracture through the laminae with associated diastasis. This finding suggests that additional reconstruction views should be obtained with particular attention provided to the posterior elements. For this purpose, parasagittal reconstruction through each pedicle and oblique reconstruction through each lamina is recommended. Both the Chance fracture and the Smith fracture have horizontal fractures through the pedicles and laminae. The spinous process is fractured horizontally in the Chance fracture but remains intact in the Smith fracture, in which the posterior force is directed through the ligaments. The ligamentous disruption that occurs with a Smith fracture leads to wide separation of the neighboring spinous processes and results in a more unstable injury than the Chance fracture.

REFERENCES

1. Chance GQ. Note on a type of flexion fracture of the spine. *Brit J Radiol* 1948;21:452–3.
2. Gehweiler JA Jr, Osborne RL Jr, Becker RF. *The radiology of vertebral trauma*. Philadelphia: WB Saunders; 1980.
3. Howland WJ, Curry JL, Buffington CB. Fulcrum fractures of the lumbar spine: transverse fracture induced by an improperly placed seat belt. *JAMA* 1965;193:240–1.
4. Rogers LF. The roentgenographic appearance of transverse or Chance fractures of the spine: the seat belt fracture. *AJR* 1971; 111:844–9.
5. Smith WS, Kaufer H. Patterns and mechanisms of lumbar injuries associated with lap seat belts. *J Bone Joint Surg (Am)* 1969;51A: 239–54.

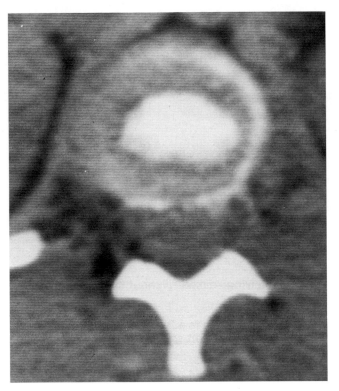

FIG. 54-1A. Axial CT scan at the level of the T12-L1 intervertebral disc. This 14-year-old patient was injured in a motor vehicle accident.

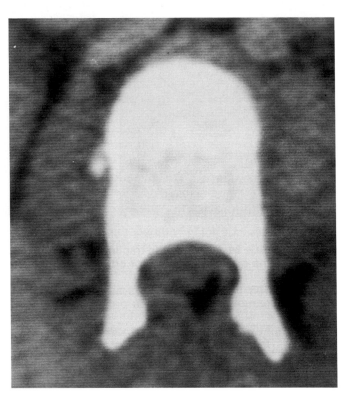

FIG. 54-1B. Axial CT scan obtained 12 mm caudad to Fig. 54-1A.

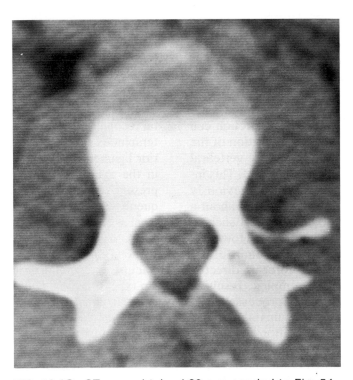

FIG. 54-1C. CT scan obtained 20 mm caudad to Fig. 54-1A.

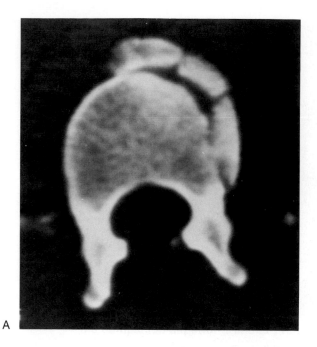

A

FIG. 54-4. Facet distraction injury. This 23-year-old was in an automobile accident. **A**: Axial CT through the L1 vertebral body reveals naked facet sign with the superior articular processes of L1 lying free of their companion inferior articular processes of T12. Fracture of the L1 vertebral body is noted. **B**: This sagittal reconstruction of the axial CT images shows wide separation of the spinous processes of T12 and L1. There is compression of the L1 vertebral body and subluxation at T12-L1. This unstable injury was surgically reduced and stabilized with rods and bony fusion.

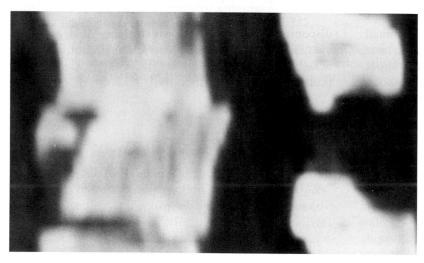

B

REFERENCES

1. Dehner JR. Seatbelt injuries of the spine and abdomen. *AJR* 1971; 111:833–43.
2. Gehweiler JA Jr, Daffner RH, Osborne RL Jr. Relevant signs of stable and unstable thoracolumbar vertebral column trauma. *Skeletal Radiol* 1981;7:179–83.
3. O'Callaghan JP, Ullrich CG, Yuan HA, et al. CT of facet distrac-
tion in flexion injuries of the thoracolumbar spine: the naked facet. *AJR* 1980;134:563–8.
4. Rogers LF. The roentgenographic appearance of transverse or Chance fractures of the spine: the seat belt fracture. *AJR* 1971; 111:844–9.
5. Smith WS, Kaufer H. Patterns and mechanisms of lumbar injuries associated with lap seat belts. *J Bone Joint Surg (Am)* 1969;51A: 239–54.

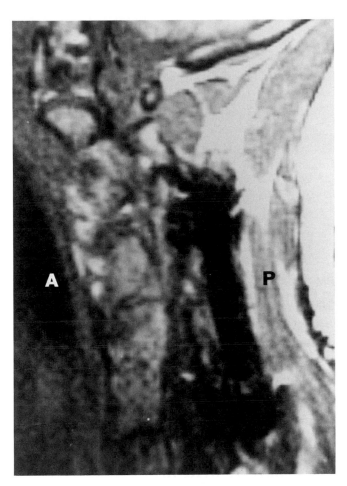

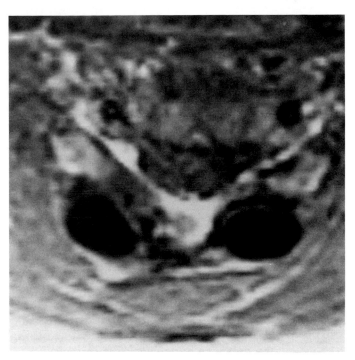

FIG. 55-1B. Axial T1-weighted SE MR image (750/15) at C4–C5.

FIG. 55-1A. A 30-year-old man had sustained severe cervical trauma 11 years earlier which left him quadriplegic. He now presented for MR imaging and CT evaluation because of clinical deterioration. Sagittal T1-weighted SE MR image (700/15) obtained 10 mm to the left of the midline. *A*, anterior; *P*, posterior.

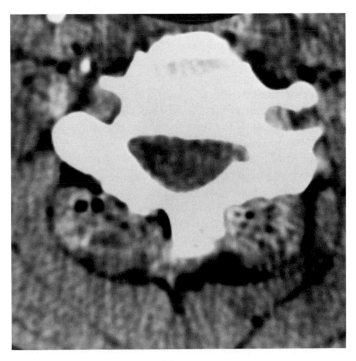

FIG. 55-1C. Axial CT at C3–C4.

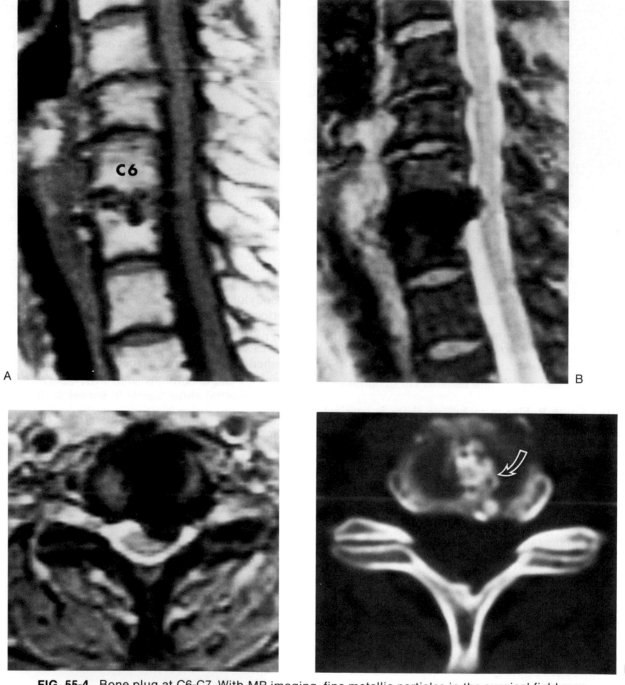

FIG. 55-4. Bone plug at C6-C7. With MR imaging, fine metallic particles in the surgical field may cause signal-void artifact that is most apparent on the gradient-echo images. **A**: Sagittal T1-weighted SE MR image (500/11) shows moderate signal void at the superior aspect of the C7 vertebra and posterior to the C6–C7 disc space. **B**: Sagittal GRE MR image (MPGR, 500/15 with 15-degree flip angle) shows much more extensive signal void because of the increased magnetic susceptibility of GRE images compared to SE images. The signal void posterior to the disc space could be mistaken for an osteophyte or a displaced bone plug. **C**: Axial GRE MR image (MPGR, 800/20 with 20-degree flip angle) at C6–C7 again shows signal void artifact to the left of the midline that has an appearance that could be confused with an osteophyte or a displaced bone plug compressing the spinal cord. **D**: Axial CT at C6–C7 obtained with bone window settings shows the bone plug (*arrow*) without displacement of the plug into the spinal canal.

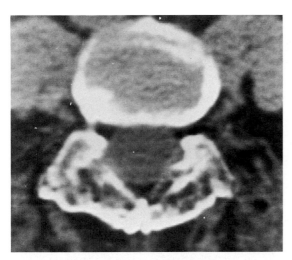

FIG. 55-5. Solid posterolateral fusion. Axial CT shows solid posterolateral lumbar fusion and ankylosis of joints. There is no osseous encroachment on the spinal canal at this level.

the solidity of a posterior or lateral fusion as well as its complications (8). Immediately after surgery, discrete isolated bone is normally seen. In time, solid fusion occurs, with increased bone mass encompassing the laminae, spinous processes, and articular processes. Ankylosis of facet joints may develop (Fig. 55-5). When there is a failure of fusion, multiple fragments of bone graft remain isolated without coalescing (Fig. 55-6). Pseudoarthrosis and incomplete facet joint fusion can be identified. Spinal stenosis may develop

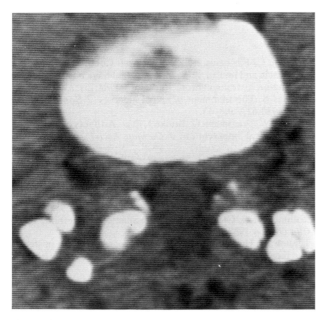

FIG. 55-6. Incomplete fusion. This patient had had an attempted fusion at L4–L5 1 year earlier. CT shows multiple small fragments of bone without evidence of solid fusion. Wide bilateral laminectomy is noted.

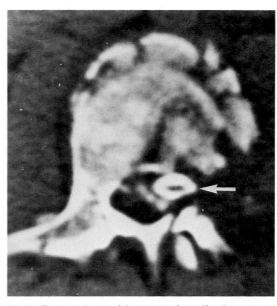

FIG. 55-7. Bone plug with posterior displacement into the spinal canal. This patient was treated for an unstable burst fracture of L3. Postoperatively, the bone plug (*arrow*) can be seen within the spinal canal on CT examination.

after surgical fusion, especially when posterior fusion has been performed. Stenosis most often occurs at the disc space level immediately above the superior extent of fusion because of a combination of disc herniation, thickening and infolding of the ligamenta flava, medial hypertrophy of articular processes, and ventral projection of the upper margin of the fusion mass (1,3). Less frequently, stenosis may occur at the level of fusion and is due to hypertrophy of the midline fusion mass causing neural encroachment. (1,3).

Lumbar interbody fusion can be accomplished by either an anterior or a posterior surgical approach. Following the removal of disc material, bone plugs are positioned in the intervertebral disc space extending from one vertebral body to the next. Early, in the first weeks after surgery, the interbody graft is not incorporated into the matrix of the host bone, and a discrete boundary between host and graft can be seen (7). As solid fusion occurs, there is obliteration of the host-graft interface. The most significant complications of interbody fusion are failure of osseous fusion with pseudoarthrosis, graft displacement, and degenerative disc disease at the level above solid fusion (2,7). When failure of osseous fusion occurs, CT shows a lack of callus and fusion between the vertebral body and the bone graft with disintegration of the graft, lucency at the involved vertebral body endplate, and loss of disc height (2,7). This may be best visualized with reformatted images. A potentially serious complication of interbody fusion is posterior displacement of a bone plug. The bone plug may be displaced into the spinal or neu-

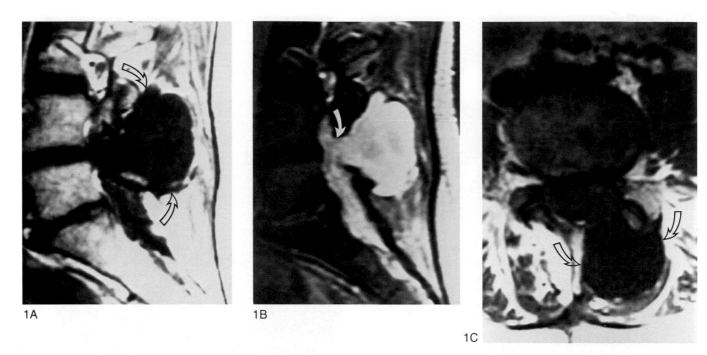

FIG. 56-1A. Pseudomeningocele. There is a pseudomeningocele (*arrows*) seen posteriorly. It is isointense relative to the thecal sac.

FIG. 56-1B. A communication between the thecal sac and the pseudomeningocele is shown (*arrow*). The bright signal of the pseudomeningocele is similar to that of the thecal sac.

FIG. 56-1C. The well-circumscribed pseudomeningocele (*arrows*) is located posterior and to the left of the thecal sac. Communication to the thecal sac is seen in the axial plane as well as in the sagittal plane.

PSEUDOMENINGOCELE

This is a pseudomeningocele, which is a posteriorly localized collection of cerebrospinal fluid usually occurring from an inadequate closure or inadvertent tear of the dura following laminectomy (4,5,8). It may also develop following lumbar puncture or after avulsion of cervical spinal nerve roots (1,4). Rarely, a pseudomeningocele occurs as a sequela of spinal trauma and may even be found at a site remote from the original injury (7). Usually pseudomeningoceles form from leakage of cerebrospinal fluid, which eventually becomes surrounded by a fibrous capsule. Less often, intact arachnoid may herniate through the tear, and enlargement of an arachnoid-lined true meningocele may occur (8). Pseudomeningocele may present from 1 month to several years following laminectomy. It is most frequent in the lower lumbar spine and least frequent in the thoracic spine. Approximately 2 percent of symptomatic postoperative patients have a pseudomeningocele; however, the relationship between the pseudomeningocele and symptoms is uncertain (8).

With MR imaging, a pseudomeningocele shows signal intensity characteristics of cerebrospinal fluid and appears as a well-defined round area of decreased signal intensity on T1-weighted images and increased signal intensity on T2-weighted images (6,7) (Fig. 56-1). Typically, a pseudomeningocele lies directly posterior to the thecal sac at the site of previous laminectomy. The extradural location can be confirmed if splaying of epidural fat is noted, a sign not described with intradural abnormalities such as an intradural subarachnoid cyst (2,7). Should blood products be present within the pseudomeningocele, increased signal intensity may be found on both T1- and T2-weighted images (Fig. 56-2).

The diagnosis of a pseudomeningocele can be accurately made with CT (4,5,8). It appears as a round, homogeneous mass of low CT attenuation similar to cerebrospinal fluid (Fig. 56-3). In the lumbar region pseudomeningocele is similar or slightly lower in density compared to the thecal sac, whereas in the cervical region it has significantly lower CT attenuation values than the thecal sac, probably because of the presence of higher density spinal cord within the sac (8). Pseudomeningoceles vary in size, are usually unilocular, and develop posterior to the sac at the laminectomy site

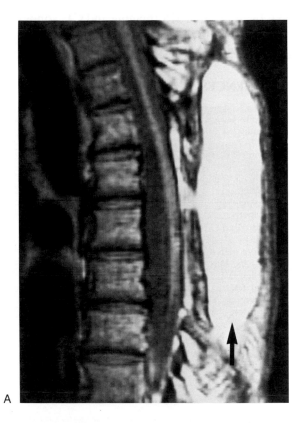

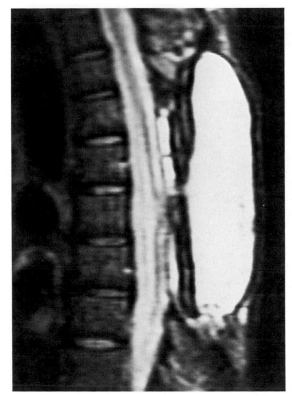

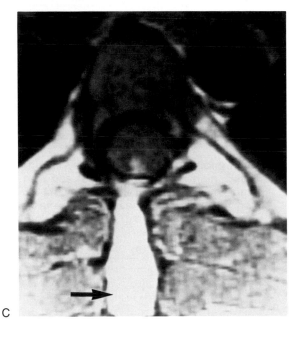

FIG. 56-2. Hemorrhagic pseudomeningocele of the thoracic spine. **A**: Sagittal T1-weighted SE MR image (857/20) shows a large pseudomeningocele (*arrow*). The pseudomeningocele has bright signal intensity rather than the typical low signal intensity of cerebrospinal fluid. **B**: Sagittal T2-weighted SE MR image (2571/70) shows bright signal intensity of the pseudomeningocele. The bright signal on both T1- and T2-weighted images is caused by the presence of extracellular (free) methemoglobin. **C**: Axial T1-weighted SE MR image (857/20) shows posteriorly located hemorrhagic pseudomeningocele with bright signal intensity (*arrow*).

(3,8). Frequently the pseudomeningocele appears to be partly or completely contained within a higher-density capsule that occasionally calcifies (1,5,8).

Conventional myelography may sometimes fail to show a pseudomeningocele (4,5); CTM may be helpful by showing even low concentrations of contrast in the pseudomeningocele that were not visualized with conventional myelography (4,5). Some authors recommend CTM scanning of patients with pseudomeningo-

cele in both the prone and the supine position in order to show the exact size of communication with the subarachnoid space (4). This additional information may be helpful to the surgeon contemplating repair of the dural tear. It should be remembered that following laminectomy in the normal postoperative patient, the thecal sac may sometimes appear to bulge slightly posteriorly. The normal posterior bulging of an intact thecal sac should not be confused with a pseudomeningocele

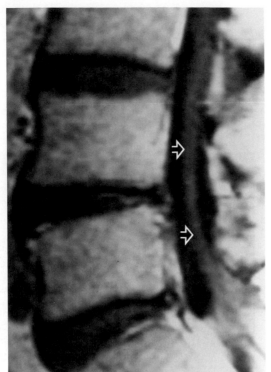

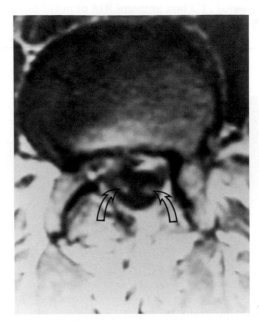

1B

1A

FIG. 57-1A. Arachnoiditis. The nerve roots of the cauda equina (*arrows*) are adherent within the thecal sac. There is narrowing of the L4–L5 disc space.

FIG. 57-1B. Clumping of the nerve roots (*arrows*) is seen within the thecal sac. In this case there was no significant change in appearance after the injection of gadopentetate dimeglumine. Note partial laminectomy defect.

ARACHNOIDITIS

Magnetic resonance imaging shows thickening and clumping of the nerve roots of the cauda equina (Fig. 57-1). These findings are caused by arachnoiditis, a noninfectious inflammation of all the meningeal layers: the pia, the arachnoid, and the dura. It is thought to be the primary pathologic process in 6–16 percent of all patients with failed back surgery syndrome (5). Patients with arachnoiditis almost invariably have low back and leg pain increased by activity. Motor, sensory, and reflex deficits often are bilateral and may occur at multiple levels (2,4). Urinary and bowel sphincter dysfunction may be present. Arachnoiditis most frequently occurs in patients who have had a history of disc herniation (12) and have had previous surgery and/or iophendylate (Pantopaque) myelography (2,9). It is thought that the disc herniation acts as a primary inflammatory focus which is then potentiated by an extrinsic process such as surgery or Pantopaque contrast (5). Other causes of arachnoiditis include spinal trauma, infection, tumor, hemorrhage, and spinal anesthesia (2,9). Some cases are idiopathic.

High-resolution, surface-coil MR imaging correlates well with CTM and conventional myelography in the diagnosis of moderate to severe lumbar arachnoiditis (10). The nerve roots of the cauda equina can be seen on T1- or T2-weighted MR images and with CTM images viewed at bone window settings. In the axial plane, normal nerve roots of the cauda equina appear as multiple small, round filling defects evenly distributed throughout the thecal sac (Fig. 57-2). The MR and CTM images of arachnoiditis may show clumping of the nerve roots of the cauda equina (see Fig. 57-1), or peripheral adherence of the nerve roots to the dural margins leading to an "empty thecal sac" appearance (7,10). With extensive arachnoiditis, nerve roots may form a single tubular mass (Fig. 57-3).

The MR and CTM findings have been compared to conventional myelograms (10). Those patients with central clumping of the nerve roots of the cauda equina as seen with MR imaging or CTM have myelograms that show thickened nerve roots with loss of definition of the nerve root sleeves (Figs. 57-4) or moderate nar-

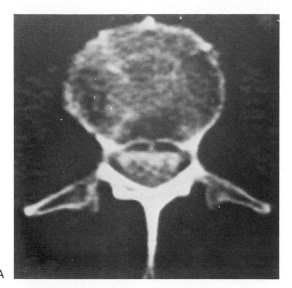 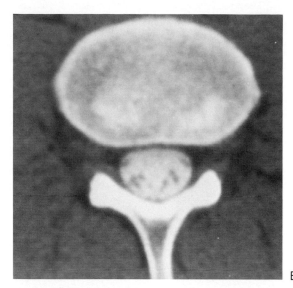

A   B

FIG. 57-2. Normal nerve roots of the cauda equina. **A**: Normal CTM at L3. The nerve roots of the cauda equina appear as multiple small, round, uniform filling defects within the contrast-filled thecal sac. Bone window settings are needed to best visualize these nerve roots on CTM examination. **B**: Normal CTM at L4–L5 in another patient. The nerve roots are less numerous and more peripheral than shown in Fig. 57-2A. Nevertheless, the nerve roots are small and rounded and are symmetrically positioned within the thecal sac.

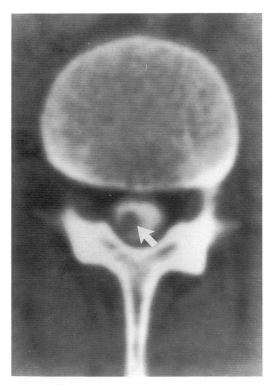

FIG. 57-3. Arachnoiditis. Axial CTM at L3 performed after a ''complete'' myelographic block; CTM study shows intrathecal contrast beyond the block. The nerve roots are matted together into a single tubular mass (*arrow*). This patient had previous surgery 3 years earlier for disc disease.

rowing or irregularity of the thecal sac. Patients with peripheral adherence of the nerve roots have myelograms showing amputation of the nerve root sleeves, absence of visible nerve roots within the sac, and a smoothly marginated amorphous appearance of the thecal sac. The MR and CTM demonstration of a soft-tissue mass within the thecal sac, obliterating most of the subarachnoid space centrally, is associated with myelographic block and a ''candle-dripping'' appearance (10).

With MR imaging, the changes of arachnoiditis can be seen on the sagittal images, but are best appreciated on axial views. In many cases, T2-weighted images provide better visualization of the nerve roots than T1-weighted images. However, the signal intensity of cerebrospinal fluid seen on T2-weighted images may obscure the soft-tissue mass effect of arachnoiditis that is seen in the more severe cases (7,10). Thus, the axial T1-weighted sequence is considered to be the most efficient sequence for imaging arachnoiditis.

In one study of one hundred patients with failed back surgery syndrome (10), twelve patients had CTM and conventional myelographic findings of arachnoiditis. Magnetic resonance findings were correlated and found to have sensitivity of 92 percent, specificity of 100 percent, and accuracy of 99 percent (10). A pitfall in the diagnosis of arachnoiditis is the appearance of normal nerve roots at the level of L2. At this higher lumbar level, the roots may have a smooth, crescentic

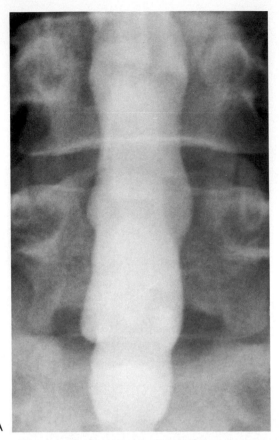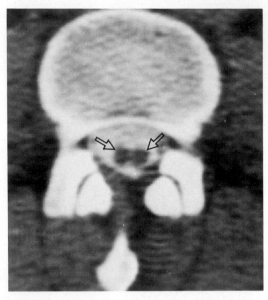

FIG. 57-4. A: Arachnoiditis. Anteroposterior radiograph of the lumbar spine from a myelogram performed with intrathecal water-soluble contrast. There is bilateral uniform lack of filling of the nerve root sleeves. **B**: Axial CTM shows marked clumping of the nerve roots (*arrows*).

appearance, lying in the dependent (posterior) portion of the thecal sac. This may be confused with peripheral adherence of the nerve roots. However, the findings in arachnoiditis tend to occur in the lower lumbar spine and extend over at least two vertebral body levels (10).

The use of gadopentetate dimeglumine in MR imaging of patients with arachnoiditis has been studied (7). After the intravenous injection of gadopentetate dimeglumine, the clumped nerve roots may lack enhancement or may show enhancement which varies from minimal to moderate. Marked enhancement did not occur in a series of thirteen patients. The enhancement that occurs is thought to be secondary to the development of a vascular network within a proliferating fi-

brous stroma (7). In some cases, contrast enhancement may make the clumped nerve roots more easily recognized. However, the enhancement does not provide additional information or alter the diagnosis which can be made as accurately on the noncontrast images (7). Thus, gadopentetate dimeglumine does not play an important role in the evaluation of lumbar arachnoiditis.

In the evaluation of arachnoiditis, myelography may be diagnostic if the radiographic and clinical findings are typical. However, MR imaging and CTM may provide important additional information, especially in patients who have a myelographic block or an inconclusive myelogram (Fig. 57-5). In one series, the myelographic diagnosis of arachnoiditis was frequently

FIG. 57-6. Arachnoiditis ossificans. **A**: CT at L5 without intrathecal contrast. There is curvilinear ossification of the arachnoid (*arrow*). Lateral recess stenosis is noted on the right. This patient had had previous iophendylate (Pantopaque) myelography and spinal surgery. Note the laminectomy defect. **B**: CT without intrathecal contrast. There is a large bony mass within the spinal canal. This ossified mass has filling defects within it which proved at surgery to be nerve roots of the cauda equina (*arrow*) entrapped within the bone. Note the surgical fixation screw.

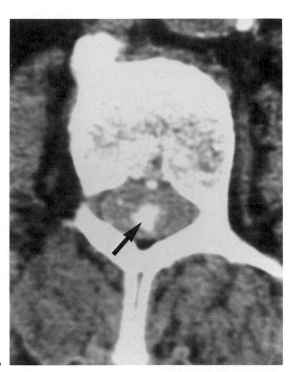

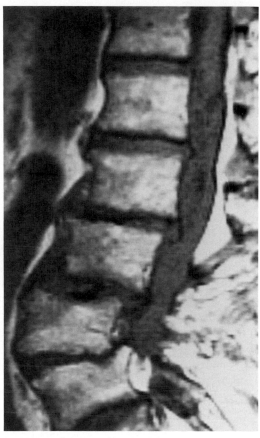

A   B

FIG. 57-5. Arachnoiditis in a 74-year-old man with low back pain and left leg pain and a history of previous lumbar spine surgery. A myelogram could not be performed successfully from the lumbar route and a C1-C2 approach was used. **A**: CTM at L2 reveals a central collection of intrathecal contrast (*arrow*) surrounded by inflammatory thickening of the meninges. There was block to the flow of contrast below this level. **B**: Sagittal T1-weighted SE MR image (600/15) shows abnormal intermediate signal intensity of the inflammatory mass throughout the thecal sac, almost completely replacing the normal low signal of cerebrospinal fluid. A small central area of low signal cerebrospinal fluid is seen. Note postoperative changes of the lower lumbar spine posteriorly, retrospondylolisthesis at L3–L4, spondylolisthesis at L4–L5, and disc bulging at several levels.

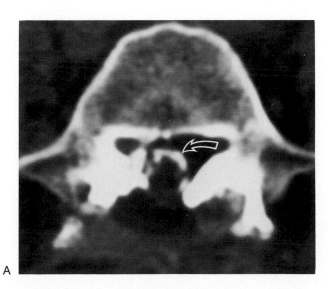

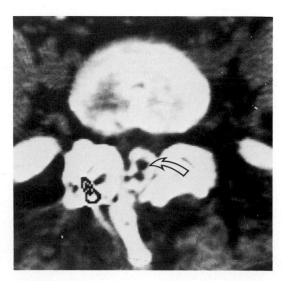

A   B

found to have coexistent pathology such as spinal stenosis, foraminal nerve root entrapment and disc herniation which, when surgically corrected, often resulted in restoration of normal function for the patient (3). Magnetic resonance imaging and CTM may play an important role in diagnosing such coexistent pathology.

Magnetic resonance imaging and CT can also be used to evaluate the sequelae of arachnoiditis. For example, patients with arachnoiditis may develop intradural arachnoid cysts or intramedullary cavities (syringomyelia) (9), best seen with MR imaging. A late sequelae of adhesive arachnoiditis is arachnoiditis ossificans, a proliferative bony metaplasia of the arachnoid which closely envelops the spinal cord and nerve roots (8). Unenhanced CT may reveal either a thin circumferential ring of calcification or ossification surrounding the arachnoid or a large thick tubular bony mass (1,6,11) (Fig. 57-6). This is a rare entity which differs from the small benign calcific arachnoid plaques frequently reported at autopsy. Etiologic factors that have been implicated include vascular anomalies of the spine, repeated spinal anesthesia, and previous history of meningitis, surgery, and trauma (1,8).

REFERENCES

1. Barthelemy CR. Case report: arachnoiditis ossificans. *J Comput Assist Tomogr* 1982;6:809–11.
2. Benner B, Ehni G. Spinal arachnoiditis: the postoperative variety in particular. *Spine* 1978;3:40–4.
3. Brodsky AE. Cauda equina arachnoiditis: a correlative clinical and roentgenologic study. *Spine* 1978;3:51–60.
4. Burton CV. Lumbosacral arachnoiditis. *Spine* 1978;3:24–30.
5. Burton CV, Kirkaldy-Willis WH, Yong-Hing K, et al. Causes of failure of surgery on the lumbar spine. *Clin Orthop* 1981;157:191–9.
6. Dennis MD, Altschuler E, Glenn W, et al. Arachnoiditis ossificans: a case report diagnosed with computerized axial tomography. *Spine* 1983;8:115–7.
7. Johnson CE, Sze G. Benign lumbar arachnoiditis: MR imaging with gadopentetate dimeglumine. *AJNR* 1990;11:763–70, *AJR* 1990;155:873–80.
8. Nainkin L. Arachnoiditis ossificans: report of a case. *Spine* 1978;3:83–6.
9. Quencer RM, Tenner M, Rothman L. The postoperative myelogram: radiographic evaluation of arachnoiditis and dural/arachnoidal tears. *Radiology* 1977;123:667–79.
10. Ross JS, Masaryk TJ, Modic MT, et al. MR imaging of lumbar arachnoiditis. *AJNR* 1987;8:885–92, *AJR* 1987;149:1025–32.
11. Sefczek RJ, Deeb ZL. Case report: computed tomography findings in spinal arachnoiditis ossificans. *CT* 1983;7:315–8.
12. Shaw MDM, Russell JA, Grossart KW. The changing pattern of spinal arachnoiditis. *J Neurol Neurosurg Psych* 1978;41:97–107.

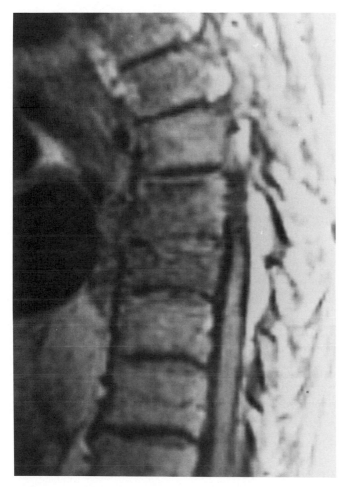

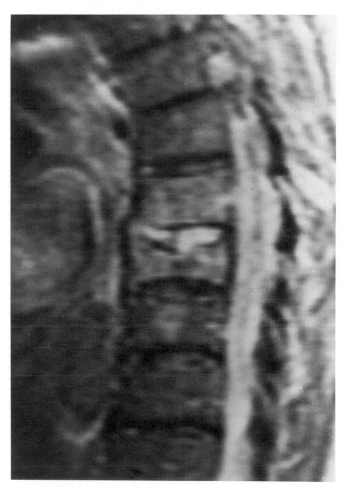

FIG. 58-1A. A 75-year-old woman with back pain had an MR examination to rule out tumor. Sagittal T1-weighted SE image (667/20) of the thoracic spine.

FIG. 58-1B. Sagittal T2-weighted SE image (2000/70).

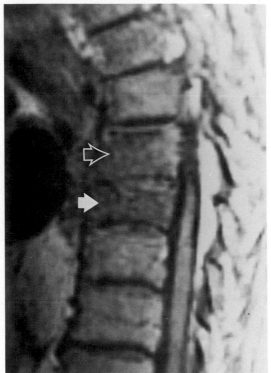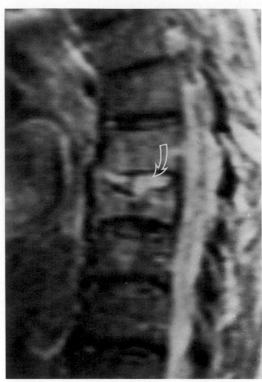

FIG. 58-1A. Pyogenic osteomyelitis. There is decreased signal intensity of the T7 (*open arrow*) and T8 (*closed arrow*) vertebral bodies. Compression of T8 is noted. The cortical margins of the vertebral endplates adjacent to the T7-T8 disc are indistinct.

FIG. 58-1B. On the T2-weighted image there is bright signal intensity of the T7-T8 disc (*arrow*) compared to the other discs. The T7 and T8 vertebral bodies show increased signal intensity caused by osteomyelitis. The patient also had aneurysmal dilatation of the thoracic aorta which was incidently noted.

PYOGENIC OSTEOMYELITIS

In this case there is decreased signal intensity of the T7 and T8 vertebrae on T1-weighted MR images (Fig. 58-1A) and increased signal on T2-weighted images (Fig. 58-1B). The vertebral endplates are indistinct and the T7-T8 disc has bright signal on T2-weighted images. This is the typical appearance of osteomyelitis.

Most often pyogenic osteomyelitis occurs from hematogenous spread of infection. Approximately two-thirds of the cases of pyogenic osteomyelitis have a known source of infection, with about one-half having a history of genitourinary tract infection or instrumentation (16). Other sources of spinal osteomyelitis include soft-tissue infections, respiratory tract infections, intravenous drug abuse, and infected intravenous sites (16).

Staphylococcus aureus is the most frequent organism causing spinal osteomyelitis and is found in over 50 percent of the cases (16). Other pyogenic organisms include *Escherichia coli, Proteus, Pseudomonas,* and group A *Streptococcus. Pseudomonas* is particularly common in heroin addicts. Hematogenous spread of infection usually begins in the vertebral body just beneath the vertebral endplate and may spread through vascular communications to involve a contiguous vertebral body, with subsequent narrowing of the less vascular intervertebral disc. In addition to the vertebral body, spinal infection may primarily involve the epidural space (epidural abscess), the disc (discitis), or the paraspinal soft tissues (paraspinal abscess).

Radionuclide scanning is a sensitive but nonspecific method of detecting early hematogenous spinal osteomyelitis. Despite its nonspecificity, radionuclide scanning is an important modality in localizing the abnormal site. Conventional radiography is typically normal in the first 2–8 weeks after the onset of clinical symptoms (13). The earliest radiographic change is blurring of the vertebral endplate. Erosions of the vertebral endplates on both sides of a narrowed disc are then seen. As the infection continues, further osteolytic destruction and vertebral collapse develop.

310

Magnetic resonance imaging is an excellent modality for diagnosing spinal infection and evaluating its extent. In one study (12), MR imaging had a sensitivity of 96 percent, specificity of 93 percent, and accuracy of 94 percent in the evaluation of patients who were clinically suspected of having vertebral osteomyelitis. The hallmarks of spinal osteomyelitis seen with MR imaging include: replacement of the normal marrow adjacent to the disc, usually involving two adjacent vertebrae; narrowing of the disc space; erosion of subchondral and cortical bone; and paraspinal or epidural abscess (19).

The involved vertebral bodies have decreased signal intensity on T1-weighted MR images and usually have increased signal intensity on T2-weighted images (12,19). The signal changes are adjacent to the affected disc in a confluent distribution in the subchondral zone and may even be quite extensive (Fig. 58-2). The T1-weighted image is almost invariably abnormal with spinal osteomyelitis, although rare cases occur in which the T1-weighted image is normal and the T2-weighted image is abnormal (5,19). Cortical destruc-

tion is best seen on proton density-weighted images (19).

Typically, the disc is abnormal in cases of pyogenic osteomyelitis. On the T1-weighted images the disc may show decreased signal intensity that leads to an inability to differentiate the margin of the disc from the margin of the vertebral body endplate (5,12). Some authors have found increased signal intensity within the disc on T2-weighted images in 87 percent of cases (12). The increased signal intensity is caused by edema (inflammatory exudate) and possibly vascular ischemia. However, signal intensity of an infected disc is variable and may also be isointense or decreased on T2-weighted images (19). Another finding described in osteomyelitis involves the intranuclear cleft which is composed of fibrous tissue and is seen in the normal lumbar discs of adults (1). Obliteration of the cleft in association with increased signal intensity of the disc on T2-weighted images suggests an inflammatory or infectious process (1,12). The configuration of the infected disc is more linear instead of biconcave because of disc collapse, and the normally visualized low-intensity in-

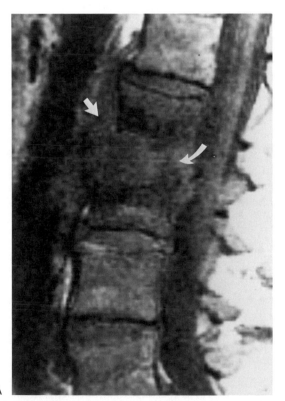

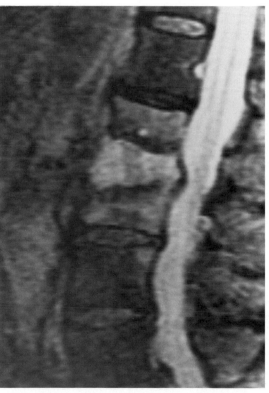

A

B

FIG. 58-2. Osteomyelitis with paravertebral abscess. This 82-year-old man had severe back pain and bilateral leg pain for 4 weeks. **A:** Sagittal T1-weighted SE MR image (600/15) shows loss of definition of the L2-L3 disc space (*curved arrow*) with destruction and decreased signal intensity of the L2 and L3 vertebrae. Prevertebral soft-tissue abscess (*straight arrow*) is seen along with some epidural extension of the inflammatory process. **B:** Sagittal T2-weighted SE MR image (2000/70) reveals marked increase in signal intensity of the L2-L3 disc and adjacent vertebrae. Posterior extension of the inflammatory process is compressing the thecal sac. Incidentally noted are degenerative changes of the other discs.

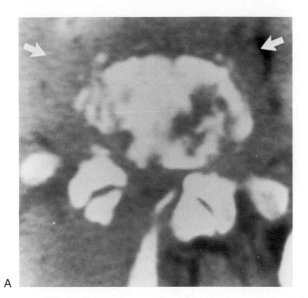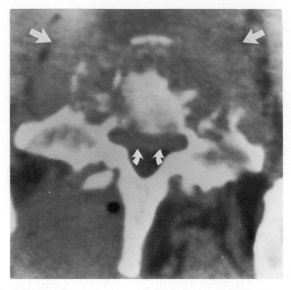

A   B

FIG. 58-3. Postoperative pyogenic osteomyelitis. **A**: CT shows destruction of the inferior vertebral endplate of L4 along with marked paravertebral extension of infection (*arrows*). Postoperative changes are seen. Note soft-tissue fullness involving the right posterior spinal structures in this patient who had persistent drainage at the operative site. **B**: CT shows destruction of the superior vertebral endplate of L5 with paraspinal (*straight arrows*) and epidural (*curved arrows*) extension of infection. Culture revealed *Staphylococcus aureus*. Gas can be seen within the posterior paraspinal structures on the right at the site of previous surgery.

tranuclear cleft is usually not evident with infection, suggesting involvement of the entire disc (12). Disc height is often diminished in cases of osteomyelitis but may be normal early in the course of the pyogenic illness or in some cases of tuberculous or fungal osteomyelitis (12,19). Rarely, the MR appearance of the disc remains normal despite disc space infection (12). Occasionally, in early cases, only one vertebra may be involved, and there may be vertebral involvement without disc involvement so that the disc does not have abnormal signal intensity (12,19). In this situation, it may be difficult to differentiate osteomyelitis from a marrow replacement disorder such as metastasis, or some cases of chronic discogenic disease.

In children with spinal infection, the disc and adjacent vertebral bodies have low signal intensity on T1-weighted images with loss of disc-vertebra margins (5). On T2-weighted images, the vertebral bodies have increased signal, whereas the disc has low signal intensity and appears flattened (5). However, vascular communications with the disc may be present in children, and an infectious process can involve the disc while sparing the vertebrae.

Adults studied by MR imaging 6 weeks to 3 months following therapy for spinal osteomyelitis show improved resolution of the disc space and less signal intensity of the disc on T2-weighted images than was evident prior to treatment (12). The abnormal signal intensity of the previously affected vertebral bodies resolves more slowly. The changes that are seen reflect the resolution of the inflammatory exudate and ischemia that leads to disc degeneration, fibrous scar formation, and reparative new bone formation. Alterations of bone fusion may be evident across an obliterated disc space late in the course of the disease. The presence of reparative sclerosis alters the signal characteristics of the vertebrae, leading to decreased signal intensity on both T1- and T2-weighted images. Some investigators (5) studying a pediatric population have reported that during antibiotic treatment, MR signal may not return to normal and that the abnormal signal may even increase in extent despite clinical improvement.

While SE T1- and T2-weighted images are usually sufficient to establish a diagnosis of spinal osteomyelitis and abscess formation, other pulse sequences and the use of contrast can sometimes provide additional information in problem cases. Gadopentetate dimeglumine may aid in the delineation of accompanying epidural and paraspinal abscesses. Rim enhancement within a vertebral lesion has been observed in tuberculous spondylitis and was correlated with an intraosseous abscess at surgery (17). However, the use of contrast may actually decrease the conspicuity of infectious lesions of the marrow since it may cause areas of low signal on T1-weighted images to appear isointense relative to normal marrow after enhancement. One should always obtain precontrast T1-weighted images in order to prevent this pitfall. Short TI inversion recovery suppresses fat signal, thus allowing water signal (pus, edema) to be clearly separated from normal tissue (2). Although STIR images are highly sensitive to abnormalities having increased water content, the images do not exhibit fine anatomic detail.

Computed tomography is also useful in evaluating patients with suspected spinal infection (4,6,22). Experimental (15) and clinical (4,6,13,22) work suggest that osteomyelitis can be detected earlier with CT than with conventional radiography. In some cases extensive destruction of cortical and medullary bone is detected by CT scanning while either no abnormality or only subtle erosions are seen with conventional radiography. In addition to osseous changes, soft-tissue extension of infection is more readily detected by CT (3,4,6,8,13,22). Paravertebral abscess or granulation tissue appears as a soft-tissue mass or swelling causing obliteration of the normal paravertebral fat (Figs. 58-3, 58-4). Gas may be seen within a paravertebral abscess. Most often, the diagnosis of osteomyelitis is made with CT when both fragmentation of the vertebral endplates and anterior paravertebral soft-tissue swelling are present (9). The CT findings of osteomyelitis in the postoperative patient are similar to those found in hematogenous osteomyelitis; however, a postdiscectomy patient may have paravertebral edema or hemorrhage, simulating infection (9). Also, aggressive curettage of the vertebral endplates during discectomy may mimic the vertebral endplate erosions of osteomyelitis (9). Never-

theless, in cases of postoperative spinal osteomyelitis, the combination of clinical data and typical bone and soft tissue CT abnormalities should lead to the correct diagnosis. Computed tomography is also used to guide abscess aspiration and to plan surgical intervention (4,6,8).

TUBERCULOUS OSTEOMYELITIS

In the evaluation of tuberculous osteomyelitis, involvement of two adjacent vertebral bodies is seen in 50 percent of the cases, while three or more adjacent vertebral bodies are involved in 25 percent (20). In the remaining 25 percent of cases, the disease is either confined to one vertebral body or has spread to involve two or more noncontiguous vertebral bodies. The intervertebral disc space may narrow secondary to vertebral destruction with subsequent collapse of the disc into the vertebral body (20); however, the disc space is maintained longer in tuberculosis than in pyogenic infection (21). With continued anterior vertebral body destruction and maintenance of the posterior elements, kyphosis occurs.

In a small series of patients with tuberculous spondylitis, the involved vertebrae had heterogeneous MR signal with areas of both increased and decreased signal intensity on T1-weighted images (19). These areas had heterogeneous increased signal on T2-weighted images. In a report of disseminated skeletal tuberculosis, there were multiple lesions that had increased signal intensity on both T1- and T2-weighted images (14). The reason for the atypical bright signal on T1-weighted images is not clear, but it was speculated that a proteinaceous material, a product of the infectious process, may cause shortening of the T1 relaxation time (14). Pathologically, there was no evidence of hemorrhage which could also account for this appearance.

An atypical finding described in patients with tuberculous spondylitis is the preservation of the disc space despite extensive vertebral disease that may involve multiple levels, thus mimicking metastasis (18,19). The disc may be isointense relative to other noninvolved discs. Extensive paraspinal involvement is another feature of tuberculous spondylitis. Paraspinal masses are present in 55–96 percent of cases, and their large size is frequently out of proportion to the osseous and disc space involvement (18).

Computed tomography has been useful in the evaluation of patients suspected of having tuberculosis of the spine; CT is more accurate than conventional radiography in showing the extent of bone destruction and the presence of paravertebral or psoas abscess (7,10,21) (Fig. 58-5). Calcification within the abscess is readily detected with CT and reflects the chronicity of the tuberculous process (11). The rim of the tuberculous ab-

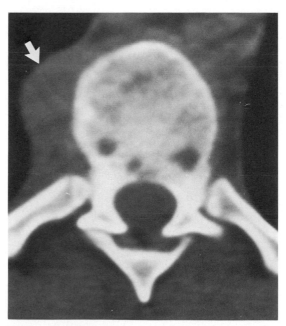

FIG. 58-4. Pyogenic osteomyelitis. This 19-year-old had back pain and fever which followed treatment for pneumonia. Computed tomography shows osteomyelitis at T8-T9 with a paravertebral abscess (*arrow*). Multiple round osteolytic lesions were seen on both sides of a narrowed disc space.

314 / CASE 58

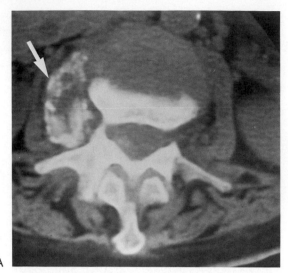 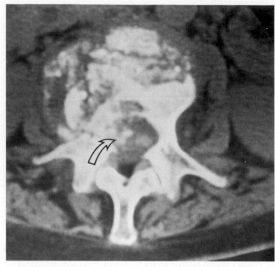

A   B

FIG. 58-5. Tuberculous osteomyelitis. **A**: Axial CT at L2–L3 disc level. This 65-year-old woman had back pain for 18 months. There is a large calcified psoas abscess on the right (*arrow*). **B**: Axial CT at L2 shows marked destruction of the L2 vertebral body and right pedicle. Extensive bony fragmentation is noted with extension into the spinal canal (*arrow*).

scess is thick and nodular. When compared to a nontuberculous paraspinal abscess, a tuberculous paraspinal abscess is more likely to be multiloculated and calcified; to spread to superficial dorsal soft tissues; and to have a thick irregular rim (21).

REFERENCES

1. Aguila LA, Piraino DW, Modic MT, et al. The intranuclear cleft of the intervertebral disk: magnetic resonance imaging. *Radiology* 1985;155:155–8.
2. Bertino RE, Porter BA, Stimac GK, et al. Imaging spinal osteomyelitis and epidural abscess with short TI inversion recovery (STIR). *AJNR* 1988;9:563–4.
3. Brant-Zawadzki, Burke VD, Jeffrey RB. CT in the evaluation of spine infection. *Spine* 1983;8:358–64.
4. Burke DR, Brant-Zawadzki M. CT of pyogenic spine infection. *Neuroradiology* 1985;27:131–7.
5. duLac P, Panuel M, Devred P, et al. MRI of disc space infection in infants and children: report of 12 cases. *Pediatr Radiol* 1990;20:175–8.
6. Golimbu C, Firooznia H, Rafii M. CT of osteomyelitis of the spine. *AJR* 1984;142:159–63.
7. Gropper GR, Acker JD, Robertson JH. Computed tomography in Pott's disease. *Neurosurgery* 1982;10:506–8.
8. Hermann G, Mendelson DS, Cohen BA, et al. Role of computed tomography in the diagnosis of infectious spondylitis. *J Comput Assist Tomogr* 1983;7:961–8.
9. Kopecky KK, Gilmor RL, Scott JA, et al. Pitfalls of computed tomography in diagnosis of discitis. *Neuroradiology* 1985;27:57–66.
10. LaBerge JM, Brant-Zawadzki M. Evaluation of Pott's disease with computed tomography. *Neuroradiology* 1984;26:429–34.
11. Maritz NGJ, de Villiers JFK, van Castricum OQS. Computed tomography in tuberculosis of the spine. *Comput Radiol* 1982;6:1–5.
12. Modic MT, Feiglin DH, Piraino DW, et al. Vertebral osteomyelitis: assessment using MR. *Radiology* 1985;157:157–66.
13. Price AC, Allen JH, Eggers FM, et al. Intervertebral disk-space infection. CT changes. *Radiology* 1983;149:725–9.
14. Quinn SF, Murray W, Prochaska J, et al. MRI appearance of disseminated osseous tuberculosis. *Mag Res Imag* 1987;5:493–7.
15. Raptopoulos V, Doherty PW, Goss TP, et al. Acute osteomyelitis: advantage of white cell scans in early detection. *AJR* 1982;139:1077–82.
16. Sapico FL, Montgomerie JZ. Pyogenic vertebral osteomyelitis: report of nine cases and review of the literature. *Rev Infect Dis* 1979;1:754–76.
17. Sharif HS, Clark DC, Aabed MY, et al. Granulomatous spinal infections: MR imaging. *Radiology* 1990;177:101–7.
18. Smith AS, Weinstein MA, Mizushima A, et al. MR imaging characteristics of tuberculous spondylitis vs vertebral osteomyelitis. *AJNR* 1989;10:619–25, *AJR* 1989;153:399–405.
19. Thrush A, Enzmann D. MR imaging of infectious spondylitis. *AJNR* 1990;11:1171–80.
20. Weaver P, Lifeso RM. The radiological diagnosis of tuberculosis of the adult spine. *Skeletal Radiol* 1984;12:178–86.
21. Whelan MA, Naidich DP, Post JD, et al. Computed tomography of spinal tuberculosis. *J Comput Assist Tomogr* 1983;7:25–30.
22. Whelan MA, Schonfeld S, Post JD, et al. Computed tomography of nontuberculous spinal infection. *J Comput Assist Tomogr* 1985;9:280–7.

CASE 59

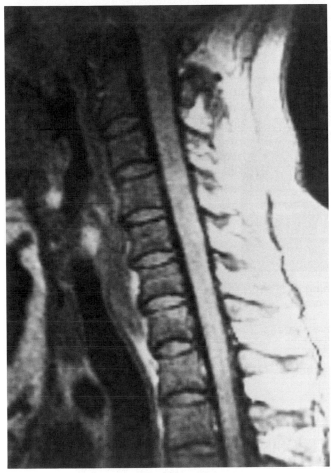

FIG. 59-1A. This 35-year-old woman presented with numbness in the left hand. Magnetic resonance imaging was performed to evaluate the patient for possible tumor or syrinx. Sagittal T1-weighted SE image (600/25) of the cervical spine.

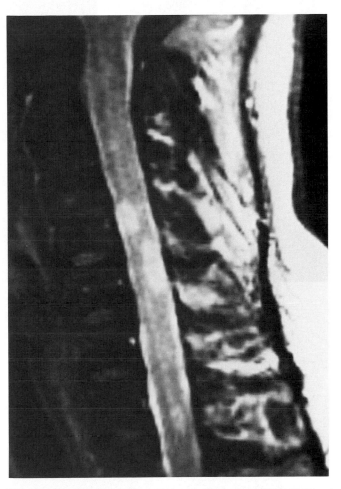

FIG. 59-1B. Sagittal T2-weighted SE image (2000/70) of the cervical spine.

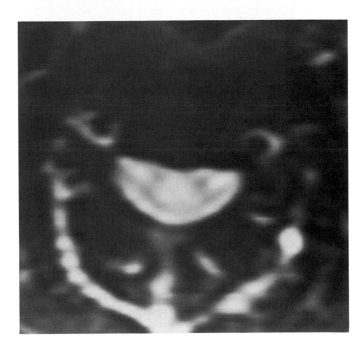

FIG. 59-1C. Axial T2-weighted SE image (2667/70) at C4.

315

lesions have increased signal intensity, often having an elongated configuration along the long axis of the cord (6,7) (Fig. 59-3). The plaques may extend for several centimeters and do not respect grey-white matter boundaries of the cord (7). Lesions of the cord are multiple in 12–40 percent of cases (1,7). In some cases a single plaque of MS may have features that are suggestive of neoplasm or myelitis with spinal cord enlargement and bright signal intensity within the cord on T2-weighted images.

Studies performed with MR imaging of the brain have shown that MS lesions are dynamic and change over time (4). Perivenous inflammatory changes found in MS, along with abnormalities of the blood-brain barrier, are factors which permit contrast enhancement. In brain studies, images obtained 3 minutes after contrast injection are most efficient for detecting enhancement (4). Magnetic resonance imaging of the brain performed with gadopentetate dimeglumine enhancement is more sensitive than clinical examination alone in detecting active lesions in patients with definite MS (4).

On the other hand, T2-weighted SE images show lesions of increased signal intensity in both clinically active and inactive stages of the disease and do not correlate with clinical activity. The use of gadopentetate dimeglumine for spinal imaging has been studied in the evaluation of some patients with clinical suspicion of demyelinating disease and elongated lesions of high signal intensity on T2-weighted images (Fig. 59-4). In one small series (6), patients with clinically active disease showed enhancement on delayed T1-weighted images obtained 45–60 minutes after injection of the paramagnetic contrast agent. No enhancement was found in those patients with clinically stable disease. Those patients with enhancement of active lesions were followed with clinical and MR evaluation. Correlation was found between clinical signs and symptoms and paramagnetic contrast enhancement, with lack of enhancement noted on follow-up studies of those patients who evolved to a clinically inactive stage.

Magnetic resonance imaging of the brain has been compared to CT, evoked potentials, and CSF oligoclo-

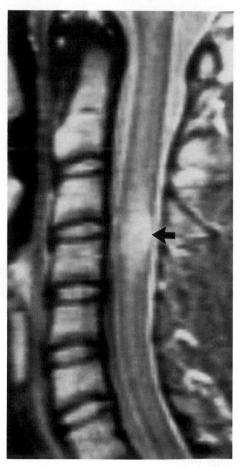 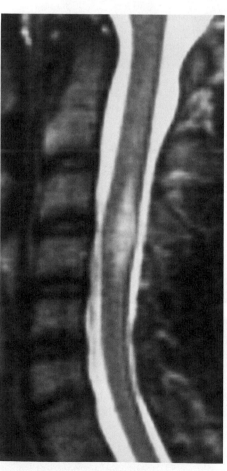

A　　　　　　　　　　　　　　　　　　　　　　B

FIG. 59-3. Multiple sclerosis. Plaque of multiple sclerosis seen with T2-weighted SE and FSE MR images. **A**: Sagittal T2-weighted SE MR image (2200/70) shows a plaque with bright signal intensity (*arrow*) within the spinal cord. **B**: Sagittal T2-weighted FSE MR image (2800/153) shows a flame-shaped plaque within the spinal cord. This FSE sequence provided excellent proton density- and T2-weighted images in 3 minutes and 5 seconds.

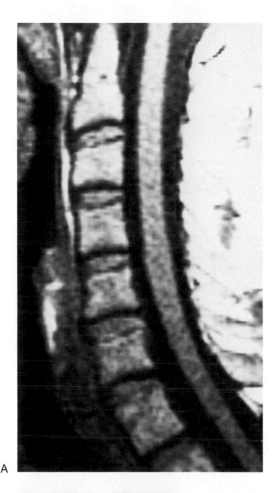

A

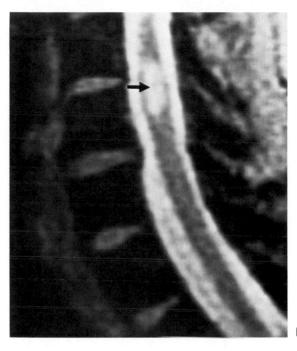

B

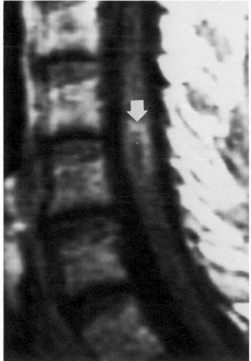

C

FIG. 59-4. Multiple sclerosis with enhancement of plaque. **A**: Precontrast sagittal T1-weighted SE MR image (600/20) of the cervical spine shows no abnormal signal intensity within the spinal cord. **B**: Sagittal GRE MR image (MPGR, 500/15 with 15-degree flip angle). A plaque is seen as a focal area of bright signal intensity (*arrow*) within the spinal cord with this GRE sequence. **C**: Sagittal T1-weighted SE MR image (500/12) obtained after the intravenous injection of gadopentetate dimeglumine shows enhancement of the plaque (*arrow*). Compare with the precontrast T1-weighted image in Fig. 59-4A. Enhancement of the plaque suggests that this is an active lesion.

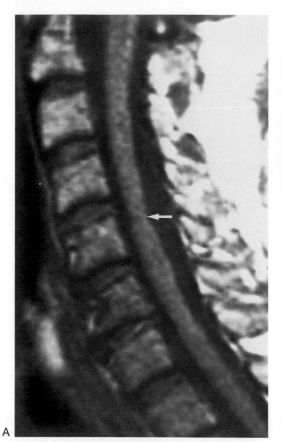 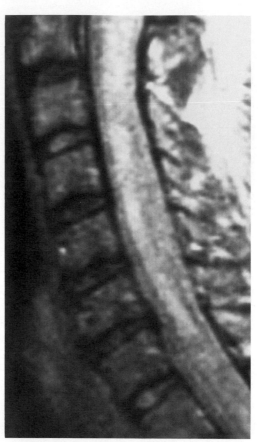

A   B

FIG. 59-5. Multiple sclerosis with spinal cord atrophy. **A**: Sagittal T1-weighted SE MR image (700/20) shows mild spinal cord atrophy (*arrow*). There is no abnormal signal within the cord. **B**: Sagittal proton density-weighted SE MR image (2432/35) shows bright signal within the cord involving several vertebral levels. The longitudinal orientation of the high-signal plaques is a frequent finding in MS, but can be seen in other disorders.

nal banding analysis in patients with suspected MS, and has been found to be the most sensitive method for diagnosing MS and the best method for demonstrating dissemination in space (8,12). Magnetic resonance imaging of the spine can also be used for this purpose. In some patients, MR imaging of the spinal cord may show lesions of MS despite a normal MR study of the brain (6). In other patients with spinal cord lesions, the MR demonstration of asymptomatic lesions within the brain provides additional support to the diagnosis.

In the chronic stages of MS, spinal cord atrophy may be present (Fig. 59-5). T1-weighted sagittal and axial images can be used to indicate the presence of spinal cord atrophy. Devic disease (neuromyelitis optica) is a form of demyelinating disease characterized by acute bilateral visual loss and transverse myelitis. In one report (11), MR imaging revealed swelling of the thoracic spinal cord caused by early demyelination associated with edema and inflammatory cell infiltration that was followed by severe spinal cord atrophy 5 months later.

Several disorders may have an MR appearance that is similar to MS. The differential diagnosis has been reviewed (13) and includes: intramedullary tumor with spinal cord swelling and increased signal on T2-weighted images; sarcoidosis with spinal cord swelling and contrast enhancement; tropical spastic paraparesis with increased signal on T2-weighted images and spinal cord atrophy similar to chronic MS; and acute disseminated encephalomyelopathy of viral origin, and vacuolar myelopathy in AIDS, with focal increased signal intensity with the cord on T2-weighted images.

REFERENCES

1. DeLaPaz RL. Demyelinating disease of the spinal cord. In: Enzmann DR, DeLaPaz RL, Rubin JB, eds. *Magnetic resonance of the spine*. St. Louis: CV Mosby; 1990;423–36.
2. Edwards MK, Farlow MR, Stevens JC. Cranial MR in spinal cord MS: diagnosing patients with isolated spinal cord symptoms. *AJNR* 1986;7:1003–5.
3. Enzmann DR, Rubin JB. Cervical spine: MR imaging with a partial flip angle, gradient-refocused pulse sequence: part II. spinal cord disease. *Radiology* 1988;166:473–8.
4. Grossman RI, Braffman BH, Brorson JR, et al. Multiple sclerosis: serial study of gadolinium-enhanced MR imaging. *Radiology* 1988;169:117–22.

5. Katz BH, Quencer RM, Hinks RS. Comparison of gradient-recalled-echo and T2-weighted spin-echo pulse sequences in intramedullary spinal lesions. *AJNR* 1989;10:815–22.

6. Larsson E-M, Holtås S, Nilsson O. Gd-DTPA-enhanced MR of suspected spinal multiple sclerosis. *AJNR* 1989;10:1071–6.

7. Maravilla KR, Weinreb JC, Suss R, et al. Magnetic resonance demonstration of multiple sclerosis plaques in the cervical cord. *AJNR* 1984;5:685–9, *AJR* 1985;144:381–5.

8. Patz DW, Oger JJF, Kastrukoff LF, et al. MRI in the diagnosis of MS: a prospective study with comparison of clinical evaluation, evoked potentials, oligoclonal banding, and CT. *Neurology* 1988;38:180–5.

9. Poser CM, Patz DW, Scheinberg L, et al. New diagnostic criteria for multiple sclerosis: guidelines for research protocols. *Ann Neurol* 1983;13:227–31.

10. Sheldon JJ, Siddharthan R, Tobias J, et al. MR imaging of multiple sclerosis: comparison with clinical and CT examinations in 74 patients. *AJNR* 1985;6:683–90, *AJR* 1985;145:957–64.

11. Tashiro K, Ito K, Maruo Y, et al. MR imaging of spinal cord in Devic disease: case report. *J Comput Assist Tomogr* 1987;11:516–7.

12. Uhlenbrock D, Seidel D, Gehlen W, et al. MR imaging in multiple sclerosis: comparison with clinical, CSF, and visual evoked potential findings. *AJNR* 1988;9:59–67.

13. Wallace CJ, Seland TP, Fong TC. Multiple sclerosis: the impact of MR imaging. *AJR* 1992;158:849–57.

CASE 60

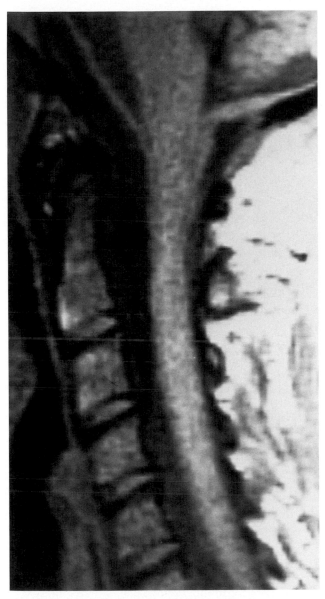

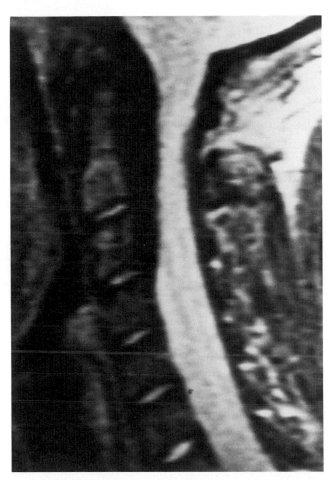

FIG. 60-1B. Sagittal SE MR image with more T2-weighting (1500/70).

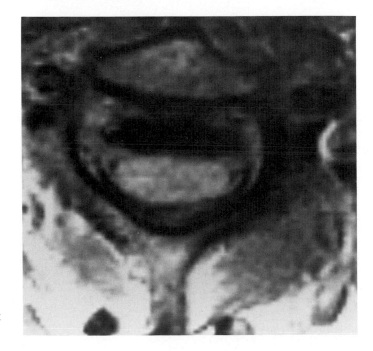

FIG. 60-1A. Sagittal T1-weighted SE MR image (600/20) of the upper cervical spine in a 24-year-old woman with a history of pain and stiffness of the neck and numbness in the fingers. There had been previous trauma to the neck from an altercation.

FIG. 60-1C. Axial T1-weighted SE MR image (600/20) at C2 level.

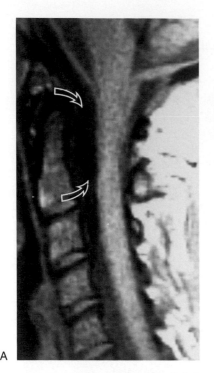
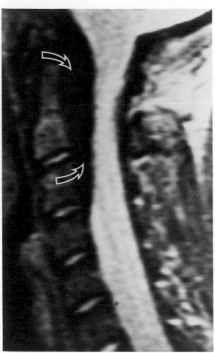
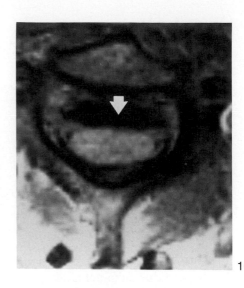

1A

1B

1C

FIG. 60-1A. Pseudotumor. A broad area of low signal intensity is seen posterior to the C2 and C3 vertebrae (*arrows*).

FIG. 60-1B. The more T2-weighted image reveals markedly low signal of the pseudotumor (*arrows*) that is composed of fibrous and granulation tissue. There is compression of the anterior subarachnoid space and the spinal cord. The degree of compression is most marked at the C2 level.

FIG. 60-1C. The axial image further shows the pseudotumor (*arrow*) causing flattening and compression of the spinal cord.

PSEUDOTUMOR

There is an anterior epidural mass at the craniocervical junction, having low signal intensity on both the T1- and T2-weighted images (Fig. 60-1). Spinal cord compression is present and is most severe at the level of the second cervical vertebra. The patient had CT studies which also showed the abnormality to have moderate enhancement after the intravenous injection of iodinated contrast. This represents a pseudotumor (inflammatory mass) composed of fibrous granulation tissue.

The craniocervical junction is ideally imaged with MR. The anatomic structures can be studied in more than one plane, free of bone-induced artifact that can be present with CT. The full extent of a pathologic process can be appreciated and the degree of spinal cord compression determined without the need for intrathecal contrast from an invasive myelographic procedure.

In this case, the mass appeared as low signal intensity on not only the T1-weighted images, but on the

T2-weighted images as well. This suggests the presence of fibrous tissue which typically has low to intermediate signal intensity on both T1- and T2-weighted images. Tumors such as metastatic disease or chordoma, which can occur in this region, usually have increased signal intensity on T2-weighted images because of increased water content. Meningiomas, on the other hand, may have a variable appearance on T2-weighted studies related to the presence of calcification and fibrous tissue.

In the craniocervical junction, inflammatory masses may be due to acute or subacute infection, or pannus secondary to rheumatoid arthritis. Pseudotumor of the craniocervical junction has also been found in patients with chronic atlanto-axial subluxations, secondary to either degenerative disease or congenital dysplasia of the odontoid process of C2 (3). In these cases, MR shows an anterior epidural mass of low signal intensity on T1- and T2-weighted images causing compression of the upper cervical cord and lower medulla. The presence of pseudotumor in patients with chronic subluxation suggests the possibility that chronic mechanical irritation is an underlying cause of the inflammatory mass. Other causes of spinal pseudotumor occur less frequently and include pigmented villonodular synovitis, epidural hematoma, gout, and fatty deposition secondary to steroid therapy (3). The pseudotumors found in these disorders typically have signal intensity characteristics that differ from those in the present case.

Magnetic resonance imaging of children with Chiari II malformation may reveal a pseudotumor of the craniocervical junction. A child with the Chiari II malformation has obliteration of the precervical cord space at birth; however, as the child grows, the spinal canal enlarges. This phenomenon, combined with dorsal displacement of neural tissue, leads to marked widening of the anterior subarachnoid space. On T1-weighted sagittal images, cerebrospinal fluid within the widened subarachnoid space at the C2 level may have slight increased signal intensity when compared to fluid seen at the other cervical levels (1). This widened space with slight increased signal intensity may simulate an intradural extramedullary mass (1).

The CSF flow void sign may in some cases simulate pseudotumor. The flow void is seen as nonuniform decreased signal intensity due to spin dephasing secondary to pulsatile cerebrospinal fluid motion (2). It is best appreciated on T2-weighted images but can also be seen on T1-weighted sagittal images when comparison is made to the ventricles of the brain. Within the spine, the flow void sign is most often seen in the cervical region since pulsatile movement of cerebrospinal fluid is greatest in this region. In MR imaging of the cervical spine performed without cardiac gating, CSF flow void was seen in 33 percent of cases and was most prominent in the upper cervical region near the foramen magnum (2). The flow void reportedly varies from 5–20 mm in length (2).

In the present case, the patient was treated with surgical decompressive laminectomy and partial excision of the inflammatory mass. No tumor was present. The MR examination provided graphic preoperative information.

REFERENCES

1. Curnes JT, Oakes WJ, Boyko OB. MR imaging of hindbrain deformity in Chiari II patients with and without symptoms of brainstem compression. *AJNR* 1989;10:293–302.
2. Sherman JL, Citrin CM, Gangarosa RE, et al.: The MR appearance of CSF pulsations in the spinal canal. *AJNR* 1986;7:879–84.
3. Sze G, Brant-Zawadzki MN, Wilson CR, et al. Pseudotumor of the craniovertebral junction associated with chronic subluxation: MR imaging studies. *Radiology* 1986;161:391–4.

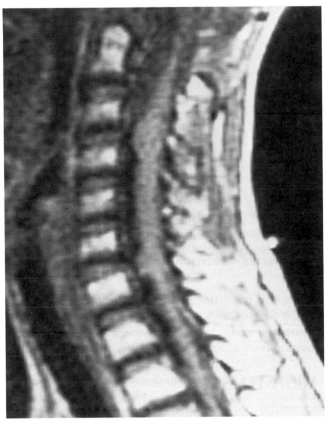

FIG. 61-1A. This 10-year-old boy had a significant past medical history which is being withheld. Sagittal T1-weighted SE MR image (800/25) of the cervical spine just lateral to the midline.

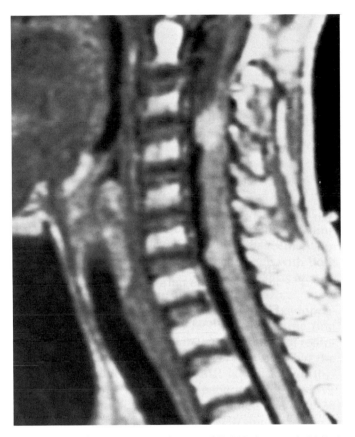

FIG. 61-1B. Sagittal T1-weighted SE MR image (800/25) obtained after the intravenous injection of gadopentetate dimeglumine (0.1 mmol/kg body weight).

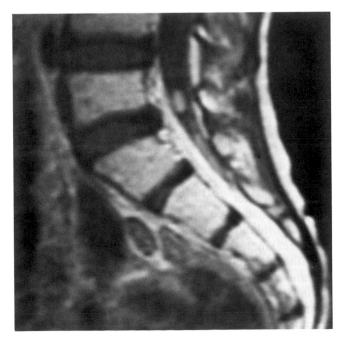

FIG. 61-1C. Sagittal T1-weighted SE MR image of the lower lumbar spine and sacrum after injection of gadopentetate dimeglumine.

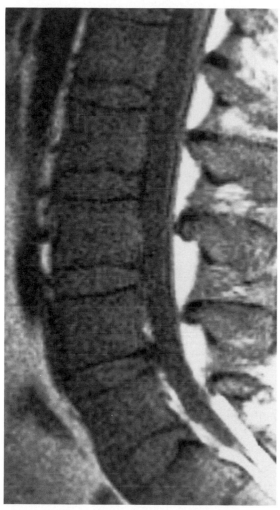

FIG. 63-1A. This 25-year-old white man has a known systemic disorder. Sagittal T1-weighted SE MR image (600/15) of the lumbar spine.

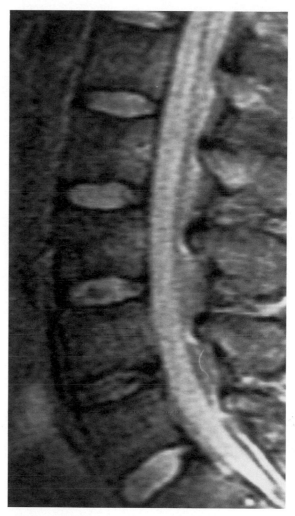

FIG. 63-1B. Sagittal T2-weighted SE MR image (2000/70).

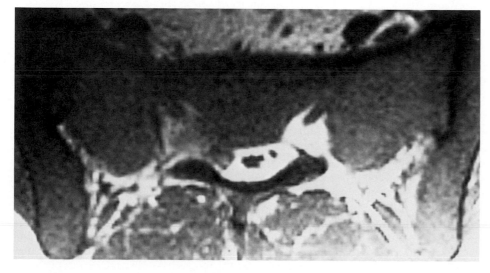

FIG. 63-1C. Axial T1-weighted SE MR image (600/15) of the sacrum.

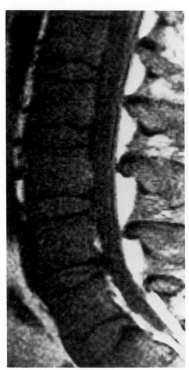
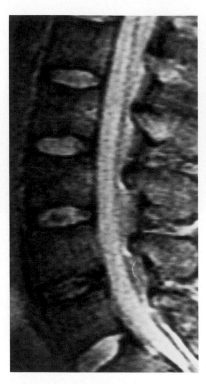
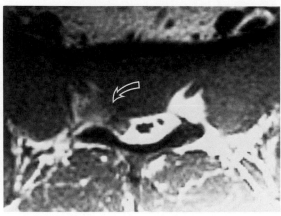

1A

1B

1C

FIG. 63-1A. Leukemia. There is diffuse decrease in signal intensity throughout the vertebral bodies. The decreased signal intensity is more than one would expect for a patient of this age and indicates marrow replacement.

FIG. 63-1B. On the T2-weighted image the bone marrow shows predominantly low signal intensity although some higher signal intensity can be seen posteriorly at several levels.

FIG. 63-1C. There is an area of intermediate signal intensity within a right sacral foramen (*arrow*) that extends into the sacral canal. This is replacing the high-signal fat and is thought to represent leukemic infiltration.

LEUKEMIA

This patient has leukemia with diffuse bone marrow replacement causing decreased signal intensity of all vertebrae (Figs. 63-1A, 1B). Leukemic infiltration into a sacral foramen and the sacral canal is seen (Fig. 63-1C).

Leukemia is the most frequent malignancy of childhood and commonly involves the axial skeleton. About 80 percent of cases in children are the acute lymphoblastic type (9). In children whose marrow is mainly red marrow, tumor invasion not only replaces red marrow but also causes existing normal red marrow to become hyperplastic to maintain hematopoiesis. In adults, whose marrow is mainly fat marrow, replacement of red marrow is met with foci of reconverted and/or hyperplastic red marrow in response to the demand for hematopoiesis. However, in more advanced cases, marrow is extensively replaced by tumor, no matter what the age of the patient.

Spinal alterations of leukemia may be difficult to detect on conventional radiography as extensive destruction of cancellous bone is required before tumor is detected. The radiographic features of leukemia vary with the type of leukemia, but usually include generalized osteopenia, vertebral collapse (3 percent of patients presenting with leukemia), focal osteolytic lesions, subchondral radiolucent bands, and (rarely) osteosclerosis.

Magnetic resonance is the imaging modality of choice in detecting the presence and extent of marrow replacement by leukemia but is not practical for screening (3). All infiltrative malignant tumors of bone marrow have intermediate to decreased signal intensity on T1-weighted images and usually have increased signal intensity on T2-weighted images (4,6,7). The appearance may vary on T2-weighted images due to the type of tissue, the amount of water content, the degree of cellularity, and the presence of necrosis, hemorrhage, edema, or fibrosis (10).

On T1-weighted images leukemic infiltration has decreased signal intensity (4–6), usually in a diffuse pattern (5) although focal infiltration may be present (6), particularly in patients with acute myelogenous leukemia (4). In some children, leukemic infiltration may appear isointense with red marrow and may not be as readily detected. Vertebral marrow in children over 10 years of age should have higher signal intensity than the adjacent intervertebral disc (3). A lower signal intensity of marrow compared to the disc in this age group suggests a diffuse marrow replacement disorder.

Those children with active leukemia have marrow which has longer T1 relaxation time than do children with leukemia in remission, or when compared to normal controls (4,5). Differences have been noted in the T1 relaxation times of those patients in remission and those with relapse, although they are not statistically significant. These observations may be helpful in staging the disease. It is uncertain what determines the prolongation of T1 in leukemia; possibilities include increased cellularity (3,4–6) or increased water content of the malignancy (10). There is evidence to suggest that MR imaging and calculation of the T1 relaxation time of the lumbar bone marrow may be helpful in determining whether treatment is effective (4). In children with acute lymphocytic leukemia, a progressive decrease in the T1 relaxation time is expected during remission, whereas after achieving a baseline of remission, lengthening of the T1 relaxation time of the marrow may indicate a relapse.

On T2-weighted images, leukemic infiltrates usually have increased signal intensity but may appear isointense (7). In some cases of leukemic infiltration, the increased signal is subtle and may not be appreciated. However, there is no significant difference in the T2 relaxation times of active leukemic marrow, leukemia in remission, and normal controls (4). The most marked MR alterations occur in patients who have acute lymphocytic leukemia and in those with chronic myelogenous leukemia, especially during the blast phase (10).

It should be emphasized that in children it is sometimes difficult to differentiate on T1-weighted images between marrow that is invaded by leukemia and normal marrow that is hyperplastic, as both may have intermediate signal intensity that may appear focal or diffuse (10). Leukemic infiltration usually has increased signal intensity on T2-weighted images, but

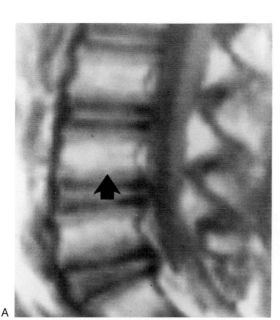
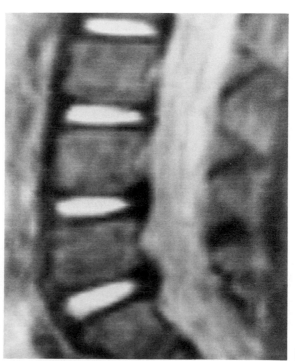

A   B

FIG. 63-2. Leukemia following marrow transplantation. Four-year-old girl four months after autologous marrow transplant. **A**: Sagittal T1-weighted SE MR image (300/30) of the lumbar spine. The typical "band" pattern (*arrow*) of intermediate signal intensity represents hematopoietic marrow adjacent to the vertebral endplates. The central portion of the vertebrae shows high signal intensity of fatty marrow. **B**: Sagittal T2-weighted SE MR image (2000/75) of the lumbar spine. The "band" pattern is not seen on the T2-weighted image because the hematopoietic marrow and the fat marrow have similar signal intensity with this pulse sequence. (Fig. 63-2 reprinted from Moore SG, et al., ref. 2, with permission).

may be isointense. Hyperplastic red marrow may have increased signal intensity on T2-weighted images to a variable degree, depending upon the amount of cellularity and tissue water present (3). The signal intensity is usually not as great as that of leukemic infiltrates.

On FSE T2-weighted images, both leukemic infiltrates and hyperplastic marrow appear as increased signal intensity. Since fat tissue also shows increased signal intensity on this pulse sequence, some form of fat suppression should be added to increase the conspicuity of leukemic tumor. Short-TI inversion recovery pulse sequences are also sensitive to the presence of leukemic infiltrates which appear as increased signal intensity. Hyperplastic red marrow also shows increase in signal intensity with STIR but to a lesser degree than leukemic infiltrates. With STIR, the suppression of fat may lack uniformity in the periphery of the field, and the central portions of the field can therefore be examined with more confidence. When leukemia

be examined with more confidence. When leukemia invades the epidural space, T1-weighted images obtained after the intravenous injection of gadopentetate dimeglumine may provide useful information.

Three months following bone marrow transplants (and as early as 1.5 months in some cases), T1-weighted images of vertebral marrow show a characteristic, broad zone of intermediate signal intensity in the subchondral region of the vertebral bodies that surrounds a central zone of high signal intensity fat (8) (Fig. 63-2). This band of intermediate signal intensity represents a zone of regenerating hematopoietic cells while the central zone of increased signal intensity represents fat marrow.

LYMPHOMA

Lymphoma invades the spine either hematogenously or by direct extension from a paraspinal tumor. Lym-

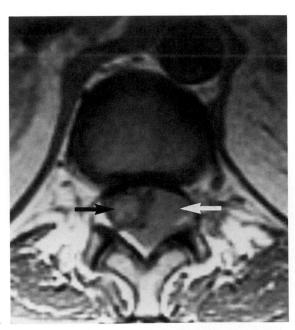
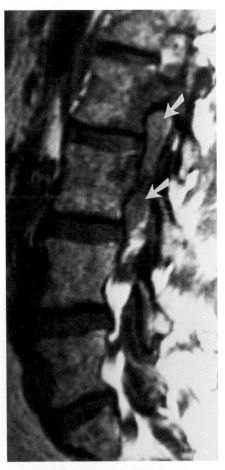

FIG. 63-3. Lymphoma with epidural and neural foraminal extension. **A:** Axial T1-weighted SE MR image (750/20) at T11–T12 shows epidural tumor on the left (*white arrow*), displacing the spinal cord to the right (*black arrow*). **B:** Sagittal T1-weighted SE MR image (700/15) of the lumbar spine obtained 10 mm to the left of midline shows low signal intensity of the posterior aspect of the L2 and L3 vertebrae caused by lymphoma. There is extension of tumor into the neural foramina (*arrows*) that is well seen with MR imaging.

phoma may rarely arise as a solitary lesion in the spine. It may also invade the spinal canal directly via the neural foramen (1) (from a paraspinal tumor) or by leptomeningeal spread. The MR signal characteristics are similar to other marrow replacement disorders; that is, focal or diffuse decreased signal intensity on T1-weighted images and increased signal intensity on T2-weighted images (1,8). Those lesions that appear osteosclerotic on conventional radiographs have very low signal intensity on T1- and T2-weighted images. Magnetic resonance imaging is helpful in depicting the extent of tumor in the epidural and paraspinal compartments (Fig. 63-3).

REFERENCES

1. Holtås SL, Kido DK, Simon JH. MR imaging of spinal lymphoma: case report. *J Comput Assist Tomogr* 1986;10:111–5.

2. Moore SG. Pediatric musculoskeletal imaging. In: Stark PD, Bradley WG, eds. *Magnetic resonance imaging*. 2nd ed. St. Louis: Mosby Yearbook; 1992:2223–30.

3. Moore SG, Bisset GS III, Siegel MJ, et al. Pediatric musculoskeletal MR imaging. *Radiology* 1991;179:345–60.

4. Moore SG, Gooding CA, Brasch RC, et al. Bone marrow in children with acute lymphocytic leukemia: MR relaxation times. *Radiology* 1986;160:237–40.

5. Nyman R, Rehn S, Glimelius B, et al. Magnetic resonance imaging in diffuse malignant bone marrow diseases. *Acta Radiol* 1987;28:199–205.

6. Olson DO, Shields AF, Scheurich CJ, et al. Magnetic resonance imaging of the bone marrow in patients with leukemia, aplastic anemia, and lymphoma. *Invest Radiol* 1986;21:540–6.

7. Ruzal-Shapiro C, Berdon WE, Cohen MD, et al. MR imaging of diffuse marrow replacement in patients with cancer. *Radiology* 1991;181:587–9.

8. Stevens SK, Moore SG, Amylon MD. Repopulation of marrow after transplantation: MR imaging with pathologic correlation. *Radiology* 1990;175:213–8.

9. VanZanten TEG, Golding RP, VanAmerongen AHMT, et al. Nuclear magnetic resonance imaging of bone marrow in childhood leukaemia. *Clin Radiol* 1988;39:77–81.

10. Vogler JB III, Murphy WA. Bone marrow imaging. *Radiology* 1988;168:679–93.

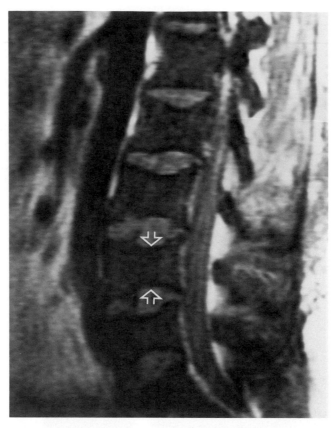

FIG. 64-1. Sickle cell anemia. There is very low signal intensity of the bone marrow of all lumbar vertebrae. Note the central depressions (*arrows*) producing the H-shaped configuration characteristic of sickle cell anemia.

SICKLE CELL ANEMIA

The T1-weighted image (Fig. 64-1) shows markedly decreased signal intensity of the bone marrow and the H-shaped vertebrae that is characteristic of sickle cell anemia (SCA), a chronic hemolytic anemia that is caused by abnormal hemoglobin S. In this disorder, (which occurs almost exclusively in the black population), red blood cells become distorted in shape when in an atmosphere of low oxygen tension. This leads to clumping of red blood cells, thrombosis, and tissue ischemia. Fragility of the cells causes hemorrhage and anemia (4).

Patients with chronic anemia, including hemolytic anemia and thalassemia, develop hyperplastic red marrow to compensate for the anemia condition. Any chronic marrow stress disorder leads to hyperplasia of existing red (hematopoietic) marrow and reconversion of yellow (fatty) marrow to red marrow in order to meet the body's demand for erythropoiesis. Thus, thalassemia, an unrelenting marrow stress disorder, and SCA, an intermittent marrow stress disorder, lead to marrow hyperplasia (3).

Magnetic resonance imaging is helpful in evaluating the marrow of patients with severe anemia. The signal changes of SCA and thalassemia are dependent upon the severity and chronicity of disease. With marrow hyperplasia, there is focal to diffuse decrease in signal intensity of the marrow on both T1- and T2-weighted images (10) as fat marrow is replaced by hematopoietic marrow. Some authors have observed slight increase in signal intensity on T2-weighted images because of the degree of cellularity and, therefore, increased water content within the tissues (8). Also, children who normally have considerable hematopoietic marrow in the spine may not show changes of marrow hyperplasia on MR images (similar signal intensities) as readily as an adult who normally has fat marrow in the vertebrae.

In some cases central depression of superior and inferior endplates, the so-called H-shaped vertebra, can be identified in patients with SCA. Repeated intermittent crises lead to arterial occlusion in the central arterial supply to subchondral bone because collateral circulation is not present after childhood. The peripheral bone continues to grow because of adequate collateral circulation, whereas growth is hindered centrally. This leads to the H-shaped vertebra, which is seen on the conventional radiograph in 44 percent of patients, almost always after the age of 10 years (4).

Patients with SCA or thalassemia who have received repeated blood transfusions or experience repetitive hemolysis may develop secondary hemosiderosis. The signal characteristic of marrow affected by hemosiderosis is extreme low signal intensity on both T1- and T2-weighted images (1,7,10). The MR appearance is caused by the paramagnetic effect of hemosiderin, which is an iron-protein complex deposited within the tissues, and possibly in part to other factors such as macromolecular-binding of water (1). Patients with thalassemia who receive repeated transfusions which relieve the stresses on the marrow system may not show such severe marrow hyperplasia as the marrow system recovers, but instead may have the findings of hemosiderin deposition with extremely low signal intensity on T1- and T2-weighted images.

APLASTIC ANEMIA

Aplastic anemia is another disorder that may have abnormality of the bone marrow on MR examination. This is an uncommon disease in which there is pancytopenia (anemia, neutropenia, and thrombocytopenia) caused by a severely hypocellular or acellular bone marrow (2). Although aplastic anemia may be caused by toxins, drugs, infection, hepatitis, radiation therapy, and chemotherapy, the etiology is not identified in about 50 percent of cases (2). The histologic pattern of marrow in patients with aplastic anemia is that of adipose tissue and areas of fibrosis (8) with occasional rests (islands) of hematopoietic marrow. The distribution of red and yellow marrow, in addition to being age-dependent (11), is related to the severity of disease and response to treatment.

The MR findings in patients with aplastic anemia are variable and reflect the relative red marrow and yellow marrow distribution (Fig. 64-2). In untreated patients, there is abundant fat because of hypocellularity of the bone marrow (2,8,13). Fat marrow in untreated patients appears as diffuse increased signal intensity on T1-weighted images (2). Contrast between fat tissue and hematopoietic tissue is maximized on T1-weighted images because of the shorter T1 relaxation time of fat compared with hematopoietic tissue (2). There is no significant difference in the T2 relaxation time of the marrow found in patients with aplastic anemia and control individuals (12). The marrow of some patients who have aplastic anemia and foci of hematopoietic marrow may resemble the marrow of normal patients (9).

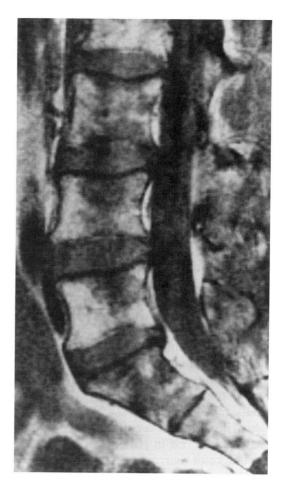

FIG. 64-2. Aplastic anemia in a 24-year-old man. Sagittal T1-weighted SE MR image (600/20) shows mottled areas of heterogeneous signal intensity of the bone marrow. The bright signal represents fat marrow that is more abundant than is expected for a person of this young age.

Magnetic resonance imaging can be helpful in the evaluation of marrow in those patients treated for aplastic anemia (2). With successful treatment, fat marrow reconverts to hematopoietic marrow and the signal characteristics between varying amounts of red and yellow marrow can be differentiated on T1-weighted images. Magnetic resonance imaging is a noninvasive method that potentially may obviate the need for biopsy to determine the degree of cellularity of marrow in patients with aplastic anemia who have undergone therapy. Early, foci of red marrow may be scattered and isolated, and later appear as a more mottled pattern. The foci may enlarge, coalesce, and become diffuse (2,13). Comparison with pretreatment images is mandatory to avoid the missed diagnosis of marrow replacement (tumor) for the islands of normal reconverted red marrow. Response to treatment may not be similar throughout the skeleton (13). Adult patients

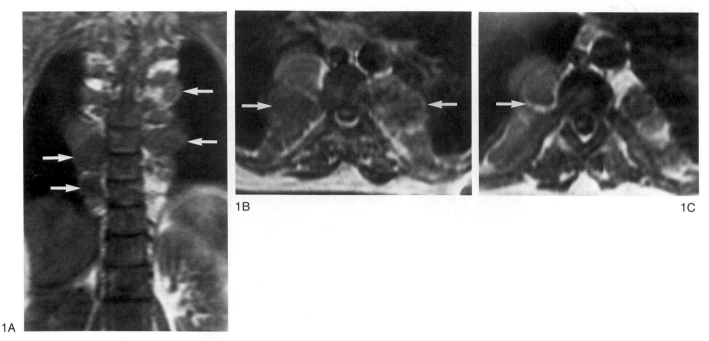

FIG. 65-1A. Thalassemia with extramedullary hematopoiesis. The bone marrow has diffuse homogeneous low signal intensity. There are large bilateral paravertebral masses (*arrows*) that are isointense or slightly hyperintense relative to the bone marrow.

FIG. 65-1B. There is marked expansion of the ribs (*arrows*) caused by hyperplasia of hematopoietic marrow stimulated by the patient's chronic hemolytic anemia. There is also extension of hematopoietic marrow beyond the ribs.

FIG. 65-1C. This T1-weighted image shows extramedullary hematopoiesis with a rim of fat that has bright signal intensity (*arrow*). The rim of fat may be characteristic of extramedullary hematopoiesis and helps to differentiate this entity from other paravertebral tumors.

THALASSEMIA WITH EXTRAMEDULLARY HEMATOPOIESIS

Extramedullary hematopoiesis is a mechanism by which the body tries to maintain red blood cell production by producing red cells outside of the bone marrow. This occurs when the marrow is severely stressed, replaced, or ablated.

Thalassemia is a disorder in which there is a hereditary defect in hemoglobin synthesis that leads to the formation of microcytic hypochromic red blood cells, ineffective erythropoiesis, and rapid hemolysis of newly formed red blood cells. In the severe homozygous form, thalassemia major (Cooley's anemia), the anemia is pronounced and compensatory marrow hyperplasia is extensive. Some patients with severe chronic thalassemia major or thalassemia intermedia, or less commonly with sickle cell anemia, develop extramedullary hematopoiesis (heterotopic marrow) when the body's need for red blood cells is not met by the activity of the hyperplastic red marrow.

Extramedullary hematopoiesis may occur in the para-spinal region of the thoracic spine (Fig. 65-1A), presacral region, or in the posterior end of the ribs (1,3, 4,5). Severe local marrow hyperplasia in the ribs causes bone expansion (Fig. 65-1B). The lesions are unilateral or bilateral and are usually multiple, resembling tumors. Proliferating marrow may extrude through the cortex of the rib or vertebral body into the subperiosteal region (2,3). With spinal involvement, marrow may rarely extrude posteriorly into the spinal canal, causing compression of neural structures.

Magnetic resonance imaging reveals paravertebral masses that are usually bilateral and symmetric, with well-defined margins (4). The masses have a rim of high signal intensity that is thought to be caused by fat and may be characteristic of masses of heterotopic marrow (4,5) (Fig. 65-1C). The central portion of the masses has relatively low signal intensity on T1-weighted images and has further decrease in signal on T2-weighted images (5). Computed tomography shows smoothly marginated, homogeneous, nonenhancing masses without bony erosion.

Extramedullary hematopoiesis may also occur focally in severe marrow replacement disorders (leukemia, Hodgkin's lymphoma); or in marrow ablative conditions (marrow toxins). In these disorders, extramedullary hematopoiesis occurs in visceral sites such as the liver, spleen, kidneys, lymph nodes, and adrenal glands, as they contain totipotential cells or embryonic rests (1). These areas of extramedullary hematopoiesis also show decreased signal intensity on both T1- and T2-weighted images.

REFERENCES

1. Chao WP, Farman J, Kapelner S. CT features of a presacral mass: an unusual focus of extramedullary hematopoiesis. *J Comput Assist Tomogr* 1986;10:684–5.
2. Korsten J, Grossman H, Winchester PH, et al. Extramedullary hematopoiesis in patients with thalassemia anemia. *Radiology* 1970;95:257–63.
3. Lawson JP, Ablow RC, Pearson HA. The ribs in thalassemia: II. the pathogenesis of the changes. *Radiology* 1981;140:673–9.
4. Papavasiliou C, Trakadas S, Gouliamos A, et al. Magnetic resonance imaging of marrow heterotopia in haemoglobinopathy. *Eur J Radiol* 1988;8:50–3.
5. Savader SJ, Otero RR, Savader BL. MR imaging of intrathoracic extramedullary hematopoiesis. *J Comput Assist Tomogr* 1988;12:878–80.

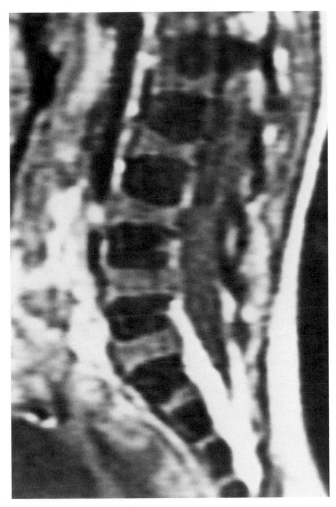

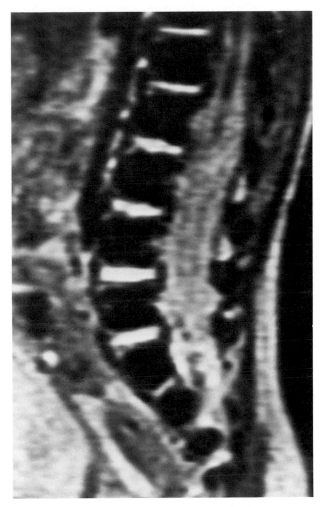

FIG. 66-1A. This 2-year-old girl was examined because of a known skeletal disorder. Sagittal T1-weighted SE MR image (800/20) of the lumbar spine.

FIG. 66-1B. Sagittal T2-weighted SE MR image (2000/60).

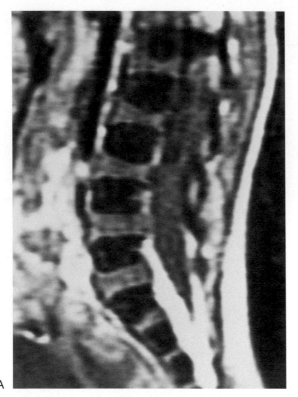
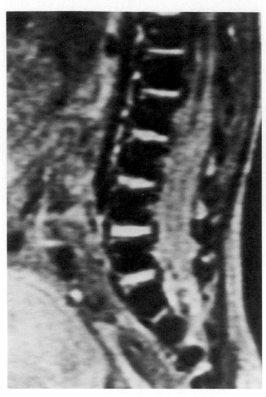

FIG. 66-1A. Osteopetrosis, congenita form. There is very low signal intensity throughout all of the lumbar vertebral bodies and the sacrum on the T1-weighted image.

FIG. 66-1B. Markedly low signal intensity of the vertebrae is seen on the T2-weighted image.

OSTEOPETROSIS

In this case there is very low signal intensity of the vertebrae on T1- and T2-weighted MR images (Fig. 66-1). The conventional radiograph shows diffuse osteosclerosis in this 2-year-old patient with the congenita form of osteopetrosis (Fig. 66-2).

Osteopetrosis is a rare, familial disorder in which osteoclasts fail to resorb bone (1). Formation of cartilage and bone continues at a normal rate, leading to a large amount of calcification of cartilage and bone (4). There are two forms of osteopetrosis. The more common form is the tarda (benign) form associated with normal longevity and without any hematologic abnormalities. It has an autosomal dominant mode of inheritance. The congenita (malignant) form is rare and usually fatal. It is inherited as an autosomal recessive trait.

Radiographically, vertebral bodies and posterior elements exhibit varying degrees of osteosclerosis. In advanced cases, marrow spaces are obliterated by unresorbed calcified cartilage and bone (2), causing marked sclerosis. In milder forms, bands of osteosclerosis are present in the superior and inferior subchondral zones. A "bone within a bone" appearance of the vertebral bodies may be seen. Interestingly, bone that develops in osteophytes in older patients with osteopetrosis appears normal histologically (2).

The appearance of osteopetrosis with MR imaging is variable and is related to the form of the disease and the amount of bone within the vertebral body. In the congenita form the vertebrae show a marked decrease in signal on T1- and T2-weighted images because of the absence of fatty marrow. On the T1-weighted sagittal images, the very low signal of the vertebrae is seen alternating with the intervening higher signal of the discs, creating a "stepladder" appearance (3). This sign is not specific and can be seen in other disorders such as hemosiderosis, or diffuse marrow replacement by metastasis or fibrosis. In patients with osteopetrosis, the lack of signal from the marrow may also be seen in broad, club-shaped ribs and iliac bones.

Patients with the congenita form may be treated with bone marrow transplantation. Those with successful marrow transplantation can show intermediate or high signal intensity within the vertebrae on T1-weighted images indicating the presence of some marrow ele-

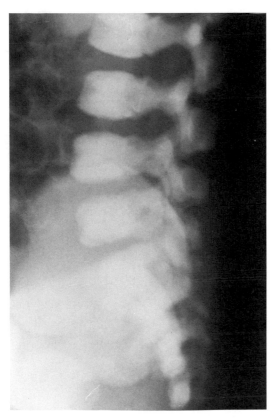

FIG. 66-2. Osteopetrosis, congenita form. Same patient as in Fig. 66-1. Conventional radiograph of the lumbosacral spine shows diffuse sclerosis of all bony elements.

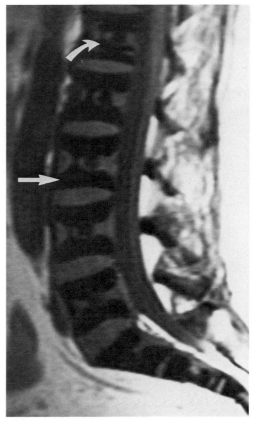

FIG. 66-3. Osteopetrosis, tarda form. Sagittal T1-weighted SE MR image (600/12) of the lumbosacral spine of a 42-year-old woman. There are thick bands of very low signal intensity at the vertebral margins (*straight arrow*). The central portions of the vertebrae are predominantly of intermediate signal. However additional sites of low signal are seen, some parallel to the endplates, creating a "bone within a bone" appearance (*curved arrow*).

ments (3). The central portion of the vertebrae may have decreased signal intensity compared to the periphery, creating a "bone within bone" appearance (3).

The MR findings in the benign form of osteopetrosis differ from the untreated malignant form. With the benign form there is intermediate or high signal intensity within the vertebrae on T1-weighted images, indicating the presence of marrow elements (3) (Fig. 66-3).

Computed tomography shows increased density within the vertebral bodies and posterior elements in patients with osteopetrosis. Dual-photon absorptiometry and quantitative CT can also be utilized to measure bone density as a follow-up for patients with osteopetrosis who undergo treatment.

REFERENCES

1. Marks SC Jr. Congenital osteopetrotic mutations as probes of the origin, structure and function of osteoclasts. *Clin Orthop* 1984; 189:239–63.
2. Migram JW, Jasty M. Osteopetrosis: a morphological study of twenty-one cases. *J Bone Joint Surg (Am)* 1982;64A:912–29.
3. Rao VM, Dalinka MK, Mitchell DG, et al. Osteopetrosis: MR characteristics at 1.5 T. *Radiology* 1986;161:217–20.
4. Shaprio F, Glimcher MJ, Holtrop ME, et al. Human osteopetrosis: a histological, ultrastructural, and biochemical study. *J Bone Joint Surg (Am)* 1980;62A:384–99.

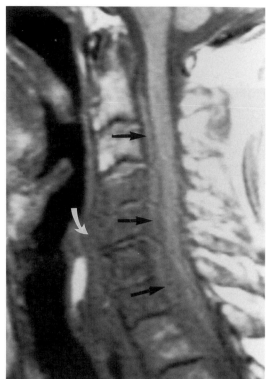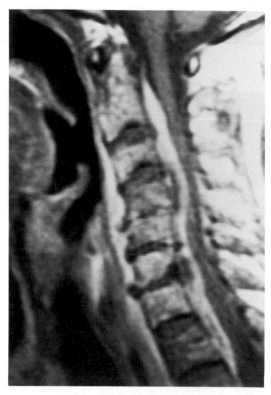

FIG. 67-1A. Epidural abscess. There is an epidural abscess (*black arrows*) and prevertebral abscess (*white arrow*) of lower signal intensity than the spinal cord on this T1-weighted image. Low signal intensity of the vertebral bodies from C4 to C7 is seen, and at surgery, osteomyelitis at C6-C7 was proved.

FIG. 67-1B. After gadopentetate dimeglumine injection there is marked enhancement of the epidural abscess which extends from C1 to T2 and is causing spinal cord compression. At surgery, the epidural abscess was comprised of extensive granulation tissue, which grew *Staphylococcus aureus.* Note enhancement of the prevertebral abscess and C4 to C7 vertebral bodies.

EPIDURAL ABSCESS

This patient has an epidural abscess, prevertebral abscess, and osteomyelitis (Fig. 67-1A). After the intravenous injection of gadopentetate dimeglumine, marked enhancement of the abscesses and the abnormal vertebrae is seen (Figs. 67-1B, 67-2A).

Epidural abscess is an uncommon disorder that may lead to considerable morbidity and even mortality if not diagnosed and treated. Frequently the diagnosis of spinal epidural abscess is not considered in the initial clinical evaluation of these patients, with the diagnosis correctly made in only 20–25 percent of cases (2,4). Other diagnoses that are considered at presentation include extruded disc, spinal tumor, vertebral osteomyelitis, musculoskeletal arthritis, meningitis, transverse myelitis, and nonspinal abnormalities such as cholecystitis, pyelonephritis, and intraabdominal abscess (4).

Typically, the clinical course of an epidural abscess

has been described as having four phases: spinal ache, root pain, weakness (including bowel and bladder dysfunction), and paralysis (6). Spinal ache, local tenderness, and spinal root weakness are frequently found. Approximately 50 percent of patients progress to paraparesis, while 20 percent develop paraplegia (2). Fever has been described in 57–95 percent of cases (2,4).

Spinal epidural abscess is classified as acute (symptoms present for 2 weeks or less prior to surgical intervention) and chronic (symptoms present for more than 2 weeks prior to surgical intervention). Patients with acute abscess may have progression from back pain to nerve root symptoms to weakness in a matter of days (2). Further progression to paraplegia can occur within 24 hours of weakness. Chronic spinal epidural abscess differs from the acute cases in that the progression of symptoms takes place over weeks or months rather than days, there is less dramatic presentation, and sep-

356

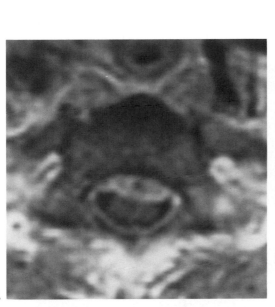

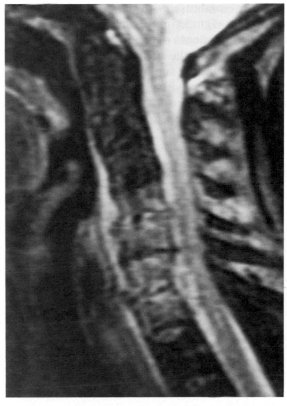

A   B

FIG. 67-2. Cervical epidural abscess and osteomyelitis. Same patient as Fig. 67-1. **A**: Axial T1-weighted SE MR image (750/20) after gadopentetate dimeglumine injection shows anterior epidural abscess compressing the anterior subarachnoid space and spinal cord. **B**: Sagittal STIR image (2300/40/165) used as a fat-suppression technique. Signal from fatty marrow is suppressed with this technique, whereas increased signal from abnormal vertebrae is accentuated from C3 to C7. Osteomyelitis at C6-C7 was proved at surgery.

sis is often absent (2,4). Regardless of the preceding course of the disease, weakness and paralysis can develop suddenly, thus making early diagnosis and treatment crucial in preventing neurologic damage or reversing paralysis of short duration (4).

Sources of infection in spinal epidural abscess include osteomyelitis, bacteremia, and postoperative infection. When hematogenous spread occurs, it is most often a result of a skin infection. Other sources such as urinary tract infection, pneumonia, pharyngitis, and dental abscess have been implicated. Epidural abscess may be found in intravenous drug abusers. Trauma to the back, which may be minor, precedes the symptoms of epidural abscess in 17–30 percent of cases (2,4).

Staphylococcus aureus is the organism most frequently present in spinal epidural abscess and is found in approximately 60 percent of cases in large series that exclude mycobacterium tuberculosis (2,4). Gram negative rods and aerobic streptococci have been implicated with gram negative organisms frequently found in abscesses of intravenous drug abusers and in patients who have undergone surgical procedures (7). In one series, mycobacterium tuberculosis accounted

for 25 percent of epidural abscesses (7). Parasitic and fungal causes are uncommon.

Conventional radiographs are frequently normal in the early stages of an epidural abscess. In patients with associated osteomyelitis, however, disc space narrowing may be seen, followed by vertebral body endplate irregularity and destruction which takes place 1–2 weeks after the initial infection. Myelography is almost always positive in cases of epidural abscess with demonstration of an epidural mass or complete myelographic block (14). Computed tomographic myelography can be used to confirm the presence of an epidural mass of soft-tissue density which replaces the normal epidural fat (11). Occasionally, gas can be seen within the epidural abscess on CT examination (8). Intravenous contrast-enhanced CT has shown rim enhancement surrounding an area of central soft-tissue density (1).

Spinal epidural abscess can be well seen with MR imaging (1,9). An epidural abscess has low or intermediate signal intensity on SE T1-weighted images and high signal intensity on proton density- and T2-weighted images (9). The abscess is hyperintense rela-

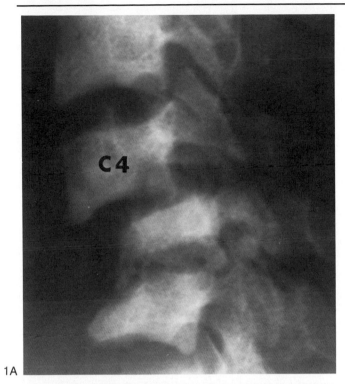

1A

FIG. 68-1A. This is a lateral radiograph of the midcervical spine of a 42-year-old man being treated with renal dialysis.

FIG. 68-1B. Sagittal T1-weighted SE MR image (500/11) of the cervical spine.

FIG. 68-1C. Sagittal T2-weighted FSE MR image (2700/ 144).

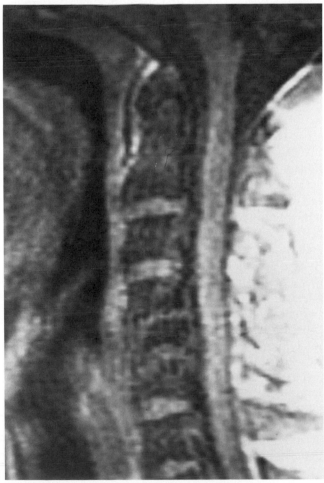

1B

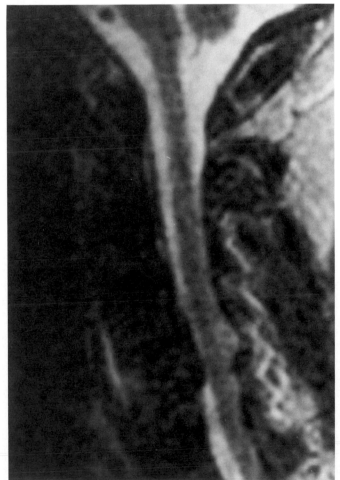

1C

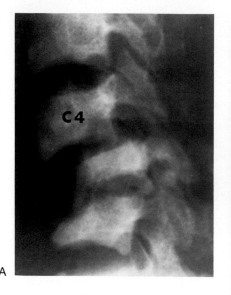

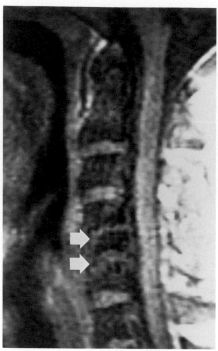

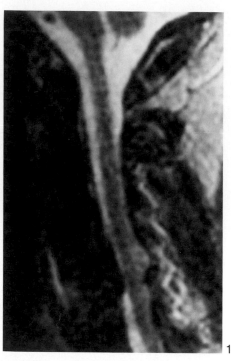

1A

1B

1C

FIG. 68-1A. Erosive spondylopathy in chronic renal failure. There is diffuse osteosclerosis of all vertebrae. There is anterolisthesis of C4 on C5. The disc spaces at C4-C5 and C5-C6 are diminished in height. The vertebral margins of C5 and C6 are partially indistinct, suggesting infection.

FIG. 68-1B. The C5 and C6 vertebral bodies are partially eroded (*arrows*) and there is diffuse decrease in signal intensity of all vertebrae compatible with the diffuse sclerosis seen in Fig. 68-1A. There is slight decrease in signal intensity of the C4-C5 and C5-C6 discs.

FIG. 68-1C. On this T2-weighted FSE image there is no evidence of increased signal intensity within the involved disc spaces, paravertebral space, or epidural compartment to suggest infection.

EROSIVE SPONDYLOARTHROPATHY IN HEMODIALYSIS PATIENT

This patient with chronic renal failure on long-term hemodialysis has cervical disc space narrowing, indistinct vertebral margins, and subluxation suspicious for infection (Fig. 68-1A). However, T1- and T2-weighted MR images do not show the typical features of disc infection or paravertebral abscess (Figs. 68-1B, 1C). Patients undergoing long-term hemodialysis for chronic renal failure may develop an uncommon complication of a rapidly progressive destructive spondyloarthropathy that may appear similar to an infectious spondylitis (2–6) as in this case. The exact etiology is unknown but possibilities include crystal deposition, amyloidosis, and hyperparathyroidism (2,3). Hydroxyapatite crystals were found in the disc of one patient (3) and calcium pyrophosphate dihydrate (CPPD) crystals were found in biopsy tissue of another patient (2). However, crystals such as CPPD, calcium hydroxyapatite, monosodium urate, and calcium oxalate are fairly common in the joints of patients with end-stage renal disease who are undergoing hemodialysis (2). Chon-

drocalcinosis of the spine usually involves the lumbar spine and occurs in older patients (3). Amyloidosis has been reported in association with a destructive spondyloarthropathy resembling osteomyelitis (7). Accumulation of beta 2-microglobulin is important in the etiology of dialysis-related amyloidosis of synovial tissue (1). It is also possible that secondary hyperparathyroidism in patients with renal osteopathy may cause subchondral resorption of bone (2) beneath the cartilage plate, leading eventually to disc and vertebral collapse.

The cervical spine is the most frequent site of erosive spondyloarthropathy, accounting for 90 percent of cases in one series (3). The most common levels are C3-C4 and C5-C6. The lumbar spine is the next most common site. In one series (4) all patients with similar spondyloarthropathy had alterations of hyperparathyroidism of the hands and wrists.

Radiographically there is marked narrowing of disc height, indistinct and irregular vertebral margins, subchondral sclerosis, and Schmorl's nodes. Collapse of

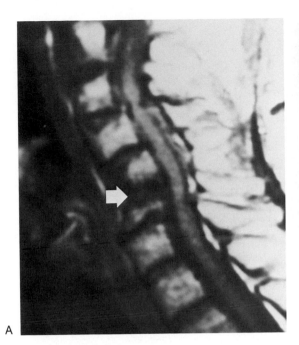
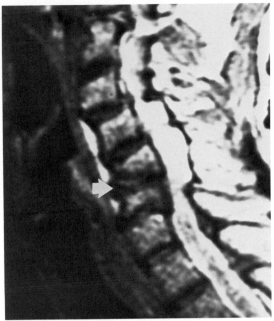

A

B

FIG. 68-2. Erosive spondylopathy. This 62-year-old man is undergoing renal dialysis. **A**: Sagittal T1-weighted SE MR image (800/20). There is erosion of the vertebral margins of C5 and C6 (*arrow*), and loss of height of the C6 vertebral body. **B**: Sagittal T2-weighted FSE MR image (3242/80) shows no increased signal intensity within the C5-C6 disc (*arrow*) and no evidence of a paraspinal mass to suggest infection. Note that the prevertebral fat has bright signal intensity with this FSE sequence.

the upper vertebra into the weakened, softened vertebra below may be seen. The process is rapidly progressive with marked alterations occurring within months (2). The conventional radiographic features of destructive spondyloarthropathy are variable and may, in more advanced cases, resemble osteomyelitis. Rapid development may even occur in patients with previously normal radiographs (3). Some investigators have observed erosions in the anterosuperior and anteroinferior margins of the vertebral bodies, almost all occurring in the thoracic and lumbar spine (6). On CT, there are multiple small destructive changes and sclerosis resembling osteomyelitis. However, there is usually an absence of associated soft-tissue mass.

Magnetic resonance imaging is an important imaging modality when this clinical problem arises, as it can aid in differentiating osteomyelitis from destructive spondyloarthropathy in patients undergoing long-term hemodialysis (Fig. 68-2). In a small series of patients (5), T1-weighted images showed decreased signal in subchondral bone marrow. The intervertebral disc is narrowed with irregular margins and isointense or decreased in signal intensity. On T2-weighted images, there is usually no evidence of increased signal intensity in the disc or subchondral bone and there is no evidence of soft-tissue mass, features that help differentiate this entity from infection. However, in one case of biopsy-proved amyloidosis involving the cervical

and thoracic spine of a patient undergoing long-term hemodialysis, osteomyelitis could not be excluded by imaging with conventional radiographs, CT, and MR (7). The involved cervical disc and subchondral bone showed decreased signal intensity on T1- and subtle increased signal on T2-weighted images (7). Abnormal soft-tissue caused spinal cord compression, both anteriorly and posteriorly. In this case, the MR findings were suggestive of infection.

REFERENCES

1. Bardin T, Kuntz D, Zingraff J, et al. Synovial amyloidosis in patients undergoing long-term hemodialysis. *Arthritis Rheum* 1985;28:1052–8.
2. Kaplan P, Resnick D, Murphey M, et al. Destructive noninfectious spondyloarthropathy in hemodialysis patients: a report of four cases. *Radiology* 1987;162:241–4.
3. Kuntz D, Naveau B, Bardin T, et al. Destructive spondyloarthropathy in hemodialyzed patients: a new syndrome. *Arthritis Rheum* 1984;27:369–75.
4. Naidich JB, Mossey RT, McHeffey-Atkinson B, et al. Spondyloarthropathy from long-term hemodialysis. *Radiology* 1988;167:761–4.
5. Rafto SE, Dalinka MK, Schiebler ML, et al. Spondyloarthropathy of the cervical spine in long-term hemodialysis. *Radiology* 1988;166:201–4.
6. Sundaram M, Seelig R, Pohl D. Vertebral erosions in patients undergoing maintenance hemodialysis for chronic renal failure. *AJR* 1987;149:323–7.
7. Welk LA, Quint DJ. Amyloidosis of the spine in a patient on long-term hemodialysis. *Neuroradiology* 1990;32:334–6.

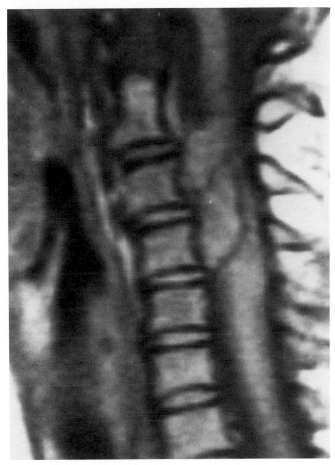

FIG. 69-1A. An 18-year-old female presented with pain in the neck and pain, numbness, and weakness of the right arm and fingers for 1 week prior to the MR examination. Sagittal T1-weighted SE image (500/30) of the cervical spine.

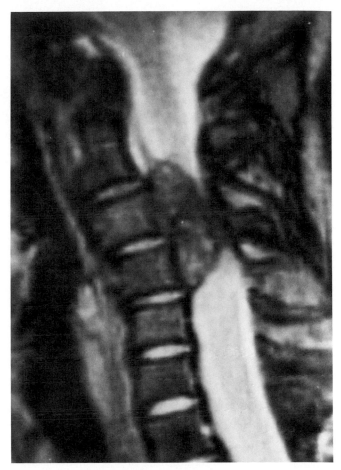

FIG. 69-1B. Sagittal GRE image (750/30 with 28-degree flip angle) of the cervical spine.

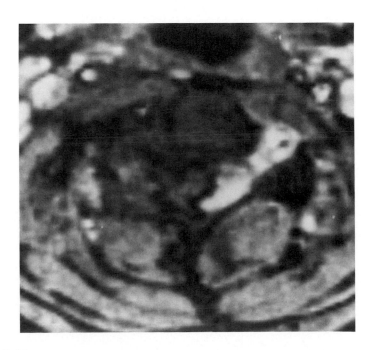

FIG. 69-1C. Axial GRE image (1000/30 with 28-degree flip angle) through the level of C3.

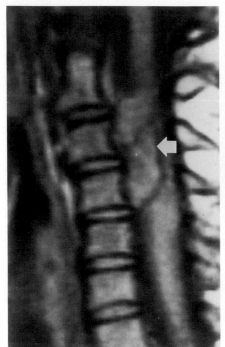
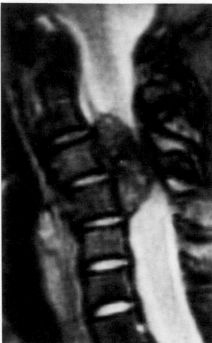
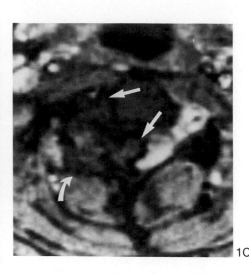

1A

1B

1C

FIG. 69-1A. Pigmented villonodular synovitis of the cervical spine. There is a large lobulated mass (*arrow*) in the spinal canal compressing the anterior subarachnoid space and the spinal cord. The mass has mainly intermediate signal intensity with foci of very low signal within the mass. A rim of very low signal intensity surrounds the mass as well. Hemosiderin deposition probably accounts for this low signal intensity in and around the mass.

FIG. 69-1B. The mass has heterogeneous, predominantly low signal intensity on the GRE image. The low-signal rim is again evident.

FIG. 69-1C. The mass (*straight arrows*) has low signal intensity and is seen within the spinal canal and neural foramen. The mass is displacing the spinal cord to the left and is eroding the lamina (*curved arrow*). Very low signal intensity hemosiderin is seen as foci within the mass and as a rim surrounding the mass. (Fig. 69-1 courtesy of Irving Erlich, M.D., Reading, Pennsylvania.)

PIGMENTED VILLONODULAR SYNOVITIS

In this case there is a mass within the spinal canal and neural foramen that has predominantly intermediate signal on T1-weighted and low signal on GRE images (Fig. 69-1). There is a rim of low signal hemosiderin. Osseous erosion is seen on the axial MR image, but was more readily appreciated on CT images. This proved to be pigmented villonodular synovitis (PVNS).

Pigmented villonodular synovitis is a slowly progressive synovial lesion of unknown etiology consisting of proliferation of synovial tissue with nodules and villous overgrowths either of a joint, bursa, or tendon (3). It may be localized or diffuse. The villonodular projections extend into the joint and are sometimes extra-articular, invading adjacent bone. There are macrophages containing hemosiderin or lipid, as well as lymphocytes, giant cells, and areas of hemorrhage.

Rare in the spine (1,5,6,9,10,12,13), PVNS occurs most often in the knee and less frequently in the hip,

ankle, wrist and elbow (8). In a review of 166 reported cases, none occurred in the spine (8). When PVNS does involve the spine, most are in the lower lumbar spine or less often in the upper lumbar or cervical spine (5). Rarely, the lesion extends over several vertebral levels (6). Pigmented villonodular synovitis of the spine is often asymptomatic. After surgery, it may recur locally.

Pigmented villonodular synovitis of the spine is difficult to detect on conventional radiographs. In some cases destruction of the posterior elements such as the pedicle, articular processes, or lamina is seen (5,9). Rarely, there are osteosclerotic changes in adjacent vertebrae (6). With CT or CTM, PVNS is seen as a soft-tissue mass in the region of the facet joint. The mass usually extends into the spinal canal and may displace the spinal cord or cauda equina. Sometimes the mass extends into the intervertebral foramen. Pigmented villonodular synovitis may show increased attenuation on CT because of the presence of iron within hemosiderin (12). Bone destruction may be evident and is easier to detect with CT than with conventional radiography (12).

The MR appearance of PVNS is variable and depends upon the relative proportion of its components which are mainly synovium, hemosiderin, and fat (4,7). Surrounding synovial fluid alters the signal characteristics as well. In addition, the field strength of the magnet influences the appearance of the lesion (2,7,11).

With MR imaging, PVNS usually has a heterogeneous appearance (4). Villous projections of synovium may not be as readily detected in the spine as they are in large joints. The synovium appears as intermediate signal intensity on T1-weighted images and as increased signal intensity on T2-weighted images because of inflammation (11). Hemosiderin deposition within the synovium appears as foci or clumps of very low signal intensity (almost absent signal) on both T1- and T2-weighted images (4,7,11). Small amounts of hemosiderin may go undetected when MR is performed with a low-field-strength magnet (7). This could be due, in part, to the overshadowing effect of high-signal fat that may be present, or to the field strength of the magnet which influences the detection of hemosiderin (7). With a high-field-strength magnet, hemosiderin within the synovium significantly alters the local magnetic susceptibility, shortening the T2 relaxation time of the synovium and therefore appearing as very low signal intensity on T2-weighted images (2). This is because over 25 percent of the iron in hemosiderin is in the ferric state and the unpaired electrons interact with adjacent water molecules, shortening the T2 relaxation of water. Since this effect is proportional to the square of the magnetic field, it is more pronounced with high-field-strength magnets compared to low-field-strength units (2). Sometimes, a rim of very low signal intensity surrounds the lesion on both T1- and T2-weighted im-

ages. This represents either hemosiderin (7) or a fibrous capsule (11). Central cystic components have been reported within the mass (7). Fluid within a joint capsule may be evident (4) but this is better appreciated in larger joints.

REFERENCES

1. Campbell AJ, Wells IP. Pigmented villonodular synovitis of a lumbar vertebral facet joint: a case report. *J Bone Joint Surg (Am)* 1982;64A:145–6.
2. Gomori JM, Grossman RI, Goldberg HI, et al. Intracranial hematomas: imaging by high field magnetic resonance. *Radiology* 1985;157:87–93.
3. Jaffe HL, Lichtenstein L, Sutro CJ. Pigmented villonodular synovitis, bursitis and tenosynovitis: a discussion of the synovial and bursal equivalents of the tenosynovial lesion commonly denoted as xanthoma, xanthogranuloma, giant cell tumor or myeloplaxoma of the tendon sheath, with some consideration of the tendon sheath lesion itself. *Arch Pathol Lab Med* 1941;31:731–65.
4. Jelinek JS, Kransdorf MJ, Utz JA, et al. Imaging of pigmented villonodular synovitis with emphasis on MR imaging. *AJR* 1989;152:337–42.
5. Karnezis TA, McMillan RD, Ciric I. Pigmented villonodular synovitis in a vertebra: a case report. *J Bone Joint Surg (Am)* 1990;72A:927–30.
6. Kleinman GM, Dagi TF, Poletti CE. Villonodular synovitis in the spinal canal: case report. *J Neurosurg* 1980;52:846–8.
7. Kottal RA, Vogler JB III, Matamoros A, et al. Pigmented villonodular synovitis: a report of MR imaging in two cases. *Radiology* 1987;163:551–3.
8. Myers BW, Masi AT, Feigenbaum SL. Pigmented villonodular synovitis and tenosynovitis: a clinical epidemiologic study of 166 cases and literature review. *Medicine* 1980;59:223–38.
9. Pulitzer DR, Reed RJ. Localized pigmented villonodular synovitis of the vertebral column. *Arch Pathol Lab Med* 1984;108:228–30.
10. Savitz MH, Katz SS, Goldstein H, et al. Hypertrophic synovitis of the lumbar facet joint in two cases of herniated intervertebral disc. *Mt Sinai J Med* 1982;49:434–7.
11. Spritzer CE, Dalinka MK, Kressel HY. Magnetic resonance imaging of pigmented villonodular synovitis: a report of two cases. *Skeletal Radiol* 1987;16:316–9.
12. Titelbaum DS, Rhodes CH, Brooks JSJ, et al. Pigmented villonodular synovitis of a lumbar facet joint. *AJNR* 1992;13:164–6.
13. Weidner N, Challa VR, Bonsib SM, et al. Giant cell tumors of synovium (pigmented villonodular synovitis) involving the vertebral column. *Cancer* 1986;57:2030–6.

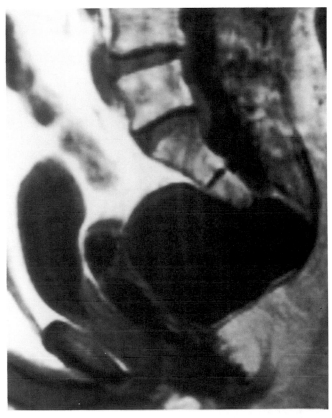

FIG. 70-1A. Sagittal T1-weighted SE MR image (800/15) in a 59-year-old man with diarrhea and possible mass.

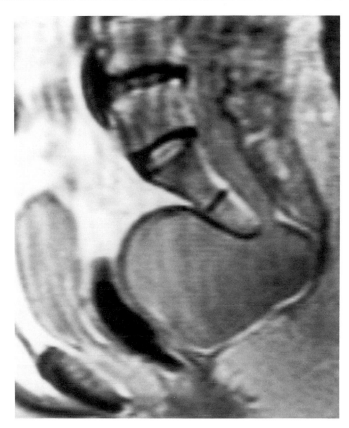

FIG. 70-1B. Sagittal proton density-weighted SE MR image (2500/40).

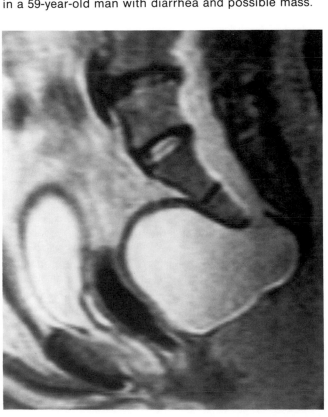

FIG. 70-1C. Sagittal T2-weighted SE MR image (2500/80).

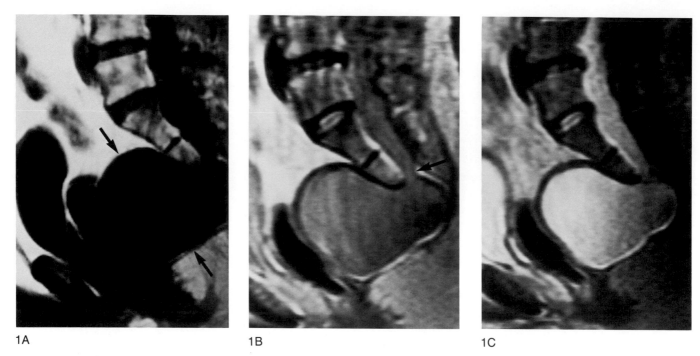

FIG. 70-1A. Anterior sacral meningocele. There is a large, rounded, well-circumscribed low-intensity mass (*arrows*) anterior to the sacrum. There is sacral dysgenesis.

FIG. 70-1B. On the proton density-weighted image the anterior sacral meningocele is of intermediate signal intensity, similar to cerebrospinal fluid. Note sacral dysgenesis with communication of the meningocele and the thecal sac (*arrow*).

FIG. 70-1C. Bright signal intensity of the meningocele is similar to that of cerebrospinal fluid. Note compression on the low-signal bowel and high-signal urinary bladder.

ANTERIOR SACRAL MENINGOCELE

This patient has a large mass lying anterior to the sacrum that has signal intensity similar to cerebrospinal fluid on all pulse sequences (Fig. 70-1). There is sacral dysgenesis, and the mass communicates with the thecal sac at the sacral level. This is an anterior sacral meningocele, a rare congenital lesion.

Anterior sacral meningocele forms as an extension of dura and arachnoid beyond the sacral canal into the retroperitoneal and infraperitoneal space (5). The meningocele contains cerebrospinal fluid and occasionally neural elements. It may occur anteriorly through a defect in the sacrum or anterolaterally through an enlarged sacral foramen. A familial association has been reported as a sex-linked trait (3).

Anterior sacral meningocele may be suspected on conventional radiographs that include the sacrum and coccyx. On these radiographs a lateral defect in the distal sacrum may be seen with associated sickle-shaped deformity of the remaining sacrum and coccyx, termed the *scimitar sacrum sign* (4,5). Other radiographic findings include enlargement of a sacral foramen, a posterior bony sacral defect, or even complete agenesis of the lower sacrum and coccyx (5). Ultrasound is also useful and shows a large fluid-filled mass posterior to the uterus and urinary bladder. Computed tomography shows a mass of fluid density and may reveal bony defects of the sacrum. The level of communication between the thecal sac and the meningocele can be shown with myelography; however, in some cases the contrast material does not fill the meningocele (1,3). Contrast filling of the meningocele is better displayed by CTM. Magnetic resonance is now the imaging modality of choice in demonstrating anterior sacral meningocele (2). When MR imaging, the location of the meningocele is well seen. The meningocele is typically isointense with cerebrospinal fluid, having low signal on T1-weighted images and high signal on T2-weighted images. Although the meningocele contains cerebrospinal fluid, in some cases the fluid has an elevated protein content (5). An intraspinal dermoid tumor with spinal cord tethering may occasionally be found in association with anterior sacral meningocele and can be shown preoperatively with CTM or MR (3). With MR imaging, the patient can be studied in several

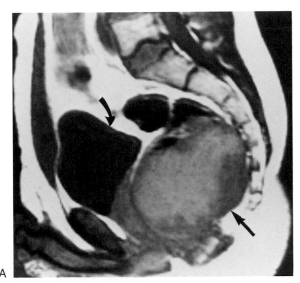
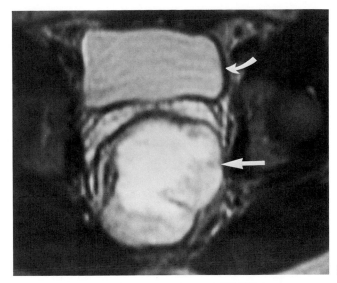

A

B

FIG. 70-2. Presacral leiomyosarcoma in a 26-year-old man. **A**: Sagittal T1-weighted SE MR image (800/20) shows a solid presacral mass (*straight arrow*) with heterogenous intermediate and low signal intensity. There is no communication to the thecal sac. Displacement of the low-signal urinary bladder (*curved arrow*) is seen. **B**: Axial T2-weighted SE image (3000/90) shows heterogenous mass (*straight arrow*) of high and intermediate signal intensity posterior to the urinary bladder (*curved arrow*).

planes, which makes it more likely that the neck of an anterior sacral meningocele will be seen. In our case, the communication between the thecal sac and the meningocele was seen in the sagittal plane, although it is sometimes best visualized on coronal images (2). Fibrofatty connective tissue with mixed signal intensity may be found surrounding the neck of the anterior sacral meningocele. Bony abnormalities can also be seen.

A review of one hundred fifty reported cases of anterior sacral meningocele (4) revealed the following associated abnormalities: presacral epidermoid, dermoid, or teratomatous tumors (9 percent); anal atresia or stenosis (9 percent); and double kidney, renal pelvis, or ureter (4 percent). Women with anterior sacral meningoceles were found to have bicornuate uterus in 13 percent of cases and double vaginas in 6 percent (4). Reported cases of anterior sacral meningocele occasionally were associated with neurofibromatosis (2 percent), or Marfan's syndrome (1 percent). Patients usually present with symptoms such as constipation, dysmenorrhea, urinary incontinence, or dystocia that are related to pressure on the pelvic organs from the pelvic mass (4). Bacterial meningitis may occur after transabdominal surgical intervention, or rarely, may be the presenting abnormality (3).

The correct preoperative diagnosis of anterior sacral meningocele is important since unnecessary morbidity or mortality may occur if the diagnosis is not suspected and aspiration is performed through a contaminated area. When the correct preoperative diagnosis is made, the results of surgical treatment for anterior sacral meningocele are good, with no reported deaths occurring in the sixty-four cases found in the literature between 1965 and 1983 (4).

Compare the appearance of an anterior sacral meningocele with that of a solid presacral leiomyosarcoma (Fig. 70-2). The leiomyosarcoma does not have signal characteristics of fluid, but instead has heterogeneous signal with intermediate and low signal intensity on T1- and high and intermediate signal intensity on T2-weighted images. There is no communication to the thecal sac.

REFERENCES

1. Dyck P, Wilson CB. Anterior sacral meningocele: case report. *J Neurosurg* 1980;53:548–52.
2. Martin B, Boyer de Latour F. MR imaging of anterior sacral meningocele: case report. *J Comput Assist Tomogr* 1988;12:166–7.
3. Quigley MR, Schinco F, Brown JT. Anterior sacral meningocele with an unusual presentation: case report. *J Neurosurg* 1984;61:790–2.
4. Villarejo F, Scavone C, Blazquez MG, et al. Anterior sacral meningocele: review of the literature. *Surg Neurol* 1983;19:57–71.
5. Wilkins RH. Lateral and anterior spinal meningoceles. In: Wilkins RH, Rengachary SS, eds. *Neurosurgery;* vol 3. New York: McGraw-Hill; 1985:2070–5.

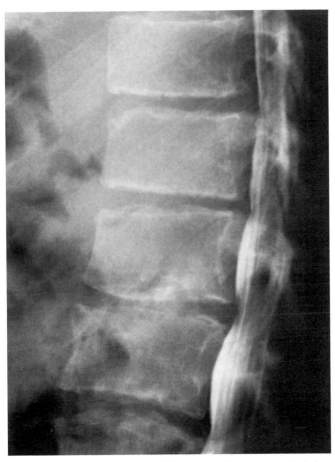

FIG. 71-1A. This 40-year-old woman has an underlying disorder and myelopathy. Lateral view of the thoracolumbar spine during myelogram performed with water-soluble contrast.

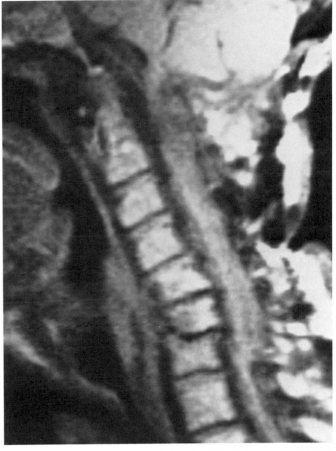

FIG. 71-1C. Sagittal T1-weighted SE MR image (700/15) of the cervical spine.

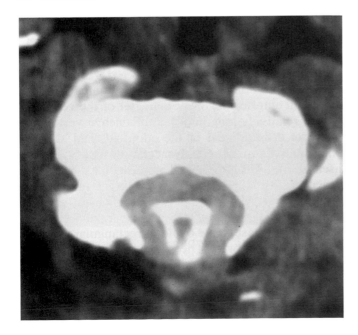

FIG. 71-1B. Computed tomographic myelography of upper cervical spine.

dient-echo images may be used to confirm shrinkage of the nidus of the AVM in the evaluation of the postoperative patient, and may help to differentiate an old hemorrhage within cord tissue from residual intramedullary AVM. Since GRE images are sensitive to magnetic susceptibility, hemosiderin within an old hemorrhage causes heterogeneity of the local magnetic field. Thus, old hemorrhage with hemosiderin has very low signal intensity, whereas the nidus of an AVM appears as increased signal intensity within the cord (2).

REFERENCES

1. Masaryk TJ, Ross JS, Modic MT, et al. Radiculomeningeal vascular malformations of the spine: MR imaging. *Radiology* 1987;164: 845–9.
2. Minami S, Sagoh T, Nishimura K, et al. Spinal arteriovenous malformation: MR imaging. *Radiology* 1988;169:109–15.
3. Moss JG, Sellar RJ, Hadley DM. Intracerebral and spinal vascular malformation in a patient without hereditary hemorrhagic telangectasia. *Neuroradiology* 1989;31:280–1.
4. Terwey B, Becker H, Thron AK, et al. Gadolinium-DTPA enhanced MR imaging of spinal dural arteriovenous fistulas. *J Comput Assist Tomogr* 1989;13:30–7.

APPENDIX: MRI SPINE PROTOCOLS

These are the protocols used with a General Electric 1.5 T superconducting magnet at the Lehigh Magnetic Imaging Center at the time of publication. Protocols vary with the field strength of the magnet and with the manufacturer, and change as new technology develops.

Study	Plane	Pulse sequence	TR	TE	Slice thickness	Gap	Matrix	NEX	FOV	Flip angle	Options	Time min·sec
Cervical disc herniation	Sag	T1 SE	500	12	3	1	256	2	24		A	4.18
	Sag	MPGR	500	15	4	0	192	4	24	15	A, B	6.26
	Ax (or)	MPGR	600	20	3	0	192	2	24	20	A, B, M	7.46
	Ax	3D GRE	35	15	1.5–2	0	128	2	20	5	B, E, M	9.35
Thoracic disc herniation	Sag	T1 SE	600	12	4	1	256	2	30		A, E, M	5.10
	Sag	PD/T2 SE	≥2000	35, 70	4	1	192	2	30		A, B, C, D	≥13.12
	Sag (or)	PD/T2 FSE	3000	18,108$_{EFF}$	4	1	256	2	30		A, E, G, H, M	6.30
	Ax	T1 SE	600	12	4	1	256	4	24		A, D, M	10.17
Lumbar disc herniation	Sag	T1 SE	600	20	4	1	256	2	26		A	5.15
	Sag	PD/T2 SE	2000	35, 70	5	1	192	2	26		A, B, E, J, M	13.12
	Sag (or)	PD/T2 FSE	3000	18,108$_{EFF}$	4	1	256	2	26		A, E, G, H, M	6.30
	Ax	T1 SE	600	20	4	1	256	4	24		A, M	10.17
	Ax	PD/T2 FSE	3000	18, 108$_{EFF}$	4	1	256	2	24		A, G, H, I, M	6.30
Postoperative lumbar spine	Sag	T1 SE	600	20	4	1	256	2	26		A	5.15
	Sag	PD/T2 SE	2000	35, 70	4	1	192	2	26		A, B, E, J, M	13.12
	Sag (or)	PD/T2 FSE	3000	18,108$_{EFF}$	4	1	256	2	26		A, E, G, H, M	6.30
	Ax	T1 SE	600	20	4	1	256	2	24		A, M	5.15
	Postcontrast Ax	T1 SE	600	20	4	1	256	2	24		A, M	5.15
	Postcontrast Sag	T1 SE	600	20	4	1	256	2	26		A	5.15
Metastasis	Sag	T1 SE	600	20	4	1	512	2	42–48		A, F, K	5.10
	Sag	PD/T2 FSE	3000	18/108$_{EFF}$	4	1	512	2	42–48		A, F, G, H, I, K	6.30
	Ax	T1 SE	600	20	4	1	256	2	24		A, F, M	5.10
Bone metastasis	Sag	STIR	1700	40	5	2	128	2	42–48		A, F, L	7.22
Leptomeningeal metastasis	Postcontrast Sag	T1 SE	600	20	4	1	512	2	42–48		A, F, K	5.10
	Postcontrast Ax	T1 SE	600	20	4	1	256	2	24		A, F, M	5.10
Total spine survey for metastasis	Sag	T1 SE	600	20	4	1	512	2	42–48		A, F, K	5.10
	Ax	T1 SE	600	20	4	1	256	2	24		A, F, M	5.15
	Postcontrast Sag	T1 SE	600	20	4	1	512	2	42–48		A, F, K	5.10
	Postcontrast Ax	T1 SE	600	20	4	1	256	2	24		A, F, M	5.15

Study	Plane	Pulse sequence	TR	TE	Slice thickness	Gap	Matrix	NEX	FOV	Flip angle	Options	Time min·sec
Intramedullary or intradural extramedullary tumor	Sag	T1 SE	600	20	4	1	256	2	24–30		A (T spine, E, M)	5.15
	Sag	PD/T2 SE	≥2000	35, 70	4	1	192	2	24–30		C spine, A, B, C; T spine, A, B, C, D; L spine, A, B, E, M	≥13.12
	or Sag	PD/T2 FSE	3000	18, 108$_{EFF}$	4	1	256	2	24–30		A, E, G, H, M	6.30
	Ax	T1 SE	600	20	4	1	256	2	24		A, M	5.15
	Postcontrast Sag	T1 SE	600	20	4	1	256	2	24–30		A (T spine, E)	5.15
	Postcontrast Ax	T1 SE	600	20	4	1	256	2	24		A, M	5.15
Multiple sclerosis (c spine)	Sag	T1 SE	500	20	3	1	256	2	24		A	4.18
	Sag	PD/T2 SE	≥2000	35, 70	3	1	256	1	24		A, B, C	≥9.54
	or Sag	PD/T2 FSE	3000	18, 108$_{EFF}$	4	1	256	2	24		A, E, G, H, M	6.30
	Ax	MPGR	600	20	4	0	192	4	24	20	A, B, M	7.43
Syrinx (c spine)	Sag	T1 SE	500	20	3	1	256	2	24		A	4.18
	Sag	PD/T2 SE	≥2000	35, 70	3	1	256	1	24		A, B, C	≥9.54
	or Sag	PD/T2 FSE	3000	18, 108$_{EFF}$	4	1	256	2	24		A, E, G, H, M	6.30
	Ax	T1 SE	600	20	4	1	256	4	24		A, M	10.17

ABBREVIATIONS KEY

TR	Repetition time
TE	Echo time
NEX	Number of excitations
FOV	Field of view
Sag	Sagittal
Ax	Axial
SE	Spin-echo
MPGR	Multi planar gradient recalled
3D GRE	Three-dimensional gradient-echo
FSE	Fast spin-echo
EFF	Effective TE

OPTIONS KEY

A	Pre saturation
B	Flow compensation
C	Cardiac gating
D	Respiratory compensation
E	Swap phase and frequency (SPF)
F	Phased array coil
G	Echo train = 8
H	Split-echo train
I	Fat suppression
J	CSMEMP pulse sequence (square-echo technique) optional, permits 4 mm slice thickness and 0.4 mm gap, no flow compensation
K	Rectangular field of view
L	TI (inversion time) = 165 msec
M	No phase wrap (NPW)

387

Subject Index